Business Aspects of Optometry

Business Aspects of Optometry

John G. Classé, O.D., J.D.
Professor of Optometry, University of Alabama at Birmingham School of Optometry

Craig Hisaka, O.D., M.P.H.
Clinical Professor of Optometry, University of California School of Optometry, Berkeley

Donald H. Lakin, O.D.
Professor of Optometry, College of Optometry, Ferris State University, Big Rapids, Michigan

Ronald S. Rounds, O.D.
Associate Professor of Optometry, Northeastern State University College of Optometry, Tahlequah, Oklahoma

Lawrence S. Thal, O.D., M.B.A.
Associate Clinical Professor of Optometry, University of California School of Optometry, Berkeley

Foreword by
Richard L. Hopping
President, Southen California College of Optometry, Fullerton

Butterworth–Heinemann
Boston   Oxford   Johannesburg   Melbourne   New Delhi   Singapore

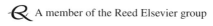

Library of Congress Cataloging-in-Publication Data

Business aspects of optometry / [edited by] John G. Classé ;
  foreword by Richard L. Hopping.
     p. cm.
   Includes bibliographical references and index.
   ISBN 0-7506-9614-1
   1. Optometry--Practice.   I. Classé, John G.
   [DNLM: 1. Optometry--organization & administration.
  2. Professional Practice--organization & administration.
  WW 704 T355 1997]
  RE959.3.T48 1997
  617.7'5'068--dc21
  DNLM/DLC
  for Library of Congress   96-50465
                                        CIP

British Library Cataloguing-in-Publication Data
A catalogue record for this book is available from the British Library.

The publisher offers special discounts on bulk orders of this book.
For information, please contact:

Manager of Special Sales
Butterworth–Heinemann
313 Washington Street
Newton, MA 02158–1626
Tel: 617-928-2500
Fax: 617-928-2620
For information on all medical publications available, contact our World Wide Web home page at: http://www.bh.com/med

10 9 8 7 6 5 4 3 2

Printed in the United States of America

To the memory of Harris L. Nussenblatt, O.D., Dr.P.H.,
in recognition of his many contributions to practice management
education and to the creation of this text

Contents

Contributing Authors

James Albright, O.D.
Clinical Instructor of Optometry, The Ohio State University School of Optometry, Columbus

Jack Bennett, O.D.
Professor and Dean, Indiana University School of Optometry, Bloomington

Jack Bridwell, O.D.
Visiting Associate Professor of Optometry, University of Houston College of Optometry

John G. Classé, O.D., J.D.
Professor of Optometry, University of Alabama at Birmingham School of Optometry

C. Thomas Crooks, III, O.D.
Assistant Clinical Professor of Optometry, University of Alabama at Birmingham School of Optometry

Paul Farkas, M.S., O.D.
Professor of Optometry, Nova Southeastern University College of Optometry, Fort Lauderdale, Florida

Neil B. Gailmard, O.D.
Clinical Assistant Professor of Optometry, Illinois College of Optometry, Chicago

Craig Hisaka, O.D., M.P.H.
Clinical Professor of Optometry, University of California School of Optometry, Berkeley

Roger D. Kamen, O.D., M.S.
Assistant Professor of Optometry, College of Optometry, Ferris State University, Big Rapids, Michigan

Harry Kaplan, O.D.
Assistant Professor of Optometry, Pennsylvania College of Optometry, Philadelphia

Donald H. Lakin, O.D.
Professor of Optometry, College of Optometry, Ferris State University,
Big Rapids, Michigan

W. Howard McAlister, O.D., M.A., M.P.H.
Associate Professor of Optometry, University of Missouri–St. Louis School of
Optometry

Gary Moss, O.D.
Associate Professor of Optometry, New England College of Optometry, Boston

David L. Park, O.D., M.S.
Private Practice, Ukiah, California

Ronald S. Rounds, O.D.
Associate Professor of Optometry, Northeastern State University College of
Optometry, Tahlequah, Oklahoma

Stuart Rothman, O.D.
Assistant Clinical Professor of Optometry, State University of New York State
College of Optometry, New York City

John Rumpakis, O.D.
Associate Professor of Optometry, Pacific University College of Optometry, Forest
Grove, Oregon

Peter Shaw-McMinn, O.D.
Assistant Professor of Optometry, Southern California College of Optometry,
Fullerton

Lawrence S. Thal, O.D., M.B.A.
Associate Clinical Professor of Optometry, University of California School of
Optometry, Berkeley

Michael Usdan, O.D.
Adjunct Professor of Optometry, Southern College of Optometry, Memphis,
Tennessee

Timothy A. Wingert, O.D.
Associate Professor of Optometry, University of Missouri–St. Louis School of
Optometry

Foreword

It is uniformly agreed that a good understanding of optometric practice management is vital to the success of a practitioner and therefore is vital to the delivery of effective patient care. Yet it is the one area of optometric education that has proved difficult to teach effectively. All optometry schools earnestly believe they provide a good series of courses in this important subject area, yet many optometry school graduates feel that their education in this area is one of the greatest shortcomings of their optometric training.

Many reasons for the lack of understanding of practice management have been proposed, since the courses are almost always taught by qualified instructors who have had or are currently operating a successful optometric practice. The students' difficulty in grasping the critical nature of the topic for their career success and the difficult task faced by the instructor in making the course materials relevant to the particular student's interest and educational level are thought to be a few of the major challenges. The realities are that the student and faculty member must deal with an already crowded curriculum, and practice management is not tested on state or national examinations. This situation almost guarantees that most students will place a lower priority on the subject matter, thereby increasing the challenge that every practice management instructor faces.

Subsequently, the graduate entering practice upon licensure is immediately confronted with the difficulties of becoming established within a competitive free enterprise system with other practitioners who may not be as scientifically up-to-date as the young graduate but who have significantly more experience in the business, communications, and administrative aspects of operating an optometric practice. Regardless of how sophisticated a practitioner is in optometric technology, if he or she is unable to deliver vision care because of ineptitude in practice management, all of the scientific and clinical training and expertise is of little or no value. In such a case, the school or college has not upheld its full responsibilities, and both the public and the optometry graduate will suffer.

For this reason, the Association of Schools and Colleges of Optometry (ASCO) and the American Optometric Association (AOA) have cooperated for a number of decades to develop an enhanced and expanded practice management curriculum for schools and colleges of optometry. At the same time, the AOA Professional Enhancement Program (PEP) was produced to help member practitioners meet the challenges of change. Because of the comprehensiveness of the materials developed and the significant success of the PEP program, an attempt was made to extract the pertinent materials and provide a series of simulated, life-like learning experiences for students in their practice management courses.

In 1986 the AOA PEP program sponsored a conference in St. Louis for practice management faculty members. A portion of the program was set aside for the instructors to exchange ideas about teaching, with Dr. Harris Nussenblatt serving as moderator. It was obvious that this dialogue was welcome and most valuable for the attendees, for collegiality quickly became the tenor of the meeting.

The faculty members requested the opportunity to meet annually for the purpose of sharing ideas, methods of teaching, and materials used in their individual practice management courses. Soon the Association of Practice Management Educators (APME) was formed. Efforts were made to find financial sponsorship for the annual meetings; Allergan provided the necessary economic support for the first 6 years, and Vistakon has continued the support for the past several years. The annual meetings of APME have seen a healthy exchange of curriculum outlines, course references, research projects, and classroom exercises. It quickly became evident that there are a number of quite talented and dedicated practice management educators who have much to offer their students as well as their academic colleagues. These faculty members regularly publish, lecture, and serve as consultants on practice management within the profession. They soon proposed that the members of APME develop a textbook for students and practitioners on the business aspects of optometry, with each practice management faculty member contributing to the book.

A review of the table of contents and a perusal of the well-organized chapters quickly demonstrates that the authors have taken a sagacious, comprehensive approach to the many vital components of practice administration and patient management. Each of the contributors is to be commended for his interest and dedication to this important aspect of optometry education. Students will benefit tremendously from the use of this textbook, as will practitioners who are in the early years of their professional career. But it is the *profession* that will benefit most from this valuable reference, as it will help optometry school graduates prepare for the new century—and new challenges—that lie ahead for optometry.

Richard L. Hopping, O.D.

Preface

This textbook represents a unique achievement in optometric education. Never before have all the educators in a subject area worked together to provide a common textbook. *Business Aspects of Optometry* represents such an effort—an effort that was motivated by the need to provide a core body of knowledge for students and to provide a common curriculum among the schools. This textbook achieves both goals, because it will be used by the practice management educators—and students—at all schools and colleges of optometry.

The cooperation to produce this book exhibited by faculty members who teach practice management has been extraordinary. It is the product of a decade of collaboration intended to improve the quality of practice management education in the schools and to elevate the standing of practice management as a discipline. The seminal event in this effort was the decision by the Association of Schools and Colleges of Optometry (ASCO) and the American Optometric Association to sponsor a meeting of practice management educators in the mid-1980s. This meeting produced recommendations for a model practice management curriculum, a curriculum that was subsequently adopted by ASCO. Financial support—initially from Allergan and then from Vistakon—allowed subsequent meetings to be held, which in turn led to the formation of an organization to promote practice management education, the Association of Practice Management Educators (APME). This organization set as one of its first goals the creation of a practice management textbook to be used at all schools. This book represents the achievement of that goal.

Business Aspects of Optometry describes the career choices available to optometry school graduates, the many steps that must be taken to initiate a private practice, and the administrative and business issues that must be understood to successfully operate such a practice. It is intended to serve as the companion volume to *Legal Aspects of Optometry*, which describes complementary legal issues. Using both books, optometry students will find the encouragement and information needed to make the large step into a professional career after graduation.

The effort to write this book was largely due to the inspiration of two individuals. The first is Dr. Richard Hopping, President of the Southen California College of Optometry. Long a champion of practice management education, Dr. Hopping not only was the individual most responsible for the decision to bring practice management educators together but who was also able to obtain the necessary financial support for annual meetings. His contributions to the advancement of practice management education have been invaluable. We must also acknowledge Dr. Harris Nussenblatt, who tragically passed away before the textbook was completed. Dr. Nussenblatt sought to create a cohesive and collegial organization of practice management educators, and his leadership led to the initiation of this project. Therefore, this book is dedicated to his memory.

It is our sincere hope that students and practitioners will find this text both informative and useful. Practice management is not a subject that can be readily taught in the classroom; to be meaningfully learned, practical experience is needed. Yet there are technical aspects of law and business administration that must be mastered before practical application is feasible. It is to those subjects, and to the broader principles of business management, that this book has been directed.

John G. Classé, O.D., J.D.
Craig Hisaka, O.D., M.P.H.
Donald H. Lakin, O.D.
Ronald S. Rounds, O.D.
Lawrence S. Thal, O.D., M.B.A.

Introduction

Lawrence S. Thal

*Those who cannot remember the past are con-
demned to repeat it.*

—George Santayana
The Life of Reason

Although optometry is a uniquely American invention, the profession's antecedents reach back to an-
tiquity and to the science of optics. The early
Greeks possessed some knowledge of optics—
Plato, Aristotle, Archimedes, and Euclid all wrote
about it. Plato's comments on optics date back to
400 B.C. Aristotle seemed familiar with what we
know today as myopia. Archimedes discovered the
relationship between a sphere and a cylinder and
was aware of the importance of this discovery, attested to by the fact that he directed that a sphere
and a cylinder be engraved on his tombstone.
(Archimedes was the ingenious Greek who is said
to have destroyed the Roman fleet by the use of
burning mirrors.)

Ptolemy of Egypt knew and wrote about refraction in the second century. He wrote 13 volumes on
the refraction of light and the function of vision.
Later, in the eleventh century, Alhazen, an Arabian
philosopher, wrote about the anatomy of the eye
and about optics. However, the clinical application
of the science of optics began in Europe. Christo-
pher Scheiner, a Jesuit priest who described the vision of myopic individuals in 1625, is often called
the "father of optometry."

The Chinese claim that the use of spectacles
began in China in very ancient times. The English-
man Roger Bacon (1214–1294) (Figure 1) was,
however, the first to write about convex lenses for
presbyopia ("old sight"), describing their use in

1276. He may have invented the use of lenses for
near vision, but Allasandre de la Spina, a thirteenth
century Italian monk, is credited with "perfecting
spectacles." However, an inscription on the tomb of
Salvino D'Armato (in 1317, the date of his death)
credits him with the invention. Although the origin
of spectacles is uncertain, it is clear that they appeared in Europe sometime between 1275 and 1285.

The ancestors of American optometrists are the
European opticians who, like other skilled crafts-
men of the time, organized guilds. The origin of the
guilds is lost in the history of the Dark Ages. It is
certain that guilds were originally organizations of
congenial people, tied together by some common
activity or background, for the purpose of ensuring
that fellow members received a Christian burial
when they died and that their widows and orphans
received adequate care. In the eleventh and twelfth
centuries, the possibility that a loved one might
spend eternity in purgatory unless he or she received proper death rites was a tremendous force in
predominantly Christian Europe.

In time, the common activity that bound members of guilds together became increasingly important and led to the establishment of craft guilds in
the fourteenth and fifteenth centuries. These guilds
set up standards and price controls for their products, to which each guild member had to adhere.
They also set up an educational system so that the
skill of the craft could be continued from year to

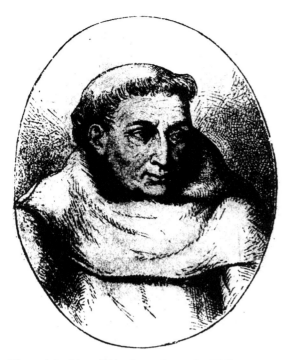

Figure 1. Etching of Friar Roger Bacon, by William H.W. Bicknell, after a painting by Howard Pyle. (Reprinted with the permission of the New York Public Library, New York, New York.)

year, and to maintain a limit on the number of skilled men in that craft. One learned a craft by first becoming an apprentice to a master. The number of apprentices each master could have was limited. The length of time and the condition of servitude as an apprentice were carefully established. When the apprenticeship was successfully concluded, the worker became a journeyman. At this point, his skill was attested to by the guild. As a journeyman he had some freedom of employment, and under certain conditions could change from master to master. After serving as a journeyman for a definite period of time, a skilled craftsman could present his masterpiece to the guild. If it was accepted and approved, he became a master and could establish his own shop.

The first separate spectacle-makers' guild was established in France in 1465, and the second began in Germany in 1577. This does not mean that there were no spectacle makers before this time, but that spectacle makers were members of other guilds. An example of a spectacle-makers' guild was the Worshipful Company of Spectacle Makers, an English guild chartered by King Charles I in 1629 (Figure 2).

In April 1628, Robert Allt, citizen and brewer, in concert with 15 other London spectacle makers—12 of whom were members of the Brewers' Company—petitioned the King in Council for a charter of incorporation. This petition reads, in part:

> To the Kings Most Excellent Majesty:
> The humble petition of Robert Allt on behalf of himself and other poor spectacle makers in and about the City of London.
> Most humbly shewing: That whereas the mystery of making spectacles hath been and still is of good esteem and repute as well in foreign parts beyond the seas as within this Your Majesty's Realm of England: and daily doth increase; and many who have served as Apprentices thereunto; and others who have remained some small time apprentices and afterwards departed from their Masters service; having by indirect and private means attained unto some small insight of the same profession, Do now use many deceipts in the said mystery in making and uttering bad and hurtful wares whereby Your Majesty's subjects are not only merely cosened, but sometimes much prejudiced; and Your Petitioners who have served 7 years apprenticeship to the same profession and are good true workmen (of whom some are charged with wives and children) much wronged in their credit, their profession vilified, and they thereby almost utterly undone, unless Your Majesty's gracious favor be extended towards them for their relief herein.
> In tender consideration whereof and forasmuch as all such trade mysteries and manufactures are incorporated into a body politic do still subsist in a comely and commendable manner and those subject to no certain ordinances, rules or government are found by experience to be in short time utterly subverted. And for that your Petitioners conceive a Corporation amongst them to be a means for redress of these their grievances.

It is apparent that little of this petition would need changing to make it suitable for placement on the agenda of an American Optometric Association meeting!

The charter granted to "The Master Wardens and Fellowship of Spectacle Makers of London" gave the company very broad powers. It established a means of government for the company, allowed the company to establish standards, and set up search and seizure provisions for substandard spectacles and for the punishment of those violating any of the rules of the company.

Generally, persons became members of the guild through apprenticeship. However, sons of members could become members directly by patrimony. Later, certain individuals were allowed to purchase membership, called redemption. During the fifteenth century, both on the continent of Europe and in Great Britain, it was almost essential that a craftsman of any kind be a freeman of the city in which he practiced his craft. The only way a person could be a freeman of the city was to become a member of a guild. Therefore, before the Worshipful Company of Spectacle Makers was formed, spectacle makers had to be members of some other guild. The Brewer's Company became the guild for spectacle makers, probably through the action of the law of patrimony. For example, it is known that the father of Robert Allt was a member of the Brewer's Company.

As the number of journeymen increased and as knowledge of the mysteries of the various crafts spread, the guilds began to lose power. Eventually they lost the ability to regulate their craft. The guilds in Great Britain gradually became social institutions, until near the end of the nineteenth century, when the old companies again began to take an interest in regulatory activities. The spectacle makers established an examination that ophthalmic opticians could take voluntarily. Those who passed the examination became members of the company, but, more important, their competency was attested to by the Worshipful Company of Spectacle Makers.

Much of the background in spectacle making was lost by the craft's mere transfer from Europe to America. In the United States, spectacles were sold primarily by peddlers, with customers selecting their own glasses by trial-and-error methods. Refractive testing of the eye did not make its appearance as a scientific application of optics until the nineteenth century. The primary advances in optics occurred in Europe.

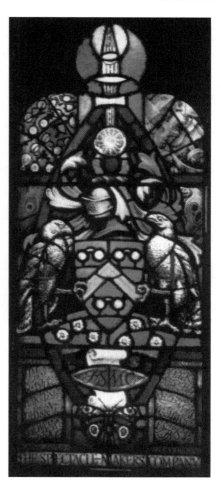

Figure 2. Coat of Arms of the Worshipful Company of Spectacle Makers, found in the Crypt, Guildhall, London. (Reprinted with permission from CJ Eldridge. The Worshipful Company of Spectacle Makers. J Am Optom Assoc 1979;50(4):481–7.)

In the early 1800s the English scientist Thomas Young (Figure 3) discovered astigmatism. In 1827 Sir George Beddell Airy, an English astronomer, expanded on Young's discovery by measuring the astigmatism in his eyes and having a cylindrical lens ground.

In 1843, Christoph Fronmüller of Germany invented the trial case, making possible the use of subjective examination and the creation of custom-made spectacles. Edward Jaeger, in 1854, published his reading card. In the middle of the nineteenth century, the principles of skiascopy were discovered

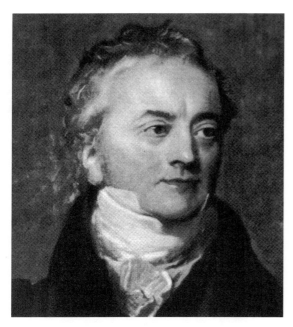

Figure 3. Thomas Young. (Reprinted with permission from CG Mueller, M Rudolph. Light and Vision. New York: Time, Inc., 1966.)

and explained, and in the latter part of the century Hermann Snellen invented his squared test type (Figure 4).

Medicine began to influence the field around 1860. In 1864, the Dutch physician Frans Donders published his seminal book, *On the Anomalies of Accommodation and Refraction of the Eye*. Until this time eye physicians—called oculists—opposed the fitting of spectacles except for "old sight." Oculists began to take an interest in refraction during the late 1800s, and it was urged by some that the important matter of fitting glasses should not be left to opticians. The jealousies that began then have yet to be outlived.

During the middle of the nineteenth century, American companies began to produce lenses and frames on a large-scale basis; leading companies included American Optical, Bausch and Lomb, and Shuron. Some of these early manufacturers set up training courses for medical and nonmedical refractionists as a means of boosting the sales of their lenses. Courses were 1–2 weeks in length, with the awarding of a gold-embossed certificate upon graduation.

Early courses in refraction were a far cry from those found in today's professional curricula. One of the most advanced courses was given by the Northern Illinois College of Ophthalmology and Otology in 1895; it required 3 months. The Johnston Optical Institute offered four courses, each complete in itself, and maintained that all four together constituted "a university course of instruction in optics" that taught "everything up to the use of the ophthalmoscope." The Klein Optical School (now the New England College of Optometry) had a tuition fee of $25 for the full term. In June 1896, Dr. Theodore F. Klein announced a course of lectures to be given in a tent in a pine grove at the edge of a lake near his summer home. A camping outfit could be purchased for $10, and fish and berries were plentiful, so the students could bring their families and incur very little expense in their quest to become refracting opticians. As with medical education, numerous correspondence courses were available, and diplomas were awarded upon successful completion of the course of study.

Despite these shortcomings, by the close of the 1800s refracting opticians had become firmly established as technical experts who were providing a needed and previously neglected service required by modern civilization. The medical profession had almost completely ignored, and even opposed, this necessary service.

Charles F. Prentice (1854–1946) (Figure 5) led the fight for the legal recognition of optometry in New York. He has been called the "father of optometry" in the United States. He was a mechanical engineer, optician, and refractionist. His efforts to establish optometry were based on the conviction that the refractive services of the time were entirely inadequate, that the refractionists, both medical and nonmedical, were, in general, incompetent and that it was necessary to found a professional group separate from medicine to take care of the needs of the public in the field of vision care.

That modern optometry's career has always been attended by controversy is not at all surprising, for the profession was born in controversy. In 1892 Prentice referred a patient to Henry D. Noyes, M.D., a leading ophthalmologist and otologist in New York City, for care of an inflammation of one eye. Noyes sent Prentice a letter, ostensibly thanking him for the referral but in fact reprimanding him for having charged the patient a fee for refractive services in addition to the charge for glasses. Noyes held this to be a serious matter that would antagonize the oculists, because they would consider Prentice's actions competitive. Noyes further objected that, by charging for services, Prentice would cause the public to assume that he had the qualifications that entitled him to a fee for advice.

The controversy gained momentum, and the New York medical society agreed to adopt a resolution to expel any member who would send patients to opticians for a refraction. When Prentice and his colleagues submitted to the New York legislature a bill to regulate the practice of optometry in the state, the medical society vigorously opposed it, ensuring that it would not pass.

Despite the bill's defeat, the idea of legislative recognition caught on among optometrists, and in 1901 Minnesota became the first state to enact an optometry law. After 12 years of continuous effort, led by Andrew J. Cross and Charles Prentice, in 1908 the New York legislature passed an optometry law. The last jurisdiction, the District of Columbia, completed the "legalization" of optometry by enacting a law in 1924. The many arguments put forth by Prentice and his colleagues during these legislative struggles are well worth reading and are as valid today as they were a century ago.

Before 1903, the American Optometric Association was known as the American Association of Opticians, an organization that included in its membership both refracting opticians (the precursors of optometrists) and dispensing opticians (known today as "opticians"). By 1903, however, the dispensing opticians had separated from the organization, and it became necessary to find a name for the refracting opticians. In 1904 the terms *optometry* and *optometrist* were adopted and a campaign was started to popularize them. In 1919 the organization changed its name to the American Optometric Association.

With the advent of the optometry laws, schools and colleges of optometry were chartered to provide students with the education and training necessary to meet the requirements set forth in these laws for the practice of optometry. Standards continued to improve as optometry elevated itself through education, organized legislative efforts, and the adoption of codes of practice and ethics.

Today, optometry in the United States has reached a position of recognition and of acceptance

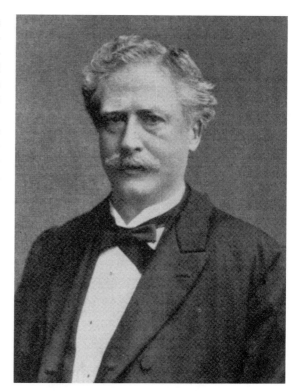

Figure 4. Hermann Snellen. (Reprinted from Graefe's Archives of Ophthalmology, 1908;67(3):379.)

that is closely equalled only in Great Britain, Australia, and Canada. Optometry is recognized as a health care profession in all of the states and by the agencies of the federal government. Use of ophthalmic drugs by optometrists for diagnosis and treatment is approved in virtually all states. Optometrists and ophthalmologists work together with increasing frequency in schools, multidisciplinary clinics, the military, referral centers, and private practice. Interprofessional referrals between members of the two disciplines have become increasingly more common. Despite the political differences between the two professions, they have in fact come to more closely resemble one another, with optometry emerging as the provider of primary care and ophthalmology continuing to emphasize training for secondary and tertiary care.

Optometrists render a vital service that was born of medicine's refusal to recognize the widespread public need for refractive care. The profession has always acknowledged an obligation to examine for

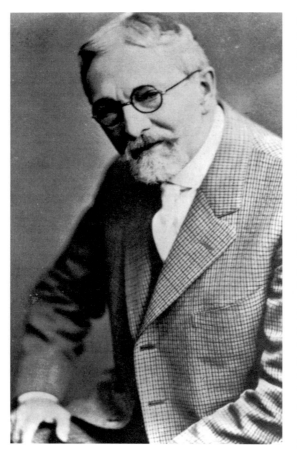

Figure 5. Charles Prentice. (Reprinted from CF Prentice. Legalized Optometry and Memoirs. Seattle: Casperin Fletcher Press, 1926.)

pathology when rendering this care, an obligation that now includes the treatment of anterior segment pathology. Optometrists have every right to be proud of the unique heritage that has led to this combination of knowledge and skills. Optometry cannot be considered a restricted form of ophthalmology; it is a primary health care profession with its own body of knowledge and unmatched expertise in the area of vision care.

Today's optometry school graduates receive an enlightened and unexcelled education in vision science and in the art and science of health care. Optometry's position that the dispensing of ophthalmic materials is an integral part of care and is best performed by the practitioner who has examined the patient has withstood the test of time. Even so, emphasis on health care services continues to grow, challenging practitioners to maintain an adequate balance between the traditional refractive services of the past and the health care services of the future. Graduates who seek to enter the practice of optometry will find career choices significantly affected by this dichotomy in services. Some career opportunities will emphasize the sale of opthhalmic materials, with vision and health care services incidental to the sale; others will emphasize eye and vision care services, with little or no attention paid to the dispensing of ophthalmic materials; still others will offer a balance between the two skills. The graduate must choose between these options, which are the hallmark of a free enterprise system.

It is the intent of this book to explore some of the vital issues necessary to the making of these choices and to consider the alternative ways by which the graduate may engage in the practice of optometry. In so doing, it is hoped that graduates will be better able to meet their responsibilities to the public and to more adequately serve the health care needs of our country.

BIBLIOGRAPHY

Arrington E. History of Optometry. Chicago: White Printing House, 1929.

Champness R. A Short History of the Worshipful Company of Spectacle Makers. London: Apothecaries' Hall, 1965.

Classé JG. Legal Aspects of Optometry. Stoneham, MA: Butterworth, 1989.

Cox M. Optometry: The Profession. Philadelphia: Chilton, 1947.

Eldridge CJ. The worshipful company of spectacle makers. J Am Optom Assoc 1979;50(4):481–7.

Gregg J. The Story of Optometry. New York: Ronald Press, 1965.

Gregg J. A History of the American Optometric Association. St. Louis: American Optometric Association, 1972.

Hirsch M, Wick R. The Optometric Profession. Philadelphia: Chilton, 1968.

Hofstetter H. Optometry. St. Louis: Mosby, 1948.

Business Aspects of Optometry

Part I
Practice Options

Chapter 1

Practice Demographics

John G. Classé and Jack Bennett

He who has begun his task has half done it.

—Horace
Epistles

To begin the study of optometric practice management, it is necessary to review the status of the profession.

Optometry is a clinical discipline, primarily composed of private practitioners. The overwhelming majority of optometry school graduates seek to enter the practice of optometry immediately after graduation. To understand the opportunities available to optometrists seeking to enter private practice, it is important to review the current demographics of the profession, including the number and distribution of optometrists, the modes of practice, the ophthalmic market, the number of eye examinations performed annually by optometrists, the types of services optometrists offer, and the income optometrists receive.

NUMBER AND DISTRIBUTION OF OPTOMETRISTS

The number of practicing optometrists has increased steadily over the past few decades. In 1978, there were fewer than 20,000 practitioners. In 1995, the number of licensed optometrists in the United States exceeded 33,000; approximately 28,900 of those were in practice. Based on surveys performed by the American Optometric Association (AOA), it is believed that 68% of practicing optometrists are in private practice, with 18% in commercial settings,

7.6% in multidisciplinary clinics or hospitals, 4.8% employed by ophthalmologists or other physicians, and 1.6% serving in the armed forces (Figure 1.1).

United States schools and colleges of optometry graduate approximately 1,100 optometrists annually. Approximately 600 optometrists retire or die each year. In 1992, the median age of optometrists was below 40 years of age—a significant reduction from the 1970s, when the median age peaked at 50.

More than half of the students enrolled at United States schools and colleges of optometry are women, and it is estimated that the percentage of female optometrists will increase from the 23% recorded in 1995 to 30% by the year 2000. This increase in the number of female optometrists represents a significant change for the profession; in 1973 only 3% of practicing optometrists were women.

MODES OF PRACTICE

The backbone of the private practice of optometry has always been the individual practitioner, an entrepreneurial individual who has begun a practice and served as its sole owner and clinician. However, over the course of the past few decades, the pre-eminence of individual proprietorships has waned. Currently, fewer than half of the optometrists in the United States are in solo prac-

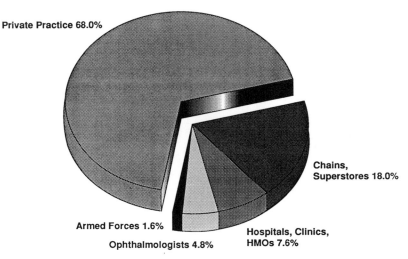

Private Practice 68.0%

Chains, Superstores 18.0%

Armed Forces 1.6%

Ophthalmologists 4.8%

Hospitals, Clinics, HMOs 7.6%

Figure 1.1. Distribution of optometrists by type of practice, 1994. (From American Optometric Association. Caring for the Eyes of America—A Profile of the Optometric Profession. St. Louis: American Optometric Association, 1996. Reproduced with permission.)

tice—down from more than 70% in the 1960s (Table 1.1). The major shift has been toward partnership, with approximately one in five optometrists now in a partnership arrangement that involves two or more practitioners.

THE OPHTHALMIC MARKET

In the United States optometrists serve approximately 55% of the population—145 million wearers of corrective lenses. It is estimated that 26 million of these individuals are full-time contact lens wearers. The need for corrective lenses in the American population is expected to increase because of the aging "baby boomers," the large group of individuals born after World War II.

Table 1.1. Modes of Practice for Optometrists, 1964–1994

Type of Practice	Percentage of Optometrists by Year			
	1964	1979	1987	1994
Sole proprietor	71	62	54	48
Partnership[a]	8	13	17	7
Group[b]	NA	3	5	14

NA = data not available.
[a]Two optometrists
[b]Three or more optometrists
Source: AOA Economic Surveys, 1964–1995. St. Louis: American Optometric Association.

In 1995, approximately 86 million primary eye examinations were performed in the United States, with optometrists conducting an estimated 70% of them. Because of the effects of presbyopia on the "baby boom" generation, it is anticipated that most growth in eye care will involve persons in the 45-year-old and older age bracket. Contact lens wearers are not expected to expand significantly in numbers; they now represent about 10% of the United States population.

The sale of eyewear in the United States produced $13.2 billion in sales in 1994. That total excludes the sale of nonprescription sunglasses and over-the-counter reading glasses. The fees from comprehensive eye examinations produced an additional $4.3 billion. The major share of this ophthalmic market of $17.5 billion was held by optometrists in private practice, who earned approximately 33% of the income (Figure 1.2). Optical chains earned 19%; ophthalmologists, 16%; opticians in private practice, 12%; optical superstores, 11%; and health maintenance organizations (HMOs) and clinics earned 9%. The 1994 figures do not represent a change in the market share for optometrists in private practice since the previous AOA survey, conducted in 1992.

NUMBER OF ANNUAL EYE EXAMINATIONS

The number of comprehensive eye examinations performed annually by optometrists has grown steadily since the mid-1980s, when "parity" legis-

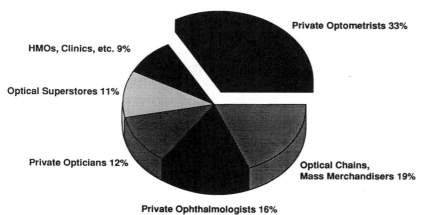

HMOs, Clinics, etc. 9%

Private Optometrists 33%

Optical Superstores 11%

Private Opticians 12%

Optical Chains,
Mass Merchandisers 19%

Private Ophthalmologists 16%

Figure 1.2. Share of the ophthalmic market, 1994. (From American Optometric Association. Caring for the Eyes of America—A Profile of the Optometric Profession. St. Louis: American Optometric Association, 1996. Reproduced with permission.)

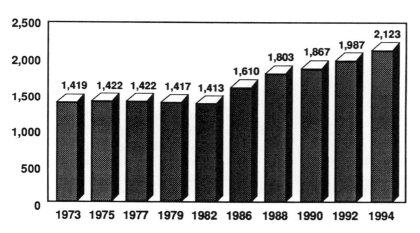

Figure 1.3. Annual number of eye examinations by optometrists, 1973–1994. (From American Optometric Association. Caring for the Eyes of America—A Profile of the Optometric Profession. St. Louis: American Optometric Association, 1996. Reproduced with permission.)

lation passed by the United States Congress gave optometrists the same standing as physicians under Medicare (Figure 1.3). This amendment of the Medicare law allowed optometrists to receive reimbursement for medical eye services performed for Medicare-eligible patients. Before the amendment, only ophthalmologists were eligible to provide these services under Medicare.

According to AOA annual surveys, as of 1994 the mean number of annual comprehensive examinations was 2,123. This is up 50% from 1982, when the total was 1,413. Use of pupillary dilation also continued to rise. The percentage of patients receiving pupillary dilation during examination was 47%. The mean number of office visits (other than for comprehensive examinations) in 1994 was 919. Because of the growing need of the United States population for eyewear, and because optometrists may provide

medical eye services to persons over 65 years of age, it is anticipated that the number of annual eye examinations will continue to rise during the 1990s.

SERVICES OFFERED BY OPTOMETRISTS

With respect to the services offered by optometrists, contact lens services are the most common, being provided by 97% of practicing optometrists. Approximately 93% of practicing optometrists provide dispensing services (e.g., spectacles). It is estimated that 50% of optometrists offer low vision services and 38% offer vision therapy. About 42% of optometrists receive Medicare reimbursement for postsurgical care rendered to patients who have received cataract surgery. More than half of all optometrists per-

Table 1.2. Mean Net Income (All Optometrists) By Year, 1958–1994

1958:	$9,970
1968:	$20,926
1977:	$37,403
1987:	$57,190
1991:	$74,845
1994:	$88,690

Source: AOA Economic Surveys, 1958–1994. St. Louis: American Optometric Association.

form some type of in-office finishing of eyewear, such as tinting, edging, or coating of spectacle lenses. This widespread use of in-office lens finishing is a recent development, thought to represent a response to consumer demands for faster delivery of eyewear.

INCOME FOR OPTOMETRISTS

The income figures for optometrists indicate that, as of 1994, the mean net income was $88,690. That figure is up 8.7% from the last survey in 1992, when the mean net income was $81,571 (Table 1.2). For individual practitioners the mean gross income was about $310,000 in 1994. That is a 20% increase from just 3 years earlier (when it was a little more than $256,000) and a 225% increase from 1978 (when it was $94,195). The 1994 survey also found that, to earn the mean net income, an optometrist had to be in practice for 11 years.

Optometric income has also kept ahead of inflation. Over the past decade the consumer price index has risen at the annual rate of 3.6%. During that same period the mean net income of optometrists rose 5.5% annually (Figure 1.4). AOA economic surveys have consistently shown that optometrists in partnership earn more gross and net income than individual proprietors, and the 1994 figures are merely the latest indication of that continuing trend. Likewise, self-employed optometrists continue to earn more mean net income than employed optometrists. In 1994, self-employed optometrists (i.e., individual proprietors, partnerships, and groups) earned $95,707; optometrists employed by physicians earned $78,373; optometrists working for optical chains earned $82,015; optometrists in multidisciplinary clinics earned $73,827; and optometrists working as employees of other optometrists earned $59,728 (Figure 1.5).

The net earnings of optometrists showed a steady increase over the course of the 1980s, particularly during the latter years of the decade. Optometrists in the East, South, and Midwest tended to report higher net incomes, with the expenses of practice slightly lower in the South than in other parts of the country.

For optometrists beginning a solo practice, 8–10 years are generally required before net income begins to reach the national mean. This length of time is usually needed to build a patient base and to pay off educational debts and the costs of initiating a prac-

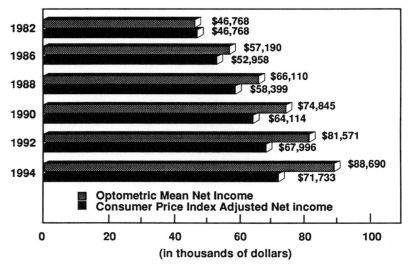

Figure 1.4. Net income adjusted for the consumer price index, 1994. (From American Optometric Association. Caring for the Eyes of America—A Profile of the Optometric Profession. St. Louis: American Optometric Association, 1996. Reproduced with permission.)

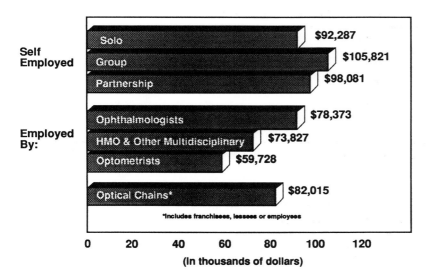

Figure 1.5. Net income by type of practice, 1994. (From American Optometric Association. Caring for the Eyes of America—A Profile of the Optometric Profession. St. Louis: American Optometric Association, 1996. Reproduced with permission.)

tice. Peak earning years generally are from 10 years to approximately 30 years in practice, at which time the average individual practitioner begins to reduce the time spent at work. Optometrists may expect to enjoy a professional career of 40 years or more.

EXPENSES OF PRACTICE

The expenses of self-employed optometrists in private practice may be divided into the following categories: laboratory costs; wages, benefits, and commissions for employees; rent or mortgage expense; and other costs of doing business. The net income is the amount remaining after these expenses have been paid. The percentage of gross income devoted to these expenses has changed relatively little over the past few years (Table 1.3). The laboratory costs range from 28% to 29% of gross income. The wages, benefits, and commissions paid to employees range from 13% to 15%. The cost of rent or mortgage payments ranges from 6% to 7%, and miscellaneous costs range from 14% to 16%. The ratio of net-to-gross income for optometrists usually ranges between 32% and 34%.

The gross earnings figures for optometrists are usually derived from three principal sources: examination fees, the sale of spectacles, and the fitting and sale of contact lenses. The approximate breakdown of these sources of income shows that the examina-

tion, diagnosis, and treatment of patients produces 45% of income; the sale of ophthalmic lenses and frames generates 35% of income; and the fitting and sale of contact lenses provides 20% of income.

An important factor affecting examination income is the emerging influence of government third-party reimbursement plans (e.g., Medicare, Medicaid, CHAMPUS) and nongovernmental vision and medical eye care plans (e.g., private vision service plans, insurance company health plans, Vision Service Plan). Although the influence of these plans varies from community to community, as of 1994 the percentage of mean gross income derived from nongovernmental third-party reimbursement plans for the average optometrist was approximately 30%; for government programs it was about 21% (Table 1.4). About two-thirds of optometrists report that they participate in managed care programs such as HMOs.

The results cited above are based primarily on AOA economic surveys and include all ages and years of practice. A somewhat different picture emerges for beginning practitioners.

BEGINNING PRACTITIONERS

Surveys conducted by the Association of Practice Management Educators (APME) during the period 1990–1995 have revealed that approximately 95% of optometry school graduates seek

Table 1.3. Cost of Conducting an Optometric Practice, 1988–1994

	1994	1992	1990	1988
Net income	32.2%	32.1%	32.7%	34.4%
Laboratory expenses	28.9%	29.0%	28.9%	29.2%
Employee wages	14.7%	14.5%	14.1%	13.2%
Rent, utilities, telephone	6.6%	6.7%	7.1%	6.8%
Contributions to retirement	1.7%	1.8%	1.8%	2.0%
Other expenses	15.9%	15.9%	15.4%	14.4%

Source: AOA Economic Surveys, 1988–1994. St. Louis: American Optometric Association.

Table 1.4. Third-Party Participation by Optometrists, 1986–1994: Mean Percentage of Gross Income From the Program (By Year)

Source of Income	1994	1992	1986
Government third-party plans	21.0	20.2	15.0
Nongovernmental third-party plans	30.8	26.4	NA

NA = data not available.
Source: AOA Economic Surveys, 1986–1994. St. Louis: American Optometric Association.

to enter the practice of optometry immediately, with the remaining 5% opting to pursue further educational training through residencies.

There is an abundance of choices awaiting graduates who are interested in entering practice—starting a solo practice, purchasing an existing solo practice, or entering into partnership; working as the employee of an optometrist, an ophthalmologist, or a commercial entity; becoming a member of a multidisciplinary clinic; serving in the armed forces or other government agency; going to work for private industry; or joining the faculty of a school or college of optometry. Based on APME survey results, most optometry school graduates seek to become private practitioners in a partnership setting within medium-size communities, and most of them believe it will require 5 years or more to realize this opportunity.

CHOICE OF PRACTICE OPPORTUNITY

One-third of graduates do not select a practice opportunity until after graduation from optometry school. The most popular choice of practice opportunity is associateship with another optometrist. Only about 10% of graduates enter immediately

into individual proprietorship, and an equal percentage choose a commercial mode of practice.

There are differences between male and female graduates. More than one-half of female graduates do not choose a practice opportunity until after graduation from optometry school, as compared to one-third of male graduates. Whereas approximately 30% of male graduates become self-employed immediately after graduation, only 12% of female graduates do so. Over 60% of males and over 70% of females enter into employment opportunities, with females more likely than males to seek residency training.

LOCATION OF PRACTICE

Two-thirds of optometry school graduates choose practice opportunities in cities that have a population of less than 100,000 persons.

ULTIMATE MODE OF PRACTICE

Approximately 70% of optometry school graduates seek ultimately to enter into partnership arrangements; about 25% wish to become individual proprietors. The majority of these graduates believe that it will require 5 years or longer for them to attain their ultimate mode of practice.

INCOME

The mean gross income for 1994 graduates in the first year of practice was approximately $47,300. The lowest income was earned by residents; the highest was earned by employees of commercial entities and of ophthalmologists. Men earned slightly more than women.

INDEBTEDNESS AT GRADUATION

Approximately 80% of optometry school graduates need to take out student loans to complete optometry school. The most common range of indebtedness is $40,000–60,000.

The process of identifying a practice opportunity should begin in optometry school, with a systematic effort to determine the personal and professional needs of the individual student. This process should come to fruition at graduation, permitting a smooth transition from student to practitioner. To realize such an ambitious goal, however, several key matters must be considered.

DECIDING ON PRACTICE OPPORTUNITIES

To successfully enter the practice of optometry, a new licensee must make several key decisions:

- Where to practice
- Whether to begin as an employer or as an employee
- How to satisfy the debts of education or of beginning a practice

Individual decisions should be based on personal preferences and an understanding of the relevant facts. Research is usually necessary to obtain information about a location or community. The status of the state law defining the practice of optometry is also an important consideration. Investigation of the community and its economic standing is important in considering the capacity of a community to absorb another practitioner or to support an op-

tometrist. Visits to the community and to individual practitioners are often crucial.

The decision to begin practice as an employee is usually based on economic necessity or recognition of the need for experience before initiating an individual practice. Graduates should consider carefully the advantages and disadvantages of employee arrangements; if employment is determined to be the best option, a systematic effort to locate a practice opportunity should be started while in optometry school. For graduates who desire immediate self-employment, meticulous planning, the use of competent advisors, and careful financial decision-making is obligatory.

Indebtedness should not be permitted to adversely influence goals and career plans. Maintaining educational debt at a minimum is a prerequisite for all graduates. Indebtedness influences earning capacity and the ability to secure loans needed to purchase equipment for the start of a practice, to buy a house and car, or to respond to unexpected financial emergencies. Planning should be initiated in school so that personal and professional goals can be attained more easily after graduation.

A wealth of reference materials is available to students or recent graduates, and they should be obtained and consulted. The AOA has a practice placement service and provides technical information to optometry students and association members. Optometry school alumni associations may also be used as a resource. The most important resource, however, is the initiative of individual students. Visiting practices, assessing communities, and compiling information about practice options are essential tasks that should be performed during optometry school. The prepared graduate is more likely to find an opportunity and to take advantage of it. That alone is reason to devote the necessary effort to the task.

In the chapters that follow, the process of beginning a practice, organizing it, and operating it efficiently are described. It should always be kept in mind, however, that the individual initiative of the clinician is the primary consideration for any practice and that success is more often dependent on it than on any other factor.

BIBLIOGRAPHY

Allergan, Inc.1994/1995 Pathways in Optometry Program Survey. Irvine, CA: Allergan, 1995.

American Optometric Association. Caring for the Eyes of America—A Profile of the Optometric Profession. St. Louis: American Optometric Association, 1996.

American Optometric Association. A Profile of the Optometric Profession. St. Louis: American Optometric Association, 1996.

Chapter 2

Self-Employment Options

James Albright, Craig Hisaka, W. Howard McAlister, and Timothy A. Wingert

Liberty means responsibility. That is why most men dread it.

—George Bernard Shaw
Maxims for Revolutionists

The majority of optometrists—approximately 70%—are in private practice (Table 2.1). Therefore, the decision to enter private practice is one that is made by most optometry school graduates. Surveys conducted in the 1990s by the Association of Practice Management Educators (APME) have revealed that approximately 60% of graduates enter private practice after graduation as employees and that approximately 30% are self-employed (the remaining 10% enter residencies). These same APME surveys have shown that most graduates who enter employee positions immediately after graduation intend to become self-employed eventually.

The basic decision that must be made by the new graduate is whether to be an employer or an employee. This chapter describes the advantages and disadvantages of entering the various types of self-employment—as a sole proprietor, as a partner, or as a member of a professional association or corporation. It also describes expense sharing. Employment opportunities are described in Chapter 4.

SOLE PROPRIETORSHIP

A sole proprietorship can be described as a nonincorporated business organization that has one indi-

vidual as its owner. The optometrist-owner may have one or more optometrists working for the practice, either as employees or as independent contractors. The sole proprietor, however, owns 100% of the practice.

To enter into sole proprietorship, a graduate may start a new practice or may purchase an existing practice.

STARTING A PRACTICE

The decision to start a practice is a major one and requires extensive planning. Usually, the greatest drawback to starting a practice is financial. Most optometrists have significant loans and debt when they graduate, and the added debt of opening a new office may prevent such an undertaking from being financially feasible. The optometrist must carefully evaluate income and expense projections for the practice, with emphasis on keeping fixed overhead expenses to a minimum. Projections for income should be conservative. When starting a practice "cold," it is essential to have outside sources of income from other employment opportunities.

In addition, the new practitioner needs to learn and develop excellent business and management skills. It will be helpful to take extra

Table 2.1. Mode of Practice for Self-Employed Optometrists, 1994

Mode of Practice	Percentage of Optometrists
Sole proprietorship	24% sole proprietorships
	24% professional associations or corporations
Partnerships	10% partnership and group practices
Professional associations or corporations	11% two or more shareholder professional associations or corporations
Optical chain franchises	1% owner of optical chain franchise

Source: Adapted from American Optometric Association. Caring for the Eyes of America—A Profile of the Optometric Profession. St. Louis: American Optometric Association, 1996.

course work in these areas. Courses in business law, financial management, and marketing are particularly useful. Developing a team of advisors—including a skilled certified public accountant (CPA) familiar with optometry, an attorney, real estate and insurance agents, and a banker—is essential.

Another key factor in starting a practice is finding the right location. An excellent location can mean more than an increase in earnings; it can be the difference between success and failure. The topic of location is discussed in Chapter 6.

If a graduate is willing to accept the responsibility of managing a business and can overcome the financial risks involved, the pride, rewards, and satisfaction of watching a practice grow and mature can be extremely gratifying. A graduate must be willing to forego immediate financial returns for the long-term benefits that self-employment provides. In financial terms, however, the rewards are much better for self-employed optometrists than for employed practitioners. The American Optometric Association (AOA) Economic Surveys (see Chapter 1) show that higher levels of income are reported by self-employed optometrists. When starting a new practice, however, about an 8- to 10-year period is needed to achieve mean income levels. Once the practice has been established, it can sustain the practitioner 30–40 years. Often a sole practitioner will take on employees or decide to form a partnership, which further increases the size of the practice. Because of the liberty the sole proprietor enjoys to make key decisions, there is considerable flexibility in this form of practice arrangement.

PURCHASING A PRACTICE

The purchase of an existing practice can be a better choice than starting a new practice. An established office will have equipment, patient flow, staff, and procedures already in place. Financial planning is much easier, because the practice has an established gross income, overhead expenses, and cash flow.

Determining the fair value of the practice is usually the most difficult aspect of the purchase agreement and is discussed in Chapter 3.

To pay for the practice, a loan can be taken from a bank or the seller can self-finance the purchase. In either event, the purchaser must pay for the practice, with interest, over a period of years. Such an arrangement can be financially advantageous, however, to starting a new practice. The sole proprietor can often do better financially during the 5–10 years of repayment than if a new practice is started. Again, financial and legal advice will be needed to determine if the arrangement is a fair one, to allocate the practice assets for tax purposes, and to draft the contract of sale.

Table 2.2 summarizes the major advantages and disadvantages of a sole proprietorship.

The largest single group of practicing optometrists—approximately half of those in private practice—are in sole proprietorships. However, the

Table 2.2. Advantages and Disadvantages of Sole Proprietorship

Advantages
  One person rule, with control over decisions and destiny
  Higher long-term income potential and greater equity potential
  Independence, control of the office schedule, time off, vacations, and similar matters
  Choice of optometric specialties to be practiced
Disadvantages
  The pressure of all decisions and management and marketing responsibilities lies on the shoulders of the practitioner
  Multiple financial risks and competitive challenges
  Lower starting income, higher start-up costs
  Lack of office coverage in cases of illness, vacation, time off, and so forth
  Fewer specialties to offer

trend is away from solo practice and toward partnership or group practice.

PARTNERSHIP

A partnership may be defined as a voluntary contract between two or more practitioners to pool their skill, knowledge, labor, and capital in a practice, with the understanding that there will be some proportionate sharing of profit and loss between them. Partnership is the most common form of group practice. In a partnership arrangement, ownership is shared, as is decision-making. Often the partners will divide partnership duties so that one partner is responsible for the management of personnel, another is responsible for financial management, and so on. Income is divided (as is loss) on some proportional basis. The most common means of division is on a percentage basis (e.g., 50%-50%), but income can also be divided on the basis of productivity (e.g., 60%-40%) or by a combination of these two techniques (e.g., 50% of income divided on a percentage basis; the other 50% on a productivity basis). The partnership agreement should specify the management of this and other matters.

The partnership terms should be described in a written agreement. Because of the complexity of these agreements and because state laws will govern certain aspects of the partnership (through the Uniform Partnership Act), an attorney will be needed to draft the partnership agreement. The agreement must describe the formation, maintenance, and dissolution of the partnership. Dissolution must be planned for because all partnerships are limited by the lives of the partners and, thus, will have to be dissolved one day. It is to be hoped that the dissolution will be due to retirement; however, the death or disability of the partners must also be considered.

Partnerships are usually formed by the assimilation of an associate into a solo practice or by the merger of two solo practices.

ASSOCIATESHIP

Most two-person partnerships are created by an established practitioner and a new graduate. There is an initial trial period, usually involving 1–2 years. The purpose of the trial period is to see if the two practitioners are compatible and can work well together.

There are significant advantages for the new graduate who chooses to try associateship in the hopes of entering into partnership. First, there is immediate earning capacity with the associate usually being paid a salary, a percentage of income produced, or a combination of the two. The associate also gains valuable experience, learning the business side of optometry and the art of practice management. To receive this income, there is little initial investment required of the associate, an especially important consideration when there are educational debts to be paid. Most important, if the associate chooses well, a partnership will be formed, providing practice and financial security for as long as the partners wish to continue the arrangement.

If the two practitioners decide during the trial period that partnership is desirable, they can begin

Table 2.3. Checklist of Issues to be Discussed by the Prospective Partners

_____	Name of partnership
_____	Purpose of partnership
_____	Location of practice
_____	Value of practice
_____	Statement of capital
_____	Division of income
_____	Additional income
_____	Partners' powers and limitations
_____	Spending of partnership funds
_____	Division of practice expenses
_____	Policy and procedure decisions
_____	Nepotism
_____	Financial records and accounting procedures
_____	New equipment fund
_____	Provisions for taking in additional partners
_____	Vacations, professional time, postgraduate courses
_____	Military leave
_____	Disability insurance
_____	Life insurance
_____	Optometric fees
_____	Prohibited acts
_____	Outside employment or business interests
_____	Arbitration clause
_____	Withdrawal of partner
_____	Retirement plan
_____	Expulsion of partner
_____	Voluntary dissolution of partnership
_____	Restrictive covenants
_____	Malpractice insurance coverage
_____	Amendment and review

the process of negotiating and reaching agreement to form a partnership. During negotiations they should discuss and reach agreement on the following key issues:

- Philosophy of practice
- Time and work load devoted to the practice
- Distribution of earnings and expenditures
- Delegation and management of support personnel
- Value of the practice

There are many items that need to be discussed before they are incorporated into the partnership agreement (Table 2.3). One important consideration is the buy-in arrangement for the associate. Often the buy-in can be achieved without the direct payment of money. After the purchase price is agreed on, the payment is made over a period

that is usually 5–7 years. The associate is paid less than the associate actually earns, with the difference constituting a payment toward the purchase price. This difference is greatest in the first year and gradually decreases over the payment period, until eventually equality is attained. The total sum contributed by the associate equals the agreed-on amount for purchase. Of course, the associate can also borrow the requisite amount from a bank, purchase the 50% interest, and repay the bank over a period of years. Whether this alternative would be preferable depends on the cost of the loan (and the ability of the associate to obtain the loan).

MERGERS

A merger occurs when two or more established practices join together and the practitioners combine resources to share in profits and losses. In some mergers, the practitioners maintain separate locations.

Considerable negotiation is often required to achieve a merger because of the increased number of assets, personnel, and operating procedures. Complicated financial arrangements are usually needed to equalize the contributions to the partnership by the partners. Accountants and attorneys are required participants of the formation process.

The more important items that must be discussed include legal and tax considerations, the premerger agreement, division of income and responsibilities, financial record keeping, administrative policies, patient records, and sharing of office space, assets, and personnel.

Legal and Tax Considerations

An in-depth analysis of the legal and tax consequences of the merger should be performed to determine the tax issues that must be dealt with by the new partnership. Tax planning is particularly important.

Premerger Agreement

It is often wise to sign a premerger agreement, particularly if the purchase of realty or other significant financial commitments are to be made. The purpose of the agreement is to protect each practitioner from the unilateral withdrawal of the other after sizable financial obligations have been incurred.

Division of Income and Responsibilities

The practitioners must discuss and agree on the financial terms of the partnership. Patient volume, fees, working hours, and percentage of ownership are but a few of the matters to be decided. The capital contributions of the partners to the partnership must also be determined. If these contributions are inequitable, adjustments must be made to equalize the accounts over time. In addition, the partners will need to divide the administrative duties of the partnership.

Financial Record Keeping

Financial matters such as credit and payment policies, the financial record keeping system to be used, and collections procedures must be determined. If third-party insurance plans are to be billed, new provider numbers may be required.

Administrative Policies

The partners will need to set the procedures for scheduling of appointments, division of patients, hours and days of work, and management of patients.

Patient Records

A filing system for patient records will have to be selected and a uniform system of recording of data will need to be devised.

Sharing the Office

If a new office will be needed to accommodate the partnership, the partners will need to determine the space needed, its location, and the layout of the fa-cility. Appropriate use of space, personnel, and patient flow will have to be determined.

Sharing Assets

The practitioners must determine the equipment, instruments, furnishings, inventories, and other items to be shared. Some assets may need to be discarded; some new assets may need to be purchased.

Sharing Personnel

The staff members to be retained, their duties, and what they are to be paid must be decided. Then, the partners must meet with their staffs to inform them of the merger and to discuss individual staff roles in the new partnership. A new office policy manual will be needed, because administrative policies are usually different between offices.

LIMITED LIABILITY COMPANIES

A relatively new development in partnership arrangements is the limited liability company (LLC). An LLC may be formed by two or more individuals, partnerships, or corporations, and, in structure, it is like a corporation. If an LLC has fewer than two members, it must be dissolved.

An LLC may be used to render professional services; thus, two or more optometrists can form an LLC. Special provisions apply to the personal liability of members and to the transferability of members' ownership to successors (these rules are similar to the rules for professional associations or corporations).

For tax purposes, the LLC is treated like a partnership. The profit (or loss) is allocated to the members of the LLC just as in a partnership. Members of the LLC are not liable as individuals for the debts or negligence of the LLC or for the debts or negligence of other members. In this respect, the LLC is like a professional association or corporation. The formation of LLCs is controlled by state law (the state's Limited Liability Company Act). Legal counsel will be needed to determine if this form of partnership is appropriate and to ensure that the LLC is properly established.

Table 2.4. Advantages and Disadvantages
of Partnerships

Advantages
  Generally higher earnings than solo optometrists
  Shared overhead, less captial outlay per partner
    compared to solo optometrists
  Office coverage during vacations, illness, personal
    holidays
  Consultation with partner for business and patient man-
    agement decisions
  Expanded hours, convenience for patients
  Investment in career protected and equity established for
    retirement, disability, or death
Disadvantages
  Loss of independence
  Personality conflicts with partners or the spouses of
    partners
  Differences in professional ideas and philosophies
  Unequal distribution of patient load
  Unequal distribution of income based on productivity of
    the partners

Table 2.4 summarizes the major advantages and disadvantages of partnerships.

SHIFT TOWARD PARTNERSHIP

The trend in optometry is toward partnership or group practices. Reasons for this trend are partially financial and partially personal. In a partnership, overhead is shared among partners, which increases earnings compared to the solo practice. There is a clear difference in earnings based on the size of the practice. Group practices (three or more partners) earn more per practitioner than partnerships (two partners), which in turn earn more than sole practitioners (see Chapter 1). There are also the personal benefits of partnership to be considered. Specialization, consultation, expanded office hours, and increased coverage are true benefits of partnership or group practice. These benefits allow partners to enjoy more time outside the practice, pursuing professional or personal activities without loss of partnership income.

The key to a successful partnership is choosing well and having a mutual admiration and respect for each other. A well-conceived partnership agreement is another essential requirement. Also, because of the complexities of partnership, establishing a competent team of advisors is important to continued viability and success.

PROFESSIONAL ASSOCIATIONS OR CORPORATIONS

Professional associations (PAs) and professional corporations (PCs) are artificial entities that are endowed by law with the capacity of perpetual succession. The PA or PC may consist of a single individual or several individuals, but, in either case, there is unity of ownership and management. Because of the unique powers that may be exercised by PAs and PCs, they are accorded a legal status that is akin to that of a separate being. The decision to form a PA or PC is typically a financial one, based on a determination that the tax and retirement benefits offset the additional cost and time involved. Tax and legal counsel are needed to make this decision.

The PA or PC must be owned by a professional licensee; laypersons may not hold an ownership interest. A PA or PC is formed by one or more licensees filing articles of incorporation or association within the state in which the practice will be located. The PA or PC is formed by the professional licensee, who, as owner, holds shares of stock. The licensee also serves as the chief officer of the PA or PC, responsible for management. Because the PA or PC is a separate entity, it may sign contracts in its own name, borrow money, own property, and exercise other rights normally accorded only to persons. In addition, the PA or PC may contract with individuals to provide services. The number one employee of the PA or PC is the licensee, who is paid a salary and awarded benefits under an employment agreement with the PA or PC. Therefore, an optometrist who forms a PA or PC will be its owner, chief officer, and most important employee.

PAs and PCs differ from partnerships in terms of their continuity. In partnerships, if a partner dies the partnership is usually dissolved. In a PA or PC, if a shareholder dies the PA or PC continues because it is a separate legal entity that may be owned by a successor shareholder. To transfer ownership, the successor purchases the shares of stock held by the previous shareholder.

Because the PA or PC is recognized as a separate legal entity, it is usually the owner of property used by the employees of the PA or PC. If a PA or PC is formed to render eye care services, the office furnishings and equipment, the computers, the ophthalmic instruments, inventories of frames and lenses, and other items are owned by the PA or PC. For this reason, tax deductions and benefits are claimed by the PA or PC, not by its owners.

The status of a PA or PC as a separate entity can also shield its owners from responsibility for debts, judgments, or other legal claims. Obligations of the PA or PC must be paid from the assets of the PA or PC and not from the assets of its owners. This differs significantly from partnership or sole proprietorship. The partners are responsible for the financial obligations of the partnership, and the sole proprietor is responsible for the obligations of the sole proprietorship.

In some circumstances it may be appropriate to form a special type of corporation, called a subchapter S corporation or S corporation. The typical example is a dispensary that is separate from the professional practice. The use of an S corporation allows ownership to be shared by laypersons (such as opticians, business people, or spouses). The number of owners is limited to 35 shareholders, but they do not have to be professional licensees. Another key difference is in income taxation. An S corporation is organized like a corporation, but it is taxed like a partnership. In a partnership, no tax is paid by the partnership; rather, the income (or loss) is shared by the partners. Because a PA or PC is recognized as a separate legal entity, if there is a profit earned by the PA or PC it must pay income tax on the profit. (The employees of the PA or PC also pay income tax on the salary and benefits received from the PA or PC.) In an S corporation, however, the income (or loss) is divided by the shareholders; the corporation pays no income taxes. Even so, the S corporation may still claim certain tax benefits, such as contributions to retirement plans, premiums paid for insurance coverage, and other tax deductions that may otherwise be claimed only by PAs and PCs.

Because of state legal requirements, the advice and assistance of a CPA and an attorney will be required whether a partnership, a PA or PC, or an S corporation is being formed.

EXPENSE-SHARING (SHARED EXPENSE AGREEMENT)

In an expense-sharing or shared expense agreement, two or more optometrists share a common location and the expenses of the practice in a manner proportionate to their usage. Each optometrist has a separate patient base, financial and patient records, and equipment and instruments. In an expense-sharing arrangement, the practitioners do not share in profits the way they would in a partnership, and they have separate bookkeeping systems to chart income. Certain expenses are shared, however, in some proportion agreed to by the optometrists. These expenses typically include rent, utilities, repair and maintenance costs, supplies, lease payments on shared equipment, insurance, and the salaries of common employees.

This arrangement falls short of partnership because neither practitioner has any ownership interest in the practice of the other. Instead, it consists of two independent businesses that have found it advantageous to share certain common expenses.

The basic requirements of expense sharing are:

- Each practitioner is an individual proprietor.
- Overhead expenses, such as the office lease, utilities, salaries of employees, insurance, and other necessary expenditures are shared on a pro-rata basis.
- Ownership of equipment and furnishings is usually separate, although certain items may be purchased and owned jointly.
- A joint bank account is established for the payment of joint expenses, and each practitioner is required periodically to contribute a certain sum to the account; individual contributions are usually a stated percentage of each practitioner's gross income.
- Records are separate and remain the property of the individual practitioners.

Table 2.5. Advantages and Disadvantages of Expense Sharing

Advantages

Decreased overhead per optometrist compared to two solo optometrists. With reduced overhead per optometrist, more financial resources available for equipment and instrument purchases and other assets.

Possibly some coverage for patients in cases of emergency or vacation, although joint coverage is not required and must be agreed on by the two practitioners

Consultation and referral to the other optometrist if the optometrist has a different area of interest or specialty

Each optometrist maintains a separate practice and controls individual policies, decisions, and management

Disadvantages

Coverage of patients by the other practitioner is not required in cases of illness, disability, vacations, and so forth, and must be agreed on beforehand

No established value for the practice and no built-in buyer as in a partnership or corporation

No sharing of profits as in a partnership or professional association or corporation

Conflicts over scheduling may occur when using a common receptionist

Shared expenses must be divided in a fair and reasonable manner or conflict will occur

Decisions about furnishings, improvements, salaries, and other matters may be sources of disagreement

Personnel must be shared on an equal or fair basis or problems can result

---

- Payment on accounts, collections, and accounts receivable are independently maintained.
- Personnel are usually jointly supervised, but a sole personnel manager can be designated by the practitioners if they so desire.
- A maximum sum is commonly stipulated for joint obligations unless both practitioners agree to the expenditure in advance.
- Adequate liability insurance is required of all practitioners.
- Arrangements may be made for coverage during absences, including compensation to be awarded for such coverage.
- Certain ethical standards or membership in certain professional organizations may be required of all practitioners.

Some provision for termination of the arrangement with adequate notice will be included in the agreement.

Table 2.5 lists the advantages and disadvantages of expense sharing.

As in all business arrangements, an attorney will be needed to draft a contract that reflects the agreement reached by the parties.

CONCLUSION

Self-employed forms of doing business offer the most long-term opportunity, flexibility, security, and financial return for optometrists (Table 2.6). They also require the most effort, investment, commitment, and risk. For graduates who do not feel prepared to enter directly into self-employment after graduation, various employment options may be considered. In a profession in which a 40-year career as a self-employed practitioner is not unusual, a year or two of employment, used to learn the art of practice administration and patient management, merely diminishes the term of self-employment to 39 or 38 years. In the long term, this short period of employment may prove to be an excellent investment. Employment opportunities for graduates are discussed in the next chapter.

Table 2.6. Differences Between Practice Arrangements

	Partnership	Expense Sharing	Association or Corporation	Associate
Assets	All shared equally	Some shared equally, some not shared	All owned by corporation	All owned by employer
Expenses	All shared equally	Some shared equally, some shared on the basis of use, some not shared	All paid by corporation	All paid by employer
Net Income	Divided equally or according to percentage of ownership	Each doctor gets what he or she earns	Each doctor gets a salary and net shared on the basis of each doctor's ownership	All owned by employer; each employee may pay a percentage
Fees	Same for all doctors	Each doctor sets his or her own	Same for all doctors	Same for all doctors
Billing	Combined bill	Separate bill from each doctor	Combined bill	Combined bill
Disability provision	Yes	No	Yes	Possibly
Death benefit	Yes	No	Yes	Usually none
Retirement benefits	Yes	No	Yes	Usually none
Provision for continuity of practice	Yes	No	Yes	Possibly, but often not
Obligations to cover for each other	Mandatory	None	Mandatory	Mandatory
Records	Merged	Separate	Merged, owned by corporation	Merged, owned by employer

BIBLIOGRAPHY

Allergan, Inc. Pathways in Optometry. Irvine, CA: Allergan, Inc., 1995.

American Optometric Association. Caring for the Eyes of America: Profile of the Optometric Profession, 1996. St. Louis: American Optometric Association, 1996.

Bennett I. Management for the Eyecare Practitioner. Stoneham, MA: Butterworth, 1993.

Classé JG. Legal Aspects of Optometry. Stoneham, MA: Butterworth, 1989.

Gailmard NB. The associate's job search: a reality check. Rev Optom 1994;(8):41–4.

Kattouf RS. Coasting to retirement. Optom Manage 1995;31(12):28–37.

Koetting RA, Kattouf RS. Closing the generation gap. Optom Manage 1995;31(5):16–28.

Lakin DH. Gradual transfer: partnership without the debt. Optom Econ 1995;5(3):40–4.

Miller PJ. What your heirs should know about your practice. Optom Econ 1995;5(1):28–31.

Chapter 3

Purchasing a Practice

Gary Moss, John G. Classé, and Stuart M. Rothman

You get what you pay for.

—Contemporary
American philosophy

For optometry school graduates who want to become sole practitioners, the purchase of a practice is an option that should be given due consideration. It can be preferable to starting a practice "cold," both for economic and for personal reasons. Of course, for graduates who aspire to enter into partnership, such a decision will require the purchase of some percentage of the equity of an existing partnership. Therefore, for a considerable number of new graduates, the purchase of a practice is a viable option that should be investigated and understood. Surveys show that 50–70% of graduates purchase an ownership interest in solo or group practices within 3–6 years after graduation.

The purchase of an existing practice has several obvious advantages and disadvantages.

ADVANTAGES OF PURCHASING A PRACTICE

A practitioner who buys an existing practice is purchasing a business with a proven track record. Although there will usually be some loss of patient base—on the average, 5–15%—losses should be offset by the new patients gained with the implementation of adequate transition procedures. With an existing practice, the assessment of projected income is more reliable than with a practice opened "cold," and an operating budget for the practice can be more accurately determined. The new practitioner can expect to have patients scheduled for examination from the first day of operation, which produces an immediate financial and emotional benefit for the practitioner. The new practitioner will initially incur significant out-of-pocket expenses, such as the down payment for the practice, closing costs, attorney's and accountant's fees, additional security deposits for the premises and for the utilities, and initial operating costs (such as payments for stationery, additional equipment, and inventory). Income from the practice helps ease this financial burden. Emotionally, the new practitioner gets the benefit of being busy, of helping and satisfying the existing patients of the practice, and of using a wide range of skills.

The purchaser of an existing practice is also purchasing an existing location. Usually, the purchaser assumes an office lease that has more favorable terms than the practitioner could have obtained through the negotiation of a new lease. Leasehold improvements probably will not be needed, but if a new practitioner wants to modify an office, it may not be necessary to do so immediately, and the cost should be reflected as an adjustment in the purchase price. Because the office has already been used to deliver patient care, any problems related to patient flow have probably been eliminated. The telephone system and other utilities are already connected and operational, and there is also a current telephone listing for the office in the telephone book. Laboratory accounts, as well as accounts for contact lenses, frames, and other materials, already will have been established, making it easier for the new practitioner to obtain credit when opening new accounts.

Purchasing an existing practice in a given area does not change the optometrist-to-population ratio in that area, because the new practitioner merely replaces the departing one. In an area that has experienced no growth, new patients will either be transfers from another practitioner or new arrivals to the area. When a practice is purchased, the new practitioner is not totally dependent on drawing these patients to the practice and can use the revenue from existing patients to supplement efforts to attract new patients. The practitioner can also devote efforts to internal office marketing, which, studies show, will yield a rate of return that is up to six times higher than external office marketing.

The purchase of an existing practice usually allows the new practitioner to assume command of an existing trained staff. The staff is familiar with the operation of the practice, the patient population, and the problems encountered by the practice. A familiar staff person answering the phone can ease a patient's fear of being seen by a new, unfamiliar practitioner. Having the selling practitioner remain in the practice for a transition period of several weeks to months will also ease the transfer of patients to the new practitioner while enabling the selling practitioner to familiarize the new practitioner with the operation of the office. The selling practitioner can also assist in the introduction of the new practitioner to key people in the area, such as bankers, accountants, lawyers, and other health care professionals.

DISADVANTAGES OF PURCHASING A PRACTICE

A purchaser's greatest risk arises from the potential loss of patients. Because it is difficult to predict whether the patients of the selling practitioner will return to the practice after ownership is transferred, there is considerable financial pressure on the new practitioner. The new practitioner usually will not want to disrupt operations or initially make drastic changes for fear of alienating the existing patients of the practice. Thus, the new practitioner will probably have to incorporate changes gradually, over time, until the practice reflects the style of the new practitioner.

If the selling practitioner is retiring after many years of practice, equipment may be older, and the physical layout of the office may need refurbishing. Equipment may have to be purchased or improvements made, requiring an outlay of capital. Management information systems incorporating new technologies, such as electronic data transmission, will quite often need to be purchased. While the new practitioner will want to keep the existing staff, if at all possible, doing so usually involves paying slightly higher wages. Staff members may require retraining or alteration of duties. It may be difficult to change habits or duties if staff members have been with the selling practitioner for any length of time. In addition, provider panels of which the seller is a member may not be easily transferrable to a new practitioner.

In summary, purchasing an existing practice affords the new practitioner the luxury of not having to perform the many tasks that are a part of opening "cold." Finding a location; leasing an office; hiring employees; purchasing equipment, supplies, and inventory; setting up accounts; arranging for utilities; and building a patient base are not necessary because these tasks have already been performed. In fact, it is this immediate viability that is at the basis of the purchase of an existing practice. Unlike the practitioner who opens "cold," however, the purchaser of an existing practice has to be able to fully evaluate its worth and determine a fair market price for its purchase.

EVALUATION OF THE AREA IN WHICH THE PRACTICE IS LOCATED

Evaluation of the area in which a practice is located will provide information about the current and future viability of the practice. This area may be defined as the probable drawing area of the practice. That can be five blocks, 5 miles, or 20 miles, depending on whether the practice is located in a city, suburban area, or rural area. The potential buyer can evaluate existing patient demographic data to determine the extent of this area. In addition, natural boundaries like highways, rivers, undeveloped land, and city limits can also be assumed to set borders around a practice. Although a practice moved from one location to another in the same drawing area will experience some loss of patients, a practice moved from one drawing area to a completely new one will lose the bulk of the patient base. Since a major portion of the payment for a practice is used to secure goodwill or active patient records, moving from one drawing area to another is not a wise idea. The drawing area should be evaluated as though the purchaser were opening up a new practice rather than maintaining an established one. The goal in buying an existing practice is to expand its patient base and to have it increase in value rather than attempting merely to maintain the status quo. In evaluating the area, the potential buyer must look to see if factors that will support new growth are present.

ECONOMIC EVALUATION

Economic factors to consider include the employment rate, the viability of other practices, population demographics, key economic indicators, and social factors.

Employment Rate

Employed people are more likely to have disposable income and health insurance. This fact makes it more likely that employed individuals will seek and be able to afford health care, including optometric care. Also, areas with large employer groups will have more managed care plans that offer vision services to employees. The employment rate of an area may fluctuate from year to year, but the trends of the area can be compared to state, regional, and national trends. This information can be obtained from local, state, or federal government statistics.

Viability of Other Practices and Businesses

A survey of other health care providers should be performed to determine the number of practitioners who have full-time and part-time practices in the area. Full-time practitioners derive all of their income from the area; part-time practitioners must supplement practice income with income from outside the area. Retail businesses should be evaluated for reinvestment. A reinvestment in new equipment, machinery, and inventory generally is undertaken when business owners are experiencing growth or when there is potential for new growth. Speaking to these health care professionals or small business owners would be time well spent on the part of the prospective new practitioner.

Population Demographics

There are three factors to consider: the optometrist-to-population ratio, the population growth, and the population age.

1. *Optometrist-to-population ratio.* It is estimated by an AOA Manpower study that one full-time optometrist is needed for every 7,800 people. This statistic may be misleading because it does not take into account the presence of ophthalmologists or opticians who may be duplicating some of the optometrists' services. A more realistic appraisal must consider the setting of the practice—rural, suburban, or urban. Minimum population requirements needed for these settings are rural: 5,000–8,000 people per optometrist; suburban: 12,000–18,000 people per optometrist; and urban: 25,000–45,000 people per optometrist. Using these ratios as a rough estimate of practice viability, a prospective buyer can evaluate the saturation level of practitioners in the drawing area of the practice. Although these ratios will not be changed by the purchase of an existing practice, the potential for new growth may be affected by an unfavorable ratio.
2. *Population growth.* The infusion of new people into an area means the arrival of prospective patients with no eye care practitioner. These people will be the most fertile source of growth for the practice. In an area with relatively flat growth, new patients will have to be obtained from the patient population of other practitioners or from new arrivals who have moved into the practice area.
3. *Population age.* The population age of an area should be favorable to the type of services that

may be added to the practice by the new practitioner. For example, a new practitioner who wants to add low vision services to an existing practice needs to have a population that is skewed toward senior citizens.

4. *Income level of population.* The per capita income of the drawing area needs to be evaluated for the type of services provided, as well as the fee structure of the practice.
5. *Key economic indicators.* There are several economic factors that should be considered:
   a. *New business starts.* New business in an area generally means that there is a favorable economic climate. The success (or failure) rates of these businesses and the turnover rate of small businesses in the area should be analyzed.
   b. *New housing starts.* This statistic indicates the movement of new people into an area. It may also signal the movement of new jobs and new businesses into an area.
   c. *Home prices.* The largest investment that most Americans make is in their homes. When real estate values are favorable, people feel more confident about the economy and are more likely to spend disposable income. Downward trends in real estate generally will mean a downward economic trend, which will exert an effect on all business in an area.
   d. *Industry.* Practicing in an area that is tied to a specific industry or to a specific company may be favorable when economic times are prosperous. However, it can be disastrous in tighter economic times when the industry or company is not doing well. The ideal situation would be to practice in an area that has a diversified economy and offers jobs in various industries.
   e. *Social factors.* While there is no rule that says a practitioner must live in the same area as the practice, there are geographic limits to the separation of primary residence and practice. Just as with any business, running an optometric practice requires time well beyond that needed to examine patients. The stress and strain of long hours spent commuting to and from the practice will undoubtedly take a toll on the practitioner and may affect the practitioner's willingness to tend to the practice beyond patient care hours. The practice area needs to be evaluated for social factors that would make the practitioner and his or her family comfortable living within a reasonable commuting distance of the practice. Examples of factors to consider include the quality of the school system, cultural and recreational opportunities, health care facilities, climate, affordability and desirability of housing, religious institutions, and the ability of the spouse to earn an income in his or her field of expertise.

GETTING THE INFORMATION

Fully investigating the economic and social factors discussed above requires a significant time commitment when a potential buyer visits the practice area. Information can be obtained from local chambers of commerce, real estate offices, banking institutions, other health care practitioners, other business owners, public service companies, local newspapers, direct mail companies, and friends and relatives who live in the area.

FACTORS DETERMINING PRACTICE WORTH

To evaluate the worth of a practice, the potential buyer should consider the gross and net income of the practice, the scope of practice offered by the selling practitioner, the practice location, the existing office lease, the patient records, the transition period, the physical resources of the practice, and the accounts receivable.

GROSS INCOME

Simply put, gross income is the total amount of money taken in by the practice for goods and services. The gross income for the 3 years before the sale should be reviewed. This information can be obtained from form 1120 and the profit and loss statement of the practice if the practice is a professional association or corporation, from form 1065 if it is a partnership, or from schedule

C of the seller's tax return if the practice is a sole proprietorship.

The gross income should be evaluated for growth from year to year. A practice with an increase in gross income that is less than the increase in the cost of living index for that same period of time has actually lost income. A decrease in the gross income from year to year indicates that there may be major changes in the area, the economy, or the perception of the practice or practitioner. If there are increases in fees, they must be considered, because an increase in gross income may be related to the change in fees, rather than to real growth of the practice.

Gross income should also be compared to the regional average gross income. This comparison may provide some indication of the economic viability of the practice and of the area. The number of hours that the practice is in operation must be considered. A practice that is only open part-time may have increased earning potential if hours are expanded; reduced hours may also indicate a practice that has peaked in its earning potential.

As the gross income of a solo practitioner increases, there will come a point at which further growth in income can only be achieved by the addition of another optometrist, extra technical support, or an increase in space. Practices with lower gross incomes may not be able to support a new practitioner who is not only required to finance the purchase of the practice but also to repay student loans.

NET INCOME

The prospective buyer should determine not only the actual net income that is realized by a practice but also the ratio of net income to gross income. Most dispensing optometric practices will have a net-to-gross income ratio of 25–35%. Nondispensing practices that are strictly service-based may have a higher net-to-gross income ratio, since the overhead expenses are usually lower. Practices that have a lower than average net-to-gross income ratio may incur higher than normal overhead expenses. This result may be caused by the area or the location of the practice, or it may indicate that there is inefficient office management. Practices with low net-to-gross income ratios also may be charging

lower than normal fees for services and materials or may have incurred considerable debt service.

In looking at a practice's net income, the itemization of office expenditures should be investigated. These expenditures can be found on the profit and loss statement of an incorporated practice or on the schedule C of an individual proprietor's tax return. Office expenses should be evaluated relative to national or regional averages. Deviations from average can indicate to the prospective buyer how efficiently the practice was run and how practice income was spent. The prospective buyer can use these figures to calculate how expenses might increase or decrease after the purchase of the practice. A useful means of obtaining an assessment of the practice's financial health is through the use of a financial ratio analysis (see Chapter 28).

When a practice is purchased, there is an inevitable loss of some existing patients. These are patients who, for whatever reason, decide not to return to the new practitioner. They will need to be replaced by new ones whom the purchaser will attract to the practice. The potential effect of a loss of patients to practice income should be determined; the economic effect of 5%, 10%, 15% and greater loss can be calculated using scenario analysis. Patient attrition will exert a direct effect on the gross income of the practice. Unfortunately, fixed expenses, such as salaries, rent, and utilities, will not be affected by the change in gross income. Variable expenses, such as laboratory costs for ophthalmic materials, will change with a decrease in gross income. By calculating the changes in these expenses, a hypothetical net income can be determined as a worst case scenario should the gross income of the practice decrease initially.

There are certain fixed personal expenses, such as rent or mortgage payments, home utilities, and student loans, that must be paid regardless of how successful the practice becomes. These expenses should be deducted from the net income of the practice. The amount that remains is the amount that the new practitioner can use to finance the purchase of the practice.

From these calculations, it should become apparent that the practice with the highest gross income may not necessarily be worth the most. It should also be apparent that a practice with a low gross income must produce sufficient net income to cover the practitioner's expenses, including the financing of the practice. If the practice cannot do so, the new practitioner will have to supplement this income by working outside of the practice.

SCOPE OF PRACTICE

The number and type of services provided in the practice and the primary emphasis of the practice (services or materials) constitute the scope of the practice. Full-scope practices, providing the highest level of optometric services and materials, generally possess more up-to-date equipment and, thus, have a higher value. Many retiring practitioners may not have practiced primary care optometry. For the recent or new graduate these practices offer an opportunity for a quick increase in the gross income of an existing practice. This can be achieved through attracting new patients to the practice or—with the addition of services or the expansion of hours to include evenings and weekends—through an increase in income derived from the existing patient population.

LOCATION AND LEASE

When an established practice is purchased, location usually is not a factor affecting the retention of existing patients. Location is a primary factor in the ability of the practice to attract new patients.

The practice location should be in an accessible, viable, professional or commercial area. In most suburban or rural areas, parking must be readily available. Handicapped and elderly patients require a location that is either on ground level or in a building with elevators. Visibility to street traffic is also desirable.

The average existing patient will return for care every 2–2½ years. Ideally, an office lease should be written for at least that long—3 years, with a minimum 3-year option—because such a term will allow patients to return to the same location at least once while it is occupied by the new practitioner. Moving the practice during this initial 2- to 3-year period would create a greater erosion in the existing patient base and would saddle the new practitioner with additional moving and renovation expenses at a time when these expenses could probably be least afforded. A favorable lease agreement would also include options to renew for specified periods after the expiration of the initial lease term. These options give the prospective buyer the security of a longer lease term, while retaining the flexibility to leave if the existing space becomes insufficient.

For the buyer to assume an existing lease, the lease must provide that the selling practitioner can assign it to a successor practitioner. When evaluating the existing lease, the buyer should be sure that the terms are at least as favorable as could be obtained if a new lease were negotiated. The more favorable the terms of the lease, the greater its value to the purchaser of the practice.

PATIENT RECORDS

Having an established patient base is the greatest advantage of purchasing a practice. In evaluating the practice, however, the most difficult factor to assess is the likelihood that patients will remain with the practice after it is sold. Patient records, in and of themselves, have no value for such evaluation. Transfer of records to a successor practitioner allows existing patients to feel that continuity of care has been obtained, while allowing the new practitioner to internally market to the existing patient base.

The likelihood that a patient will return to the practice for care is greatest for active patients. Since most patients will return for eye care approximately every 2 years, the greatest value is given to those patients who have received care within that period. Patient records with no activity for more than 2 years but less than 5 years have significantly reduced value. Patient records with no activity for more than 5 years have little or no value to the new practitioner; most of these patients are likely to have moved, passed away, or selected another practitioner.

A healthy practice will have a 25–35% rate of new patient visits each year. This rate can be calculated by determining the number of new patients seen over the preceding 2 years. Appointment books or patient records may be used to make this analysis. A certain number of patients examined in prior years should have returned to the practice for subsequent care. This return rate should also be evaluated to determine how well the practice has been retaining patients.

Patient records should also be sorted by the percentage paid by third-party payers and those paid directly by patients. Third-party payments will not generate the same gross revenue for the practice as fees for service. Practices that have a large percentage of third-party payments need a larger patient base and can only be transferred successfully if the new practitioner will be able to serve as a provider under the third-party plan. These patients will generally have less loyalty to the selling practitioner than fee-for-service patients. Their primary loyalty is to the practitioner who continues to provide them with the same benefits.

The average primary care practice will provide in excess of 2,000 examinations per practitioner per year. This statistic can be used as a yardstick by which to measure the patient flow of a prospective practice. Practices with fewer than this number of examinations will need to have higher fees to generate the average gross income. Practices with higher than average examination fees but with average gross incomes are either seeing fewer patients or are treating more third-party patients.

The age range of the patient population should be closely representative of the area in general. If the average age of patients is higher than the average age of the population in the area, it could indicate that the practitioner has done little to attract new patients to the practice.

TRANSITION PERIOD

The transition period allows the selling practitioner to acquaint the new practitioner with the management of the practice. This process includes review of office procedures, ordering of ophthalmic materials, meetings with suppliers, and working to transfer the loyalty of staff members. It also means introducing the new practitioner to key people in the area, including the main referral sources of the practice.

The transition period also applies to staff. In some instances, having existing staff members remain in the office can be more valuable than having the selling practitioner remain. This is especially true when the staff member has been working in the office for many years and knows all of the patients. Since staff members will be the first source of contact for patients both on the telephone and in the office, they can be a vital part of easing patient apprehension about seeing a new practitioner and can reassure patients who are hesitant about returning.

The selling practitioner should be provided with financial remuneration for assisting during the transition period. Payment is usually provided on a per diem or weekly basis. The new practitioner should also expect to increase the salaries of those staff members who are to be retained. This gesture demonstrates good faith on the part of the new practitioner and will pay for itself many times over in goodwill from the staff members.

PHYSICAL RESOURCES

The physical resources of a practice include tangible ("hard") assets, a category that consists of but is not limited to equipment, furnishings, office supplies, inventory, and leasehold improvements. "Hard" assets are those items with a value that can be accurately calculated.

Older, fully depreciated equipment will have some fair market value but must be evaluated as to its usefulness. Equipment that is in good working order and is not obsolete can be used by the new practitioner and replaced when practice revenues allow it. Obsolete or nonfunctional equipment that needs to be replaced is usually included when determining the value of the practice. This same consideration applies to furnishings, office supplies, inventory, and leasehold improvements.

In evaluating inventories of frames and contact lenses, the purchaser must be assured that the seller actually owns the inventory. Many contact lenses are supplied on consignment, and the new practitioner assumes responsibility for the consigned material. Frames usually are not consigned, but frames transferred to the new practitioner may not always be returnable if they were originally purchased by the seller.

ACCOUNTS RECEIVABLE

The accounts receivable are any fees for services or materials owed to the practice. The longer a debt is outstanding, the less the chance of its ultimate collection. For this reason, accounts receivable are often sold on a discounted basis, calculated on the age of each account. For example, accounts that are less than 30 days old may be purchased for 70–80% of their value; accounts 30–60 days old, for 50–60% of their value; accounts 60–90 days old, for 20–40% of their value; and accounts 90–120 days old, for 5–15% of their value. Accounts in excess of 120 days would not have any value. An alternative method is to pay a flat percentage rate, such as 50–70%, for all the accounts receivable.

If possible, it is preferable for the new practitioner not to purchase the existing accounts receivable but, instead, to allow them to be collected by the selling practitioner during the transition period. If the transition period is very short, the new practitioner may agree to transfer the amounts collected over a specified period of time to the seller.

FACTORS DECREASING PRACTICE VALUE

There are several factors that can significantly reduce the value of the practice to a potential buyer. Some of the most common are:

- Cutting back on the time spent in the office, which reduces the gross and net income of the practice
- Failing to have a working recall system that assures the buyer of a continuous patient flow
- Inadequate computer and office management systems
- Continuing to use old equipment that will have no value to a buyer
- Failing to participate in third-party vision and eye health reimbursement plans. This diminishes the patient base of the practice.
- Inadequate use of Medicare

The cumulative effect of these factors not only reduces the value of the practice but also limits the number of potential buyers. A selling practitioner should plan for the sale well in advance and should maintain the practice at a reasonable level of activity so that a fair value may be obtained. The equity acquired in the practice by the selling practitioner should be used as an important retirement asset, and an optometrist who does not take advantage of the opportunity to transfer the practice to a competent successor has not only lost the economic benefits of decades of effort but has also failed to provide continuity of care. The profession suffers too, as patients who were well-served by optometrists may readily turn to other types of eye care providers for care.

Despite all of the factors that have been described, the "bottom line" in any transfer of property is the law of supply and demand. The greater the demand for an existing practice, the more valuable it becomes. As a corollary rule, the greater the need and urgency to sell, the lower the price for which the practice will sell. Even so, there is a way of determining if a proposed price is reasonable.

DETERMINING IF A PROPOSED PRICE IS REASONABLE

Formulas have often been used to calculate the value of a practice. With such an approach, the items of purchase are divided into categories, and value is then attributed to each category. The sum of the various categories produces a total. This approach may be used to determine if a proposed price is reasonable.

To calculate the value of a practice using a formula, it is first necessary to consider what, in fact, is being sold.

The most obvious assets of a practice are its tangible items: equipment, instruments, records, furnishings, supplies, inventories, real estate, and so forth. These items can be assigned a fair market value with a reasonable degree of accuracy.

Another asset, the accounts receivable, can also be assigned a discounted value—based on the age of the account—or paid to the seller as collected.

It is the intangible value of the practice that is the most difficult asset to calculate. This intangible value, which is often described as being the likelihood that the buyer will be able to enjoy the same economic benefits as the seller, is known as "goodwill." One accepted way of establishing a value for goodwill is to base it on the practice's net income. To guard against fluctuations in income (large increases or decreases) the net income for the 3 years preceding the sale should be determined, and an average value used for purposes of the sale. This net income should reflect the practice's true economic value to the seller, not an artificial value such as is found on a tax return.

Therefore, the proposed price of a practice should be approximately equal to the fair market value of all tangible assets and the average of the net income for the 3 years preceding the sale, assuming that the accounts receivable are paid on a discounted basis or as received. This calculation may be used to quickly assess the reasonableness of a proposed purchase price.

The price paid for an optometric practice is typically in the range of 40–70% of the practice's past gross income for the year preceding the sale. This price may be higher if the net-to-gross income ratio is high or if the practice has exceptional assets, such as a considerable amount of up-to-date equipment. The price may be lower if the net-to-gross income ratio is low or if there is little usable equipment.

In the usual case, the proposed buyer and the selling practitioner must negotiate the terms of sale themselves. Because most optometrists are not knowledgeable about the legal, tax, and accounting issues that are part of such a sale, it is necessary to use a team of consultants so that needed technical advice can be obtained.

ASSEMBLING A TEAM OF CONSULTANTS

The purchase of a practice may be the single largest investment that an optometrist makes. An investment of this magnitude should not be attempted without consulting various experts, including an optometric advisor, an attorney, and an accountant.

1. *Optometric advisor.* This practitioner will have personal knowledge of the demographics of vision and eye care in the area; the value of equipment, inventory, and supplies; and the reputation of the seller and the practice. This advisor will be able to provide unique support in the transition after the sale. Advisors may be found through local or state optometric societies, through schools and colleges of optometry, or independently through advertisements in professional journals. A qualified practice appraiser will be able to evaluate all of these factors and arrive at a fair price for the value of the practice.

2. *Attorney.* The prospective purchaser should hire an attorney who has had experience in the sale of optometric practices. The attorney will prepare the contract for the purchase of the practice and will provide any needed documentation. The attorney usually will not negotiate the contract but may provide legal or tax advice concerning the sale.

3. *Accountant.* The accountant will review the financial records of the practice and, along with the optometric advisor, will determine its fair market value. The accountant will also evaluate the potential payment terms of the purchase, including the allocation of assets for tax purposes. It would be ideal for the accountant to have some experience with optometric or professional practice sales.

LEGAL AND TAX CONSIDERATIONS OF PURCHASING A PRACTICE

Most practice sales are self-financed. The purchaser pays a certain amount down, and the balance is paid over the course of years to the selling practitioner, who holds a note from the purchaser. Because of this long-term relationship between buyer and seller, the sales agreement needs to be fair. Otherwise, the arrangement will fail, and the selling optometrist—who is usually retired—will not receive the bargained for value from the buyer.

The note held by the selling practitioner should specify a reasonable amount of simple interest to be applied to the unpaid balance. Over the course of years, the interest adds significantly to the total amount received by the seller. It is a tax-deductible expense for the buyer.

The major steps involved in the sale of a practice are the determination of the practice's worth, the location of a proposed purchaser, the negotiation of the sales price, the allocation of the assets for tax purposes, and the drafting of a contract of sale. Professional advice and assistance is needed to perform most of these tasks. A written contract of sale must be drafted and signed by both parties.

Payment to the selling practitioner may be made monthly, quarterly, or at some other reasonable period determined by the parties. Usually a fixed dollar amount is specified, but the practitioners may choose to have a percentage of the gross income paid instead. Payment continues until the agreed sales price has been realized. Federal regulations concerning practice sales (e.g., Stark I and II laws, safe harbor laws, and the Medicare "anti-kickback" statute) have been changing rapidly in recent years. For this reason, a knowledgeable advisor should be consulted to ensure compliance with these rulings.

Table 3.1. Allocation of Assets for Tax Purposes

Practice Asset	Tax Ramifications for Buyer
Land	Not depreciable or deductible
Goodwill	Depreciable over 15 years
Building	Depreciable over 39 years
Equipment, instruments, furnishings, and similar capital assets	Depreciable over 7 years
Patient records	Amortizable over 15 years
Computers, copiers, typewriters, and vehicles	Depreciable over 5 years
Covenant not to compete	Amortizable over 15 years
Supplies and inventory	Deductible in the year of sale

One important aspect of the sale of a practice is the tax ramifications of the sale. Technical rules must be followed, particularly when allocating value to the practice assets for tax purposes. If the seller is not incorporated, each of the tangible assets being sold must be given a fair market value, and any remainder—the difference between the practice sales price and the fair market value of all tangible assets—must be allocated to goodwill. The Tax Reform Act of 1986 established 5- and 7-year depreciation periods for these assets, except for goodwill, which could not be depreciated. In 1993, however, federal tax reform allowed goodwill to be given a 15-year depreciation period; a similar period was also attributed to covenants not to compete and to patient records. Current depreciation periods are described in Table 3.1.

Optometrists who are incorporated as professional associations or corporations sell the stock rather than the individual assets of the practice. The buyer claims no tax deductions; they remain with the corporation. In most instances, however, the buyer of the practice will choose not to buy the corporation but will, instead, purchase the practice assets from the corporation. In such a case, the assets that are sold must be allocated a value, in the same manner as the sale of a sole proprietorship.

For the selling practitioner, the major tax concern is depreciation recapture income. If depreciated assets are sold, the difference between the sales price and the book value (i.e., the value of the asset after it has been depreciated) is taxed in the year of sale. If assets have been depreciated to zero under the Accelerated Cost Recovery System and are sold for their fair market value, the seller must pay the tax—usually 28% of the sales price—in the year of sale. That is one reason that selling practitioners often demand a substantial down payment from the buyer, in order to cover the first-year tax payment for depreciation recapture income. The ideal compromise agreement will fairly allocate the assets for the purchaser and provide an adequate down payment for the seller. The allocation of assets, as well as the conditions of sale, must be reported on form 8594 for the tax year in which the transaction occurred.

To illustrate the various economic and tax considerations of a practice sale, a sample transaction is included (Table 3.2).

BIBLIOGRAPHY

American Medical Association. Buying and Selling Medical Practices: A Valuation Guide. Chicago: American Medical Association, 1990.

American Medical Association. Valuing a Medical Practice: A Short Guide for Buyers and Sellers. Chicago: American Medical Association, 1987.

American Optometric Association. General Guidelines for Establishing the Worth of an Optometric Practice. St. Louis: American Optometric Association, 1988.

Brown R. Valuing Professional Practices and Licenses. Clifton, NJ: Prentice-Hall, 1987.

Desmond GM. How to Value Professional Practices. Marina Del Rey, CA: Valuation Press, 1980.

Horvath JL. Valuing Professional Practices. Ontario, Canada: CCH Canadian Ltd., 1990.

Jackson J, Hill R. New Trends in Dental Practice Valuation. Chicago: Quintessence Publishers, 1987.

Lane MJ. Purchase and Sale of Small Businesses. New York: Wiley, 1991.

Moss G. Financial decisions in a managed care era. Optom Econ 1996;2(1):25–30.

Pratt S. Valuing Small Businesses and Professional Practices. Chicago: Irwin Publishers, 1993.

Table 3.2. Sample Purchase Arrangement and First-Year Adjusted Cash Flow Analysis

Dr. Seller agrees to sell the practice for $200,000, with a 15% down payment, to Dr. Buyer. Dr. Seller will finance the balance due (85% of the sales price) over a 6-year period at a 10% simple interest rate.

Dr. Buyer has inspected Dr. Seller's schedule C (the practice is not incorporated) for the past 3 years and is satisfied that the financial data and ratios are favorable. Based on this information, Dr. Buyer is projecting the first year's gross revenues to be $300,000. The relevant variables in this analysis are:

Anticipated gross revenue	$300,000
Less fixed costs of operation	–$121,000
Less variable costs of operation	–$75,000
Less depreciation	–$16,000
Less personal income	–$55,000
Pretax income	$33,000
Multiply by applicable tax rate	× 0.28%
Tax payment due	$9,240
After-tax income	$23,760
Add back depreciation	$16,000
Net practice cash flow	$39,760
Less note payments to seller	$37,800
Adjusted cash flow for the practice	$1,960

The fixed costs for this practice include an office lease of $2,000 per month, an optician who is paid $35,000 per year, a secretary-receptionist who is paid $19,000 per year, and an ophthalmic technician who is paid $22,000 per year. The telephone bill is $750, a sum that includes an advertisement in the Yellow Pages. The cost of utilities (i.e., water, electricity, and gas) and janitorial services is $12,000 per year. Variable expenses for the practice include laboratory costs, which average about 25% of gross revenues.

Dr. Buyer plans to draw a first-year income of $55,000, with $5,000 annual increases thereafter. Dr. Buyer believes that the previous year's annual growth rate of 5% can be sustained for the next 6 years, creating a stable practice income.

Purchased assets are valued at $80,000 and will be depreciated using a 5-year straight line depreciation schedule (although other tax strategies are available and could be selected as necessary). Based on this strategy, the first-year adjusted cash flow will be $1,960. This "positive" result indicates that there will be a financial cushion for the first year; a "negative" result would necessitate revision of financial projections because there will be a shortfall of cash for the payment of obligations.

Chapter 4

Employment Options

James Albright, Craig Hisaka, W. Howard McAlister, and Timothy A. Wingert

Work expands so as to fill the time available for its completion.

—Cyril Parkinson
Parkinson's Law

Approximately 60% of the graduates from optometry school enter the practice of optometry as employees, even though the majority of these graduates ultimately intend to become self-employed. Surveys performed in the 1990s by the Association of Practice Management Educators indicate that 50% of optometry school graduates enter a practice setting that is not intended to be their ultimate choice and that they expect to spend 5 years or more in that setting before switching to the desired form of practice. These graduates invariably choose employee positions rather than starting or purchasing a practice. The usual reasons that graduates cite for choosing employment are inadequate business experience, significant debt at graduation, and overriding family obligations or commitments.

Lack of meaningful business experience is a common concern among optometry school graduates. When working for others, employees participate in optometric practices but are not financially accountable for them. Many students can overcome this lack of experience by working with private practitioners during summers or vacation periods and by planning externships in practice settings that are similar to the setting desired at graduation. During these periods, patient care and practice administration should be learned so that the student is able to feel confident about both types of management skills at graduation.

Another common concern of graduates is lack of the financial resources needed to start a practice, usually because of educational debts. Although the cost of schooling can be high, and loans may be required to pay for the years of professional education, students can and should limit debt as much as possible. Surveys conducted at schools and colleges of optometry have shown that some groups of students are good at minimizing debt while other groups are not. These surveys indicate that the degree of debt at graduation is related to careful planning and stringent use of borrowed money and that motivated students can graduate with significantly less debt.

A third reason that optometry school graduates seek employment is because of personal or family obligations that make it necessary to remain in a certain location or to provide financial support for a period of time. These obligations can be overriding if a student does not have adequate time to investigate options and identify the best opportunities. Again, time during school must be used to explore the choices that are available and to select the best available option so that the graduate will not be forced to choose a less than desirable option.

Optometry school graduates seeking employment opportunities usually look to associateship with optometrists or ophthalmologists, residencies, corporate optometry, the uniformed services, the

Table 4.1. Advantages and Disadvantages
of Optometry Employment Options

Advantages

Stable income and employee benefits available and paid by
employer (e.g., paid vacations, health insurance, malpractice insurance premiums, continuing education expenses)

Gain experience from other practitioners, learn the "art of
optometry," and increase business knowledge and skills

Minimum or no start-up costs and minimal or no investment required

Minimum management decisions required

The appropriate opportunity could lead to a future partnership

Disadvantages

Average income, limited earning potential, limited upward
mobility

Minimum or no equity acquired in a practice

Dictated office policies and minimal independence

Very few good long-term arrangements unless they lead to
partnership

After several years of employment, employees are at risk
for termination because of high salary and benefits;
thus, there is poor long-term security

A limited scope of practice may be found in certain settings
due to the volume of patients who must be seen

Veterans Administration, academia, and health
maintenance organizations. This chapter briefly discusses these employment options (Table 4.1).

ASSOCIATESHIP

An associate is an employee and, as such, holds no
ownership interest in the business entity for which
the employee works. An associate does not share
in the profits and losses but, rather, is salaried and
may receive additional employee benefits. The ultimate responsibility for the practice belongs to the
employer; the associate is not responsible for its
financial status. An associate may participate in
management decisions only to the extent permitted by the employer and will receive only a few of
the tax breaks available to persons in small businesses. Despite these limitations, associateship
can be used as a stepping-stone to partnership or
sole proprietorship. For many newly graduated
optometrists, it has proved to be an ideal means

of making the transition from an academic environment to the business world. In selecting associateship, a graduate may work for an optometrist
or an ophthalmologist.

Employment by an Optometrist

Many graduates begin their practice experience as
the employee of an optometrist in private practice.
Often the motivation for the associateship is the
hope that employer and employee will agree to
form a partnership. The associateship, which is usually for 1–2 years, serves as a trial period during
which the optometrist and the associate determine
their compatibility and the feasibility of partnership
(see Chapter 2).

Because the usual associate is a recent optometry school graduate with relatively little practice
experience, the earnings of optometric associates,
when compared to other types of employment,
tend to be toward the bottom of the scale. Figures
from surveys, such as those conducted by the
American Optometric Association, reflect this fact
(Table 4.2).

These results are misleading, however.
Other types of employment have a higher proportion of individuals who have been out of optometry school for more than 3 years and who
are therefore higher wage earners by virtue of
their years on the job. These surveys also do
not recognize the long-term potential of optometric associateship, which frequently results
in a partnership arrangement.

If associateship is contemplated, the practice
should be evaluated to determine if it is large
enough to support two optometrists. General
guidelines should be used to assess practice income, growth, and number of annual examinations.
For example, the gross income should be equal to
or greater than the average gross income for similar
practices in the region. (As of 1995, the mean gross
income for all optometrists in private practice was
\$285,000 and the median gross income was
\$305,000.) Ideally, the practice should be busy and
growing at the rate of 10–15% per year. The sole
practitioner should be performing more than 2,000
full-scope examinations annually. There should be
appropriate delegation of responsibilities to technical staff, and up-to-date management techniques

Table 4.2. Mean Net Income for Employed Optometrists, 1994

Employer	Mean Net Income
Optometrists	$59,728
Multidisciplinary clinics	$73,827
Ophthalmologists	$78,373
Optical chains	$82,015

Source: American Optometric Association. Caring for the Eyes of America—A Profile of the Optometric Profession. St. Louis: American Optometric Association, 1996.

should be employed by the practice. The office should be large enough to accommodate another practitioner, and adequate equipment and instrumentation should be available.

If an associateship is agreed on, the associate and employer should negotiate and sign an associateship agreement. This agreement provides for the employment of the new graduate during the trial period. The agreement should be in writing and should provide for:

- Duties, working hours, and place of employment
- The term of employment
- A base salary and, if agreed on, bonus income
- Benefits (e.g., health insurance, license renewal fee, professional association dues, continuing education fees, paid vacation)
- Malpractice coverage
- Death or disability of either of the parties
- Termination of the agreement

Benefits are of particular importance to associates because, if paid for by the associate, they cannot be fully deducted for tax purposes, while they can be deducted fully as legitimate business expenses by the employer. The benefits to be provided by the employer should be specified in the associateship agreement.

The associateship allows both parties to consider and discuss the prospect of partnership. If the associateship results in the decision to form a partnership, the typical buy-in period is 5–7 years, which means that the associate becomes a full partner within a few years after graduating from op-

tometry school. If the practice is maintained, it will support the new partner for the next 30–40 years, or until retirement is planned. If the associateship does not result in partnership, the associate usually leaves the practice to pursue other opportunities.

Employment by an Ophthalmologist

Increasingly, optometry school graduates are finding employment opportunities with ophthalmologists in private practice. The reason for this trend may be found in the primary care orientation of optometry. Ophthalmologists have found that employee optometrists can provide refractive care, contact lens services, management of a wide range of ocular pathology, and specialized services such as those needed by children, senior citizens, and people seeking low vision rehabilitation. Employing optometrists to provide these services allows ophthalmologists to concentrate on ocular surgery and other secondary and tertiary services.

Because ophthalmologists earn, on the average, a higher mean income than optometrists, they provide, on the average, a higher salary than that paid by optometrists (Table 4.2). Part of the reason for this difference in remuneration is the ability of ophthalmologists to offer more benefits (e.g., moving expenses, allowances for use of an automobile, group term life insurance, disability insurance) than optometrists.

There can be some significant drawbacks, however, to ophthalmologic associateship. The duties assigned to the associate may not be ideal. An associate who would prefer to treat ocular pathology may have to provide refractive care or perform work-ups for the surgeon rather than manage a wide variety of patients with ocular disease. For this reason, it is important to determine if the duties of the associateship match the graduate's practice goals. Another drawback is that ophthalmologic associateship does not offer much opportunity for long-term advancement. It is rare for ophthalmologists to join into partnership with optometrists. In fact, in many states optometrists and ophthalmologists are prohibited by law from jointly forming a professional association or corporation for that purpose. Therefore, optometrists employed by ophthalmologists tend to either remain employees or to leave the practice to begin or join an optometric practice.

Whether a graduate wishes to work for an optometrist or an ophthalmologist, the likelihood of finding an associateship opportunity is directly related to the effort put into the search and the graduate's ability to form a personal relationship with the potential employer prior to graduation. The associateship market is a competitive one, and students who begin early, meet potential employers, and work in their practices before graduation are the ones who graduate with opportunities awaiting them. To wait until the fourth year of optometry school to solicit an invitation to interview by mail, and to have but one opportunity to make a favorable impression, is to invite disappointment. If associateship is desired, the process of looking for a potential employer should begin as soon as possible, and when opportunities are found, the student should try to visit the practitioner frequently. The better the personal relationship the more likely it will result in a successful associateship.

RESIDENCY

There are approximately 120 accredited residency positions that provide postgraduate education for optometrists. These positions may be found in a variety of practice locations, including schools and colleges of optometry, Veterans Administration hospitals and outpatient clinics, Indian Health Service facilities, eye care surgery referral centers, and U.S. military posts. They offer a wide range of experiences and environments for learning, providing a year of intense clinical and educational experience in a particular area of optometry. Residency programs are currently available for training in family practice optometry, binocular vision therapy, contact lens practice, low vision rehabilitation, pediatric care, and diagnosis and treatment of ocular disease. To apply for a residency program, the applicant must have graduated from an accredited school or college of optometry. Because there is only one residency program available for every 10 graduates, residency positions are highly competitive. It is important for applicants to take and pass parts one and two of the examination given by the National Board of Ex-

aminers in Optometry (NBEO). Excellent academic records are also advisable.

Residency programs offer a concentrated clinical experience, with some time devoted to other activities, such as didactic education, research, and teaching. The range and extent of nonclinical activities varies from program to program. Residents can expect to work full days and to serve as necessary providing emergency and on-call care. Salaries for residents are standard and provide essentially subsistence level wages. Pay can be an issue for residents who must live in expensive metropolitan areas.

Optometrists who have recently completed a residency are the individuals best able to discuss a particular program's strength and weaknesses. They should be consulted by students interested in applying for a specific residency position.

Veterans Administration

The Veterans Administration (VA) was organized in 1930 and is one of the largest independent agencies within the U.S. government, operating the world's largest system of hospitals and clinics as part of its overall responsibility for the nation's veterans. The VA also plays an important role in the education of health care professionals. It is estimated that, in any given year, over 25% of all U.S. medical and surgical residents receive training at VA hospitals.

The involvement of optometrists in VA education and patient care has a much shorter history. Optometrists were not eligible to serve in VA staff positions until 1957, and the first VA residency position for optometrists was not created until 1972. Today, opportunities may be found both for VA staff optometrists and for residency positions.

To be selected for an entry-level VA staff position, the applicant must have a doctor of optometry degree from an accredited school and an optometry license from one state and must pass a physical examination. These qualifications allow an optometrist to apply for an associate grade position. A limited number of entry-level positions are available, however, and, to be competitive, applicants should also have completed a residency or have experience as a practitioner. To be selected for the next level, full grade, the optometrist must have served in a residency program or served 2 years as a practitioner. There are three more levels—intermediate, senior, and chief—which require increasingly stringent qualifications. There are numerous benefits, such as health and disability insurance, paid vacations and similar entitlements, and a generous retirement plan.

There are presently over 150 staff positions in the VA system, located in hospitals or outpatient clinics. Staff and clinic sizes vary from facility to facility, as do practice privileges, because the scope of practice for each practitioner is determined by the facility rather than by state law (VA facilities are subject to federal rather than state regulation). Primary care is offered to a diverse population of veterans, and there is ample opportunity to participate in research projects. VA staff optometrists frequently contribute to the professional literature and provide postgraduate education. They also contribute to the education of optometrists through VA residency programs.

There are about 50 residency positions at VA facilities, providing excellent clinical postgraduate training for young optometrists. To be eligible to apply, applicants must have graduated from an accredited school of optometry. Although not a requirement, it is highly desirable for applicants to have passed the examination given by the NBEO. Because there are a limited number of VA residency positions, there is significant competition for these positions. The pay for VA residency positions, like all residency positions, is low. Days are full, and there are after-hours responsibilities as well. The year of training, however, enables residents to qualify for VA staff positions, to apply for positions in academic institutions, or to provide improved skills in a private practice setting.

CORPORATE PRACTICE

Ophthalmic companies employ optometrists to provide services in several types of practice settings, including "next-door" or mercantile lease arrangements, as part of a trademark chain, or within a "superstore." Although the financial arrangements vary among these types of employers, optometrists in corporate settings serve as "independent contractors" rather than as employees. An independent contractor is someone who contracts to perform work by his or her own methods and without being subject to the direct control of the employer. The advantage to the corporate employer of such an arrangement is that the employer is not responsible for the negligence of the independent contractor and does not have to contribute half of the independent contractor's social security payments to the federal government. Thus, the independent contractor is liable for any liability claims arising from employment and is solely responsible for the withholding and payment of the independent contractor's income tax and social security contributions.

The advantages to corporate practice are that there is little investment, the beginning income is very good (see Table 4.2), and positions are available for new graduates. In the typical situation, the employer provides the office, staff, and equipment and uses advertising to attract a patient base. As payment, the optometrist receives all fees charged for services or a percentage of fees charged for services, with a minimum salary usually guaranteed. In rare instances, the optometrist may share in the fees received from the sale of ophthalmic materials, but typically these fees are paid solely to the corporate employer. The lease arrangement between employer and optometrist is inevitably favorable, with the optometrist paying nothing or a nominal fee for the rental of the office space. The lease arrangement is for a limited period, however, and may be cancelled at the option of the employer. The arrangement may also assert that the patient records are the property of the corporate employer and must remain in the office after the relationship with the optometrist has ended.

The disadvantages of corporate practice are a lack of security, limitations in the scope of practice, and a ceiling on earnings. Because an optometrist working in a corporate environment has no ownership interest, there is no long-term security. Unlike a private practitioner, at retirement there is nothing to sell to a successor practitioner. In a corporate setting, the scheduling of patients often does not permit a full scope of practice to be enjoyed, and the optometrist may not be able to develop specialized skills because so much time must be devoted to routine examination. Although the optometrist receives a minimum salary and is remunerated based on fees for services, there is a ceiling on earnings that is based on the corporate employer's profit margin. If profits get too low, the optometrist gets no further increase or is discharged so that a newer optometrist can be employed at a lower pay rate. As a consequence, the optometrist in a corporate setting does not achieve the job security or the income earned by self-employed optometrists in private practice.

New graduates often look to corporate practice as a means of obtaining practical experience while reducing the debts of professional education. Although these goals can be accomplished, employment for a period of years is required. Unfortunately, after several years it can be financially difficult for the optometrist to leave a steady income for the uncertainties of beginning a new practice or purchasing an existing practice. Regardless of the practice option chosen, debt must be incurred (to open or buy the practice), and this indebtedness may conflict with other financial needs or priorities. The longer the optometrist remains in the corporate setting, the more difficult it becomes to leave.

UNIFORMED SERVICES

Employment positions exist for optometrists within the U.S. Army, U.S. Air Force, U.S. Navy, and U.S. Public Health Service. The majority of these positions are in patient care, although some are purely research and some are purely administrative. Most of these positions require optometrists to be commissioned officers, but in a few positions, optometrists are civil service employees.

There are more than 400 optometrists serving in the armed forces. Optometry school graduates entering military service enter with the rank of O-3. If they enter the Army or Navy, they will serve in the Medical Service Corps; in the Air Force, they will serve in the Bioscience Corps. A limited number of optometry school graduates enter military service each year through the Health Professions Scholarship Program, which pays for 1–4 years of the graduate's professional school education.

Optometry officers provide patient care in multidisciplinary environments such as medical centers, community level hospitals, and clinics. Though the scope of practice varies between installations, in general it is broader (particularly with respect to the management of ocular disease and trauma) than the scope of practice traditionally seen in the civilian optometric community. For the new graduate, the patient care experience in the

first few years of military service practice is usually more extensive than the experience enjoyed by contemporaries in private practice settings. Since the dependents of military active duty personnel, retirees, and their dependents are eligible for care from military health care providers, the optometry officer will see patients of all ages.

Over 80 optometrists serve as officers in the Public Health Service (PHS). The vast majority of patient care positions within the PHS are in the Indian Health Service. Most optometrists serve as commissioned officers, and, like the military services, the entering rank is O-3. A few optometrists serve as civil servants. Eligible beneficiaries in the Native American patient population also include all age groups, although almost half of the beneficiaries are under age 21. Many health care facilities of the uniformed services provide clinical training to optometry students, thereby allowing clinicians of the uniformed services an opportunity to teach.

Commissioned officers and civil servants receive a salary, tax-free housing, and subsistence allowances and do not share in the cost of operating a practice. In general, the patient care equipment and facilities are very good. A retirement plan, health care coverage, protection against disability, and malpractice coverage are provided. Junior officers usually have few administrative requirements related to operating the practice. All members of the uniformed services receive 30 days of paid vacation each year.

For mid-career practitioners, several opportunities exist to enter graduate degree programs or residencies, at government expense, while remaining on active duty and drawing full pay and allowances. The number and type of positions vary from time to time and between services. There are also a limited number of career broadening assignments in administrative areas, as well as research.

Military officers may be assigned to different facilities all over the world, allowing for the opportunity to travel to many exotic locations. Time off and funding for continuing education are generally provided to meet credentialing and state license requirements.

In the multidisciplinary environment of the uniformed services, commanders will nearly always be medical officers (M.D. or D.O.). In most locations, if an ophthalmologist is present, the optometrist will be part of the ophthalmologist's service. Though relations are often cordial, when they are not, the optometrist is at a decided disadvantage. Though trained and licensed as an independent health care practitioner, the optometry officer may not be able to function as such.

Most assignments allow for a varied patient population, but in some locations the patient census consists mostly of young, healthy males. These locations are generally in training centers, where the practitioner may provide only very limited basic care to a large volume of patients each day. Due to the chronic shortage of optometrists in the uniformed services, the opportunity to provide specialty care, such as contact lenses, low vision rehabilitation, and binocular vision therapy, may be very limited.

The salary received by both officers and civil servants is not competitive with that of most other positions available to new graduates. Also, the special pay for optometry officers is a small fraction of that paid to medical and dental officers. Though the retirement pension is very good, it is only authorized for those with at least 20 years of service. Under the current downsizing of the military, many officers with several years of service risk being involuntarily separated from the service and receiving no retirement benefits.

Many officers complain of being required to perform nonpatient care duties such as administrative officer of the day, linen inventory officer, and so forth. Administrative performance is often perceived as being more important to promotion and success than is patient care. Usually, most officers of equivalent education, such as physicians and dentists, are not required to serve in such nonprofessional capacities.

Many Indian Health Service locations are in remote locations and require extensive travel. Moving is required of military officers on a frequent basis. This obligation can cause considerable disruption in family life. Although many positions are in exotic locales, there are also a number of hardship tours, including assignments in combat areas.

ACADEMIA

Fewer than 600 full-time faculty positions exist within schools and colleges of optometry for clini-

cal and classroom teaching and for clinical and basic research. Academicians progress through various academic ranks, beginning with instructor, assistant professor, associate professor, and culminating with professor. Promotion depends on the faculty member's contributions to teaching, scholarly activities, and service.

Accepting a faculty position requires no investment of capital and does not incur the same type of time demands found in a private practice setting. There are far fewer administrative tasks generally required of junior faculty when compared to optometrists in a private practice. Optometrists in academia receive a guaranteed salary as well as such benefits as health, disability, and malpractice insurance, vacation, and a retirement plan. Time and stipends are usually provided for attending professional conferences. Optometrists at schools and colleges of optometry have opportunities to pursue areas of special interest in an intellectual environment. In many cases income can be supplemented by offering continuing education as well as providing patient care outside the academic institution. Excellent job security is obtained when a faculty member achieves tenure. Eligibility for tenure occurs 7–10 years after being placed on a tenure track.

From an economic viewpoint, academia provides a relatively low level of remuneration for doctors of optometry. Although there is no development of equity, as is found in private practice, retirement plans are usually generous. To gain a position as a faculty member, additional professional or graduate degrees or a residency are usually required. Thus, the educator must train longer to be paid relatively less than contemporaries in other settings. Faculty members have minimal independence, and junior members have very little ability to affect academic policy. If a faculty member is on a tenure track but not awarded tenure, other employment must be sought.

HEALTH MAINTENANCE ORGANIZATIONS

HMOs provide comprehensive health maintenance and treatment services for a voluntarily enrolled group of patients who pay a periodic fixed rate for services. These patients may also pay a small co-payment fee at each office visit. There are two types of HMOs: staff models and independent practice associations (IPAs).

Staff model HMOs provide services to members through their own professional staff, which is employed by the HMO. An optometrist working for a staff model HMO is usually paid a salary with the workload being an additional consideration.

IPAs contract with a private practitioner to have that practitioner deliver health services to its members. These practitioners are usually paid either on a capitation basis or on a fee-for-service basis.

Staff model HMOs offer an immediate income with no startup cost (see Table 4.2). While a staff optometrist does not have to be concerned about clinic coverage for patients when the optometrist is out of the office, the daily schedule of office hours is usually beyond the optometrist's control. To compensate for the moderately attractive salary offered to optometrists, many HMOs offer a good fringe benefit package that includes paid time off for continuing education, a monetary stipend for continuing education expenses, health insurance, life insurance, disability insurance, sick leave, and a retirement plan.

Staff model HMOs require minimal management time and require few management decisions from the optometrist. The optometrist, as a primary care provider, usually operates as the gatekeeper of the system for all patients with vision problems. There is no limit to the age of patients seen in this setting, and with the optometrist as the entry point into the system, there is diversity in the types of cases the optometrist will encounter. It is a multidisciplinary practice environment, and the optometrist often practices side by side with the primary care physician.

As an employee, the optometrist will build up little or no equity in the practice. Depending on the organization of the HMO, medical practitioners may control the administration of the optometrist's department. Under medical control, the optometrist may not be used as the gatekeeper of the system. It may also result in the optometrist not being allowed to practice the full scope allowed by state law, seeing a restricted age of patients, and being allocated a decreased amount of examination time per patient.

CONCLUSION

The choice of an employment option after graduation from optometry school is usually based on a decision by the graduate not to become an employer but to obtain practice experience as an employee. In making such a decision, graduates should always consider whether the employment opportunity possesses the flexibility to allow changes in career direction. Because so many graduates enter employment positions thinking that they will provide a short-term experience, it is important that the option chosen provide an opportunity to change direction when it is appropriate and timely to do so.

BIBLIOGRAPHY

American Optometric Association. Optometry and HMOs. Washington, DC: American Optometric Association, 1989;4–5.

Anonymous. Federal service optometry, part II. AOA News 1990;29(1):9–10.

Anonymous. Optometry in the Alaskan bush. AOA News 1990;28(24):1,13–14.

Anonymous. Military optometry makes problem-solving strides. AOA News 1990; 28(24):1,8.

Anonymous. Special report: federal service optometry. AOA News 1989;27(23):1,3–4,13.

Berman MS. Challenges for optometric education. J Optom Ed 1992;17(4):105–6.

Catania LJ. Optometry in group practice. Group Practice 1975; 5(Sept/Oct): 21–2.

Classé JG. Legal Aspects of Optometry. Stoneham, MA: Butterworth, 1989.

Clausen LR. Advanced education. J Optom Ed 1992;17(4):107–10.

Department of the Army. The Medical Service Corps, The Army Medical Team. 587–204. Falls Church, VA: U.S. Government Printing Office, 1988.

Department of the Navy. Navy Recruiting Command: Navy Medical Service Corps. 953-1754(20) 1988. Falls Church, VA: U.S. Government Printing Office, 1988;953–1754.

Grosvenor T. The Clinical Master of Science degree. Optom Vis Sci 1992;69(3):255–6.

Kaminski A, Pennington JA. Vision care model within a prototype HMO. J Am Optom Assoc 1975;46(9):875–80.

Kaz MA. Five steps that determine your practice's true value. Rev Optom 1995;132(12):33–8.

Luft, H. Health Maintenance Organizations: Dimensions of Performance. New York: Wiley, 1981.

McAlister WH, Davidson DW. A 1988 survey of federal service optometrists. J Am Optom Assoc 1992; 62(7):500–3.

Newcomb RD, Marshall EC (eds). Public Health and Community Optometry (2nd ed). Stoneham, MA: Butterworth, 1990; 262–3, 267–70.

Robert B. View of optometry in Southern California Permanente Medical Group. Opt J Rev Optom 1974; 5(1):27–34.

Scerra CA. Seeking the substance of practice valuation. Optom Econ 1995;5(2):42–6.

Schwartz C. Optometry and HMOs: the view from inside. Optom Econ 1995;5(2):17–19.

Shipp MD, Talley DK. A 1987 survey of military optometrists: activities, roles and attitudes. J Am Optom Assoc 1988; 59(10):802–14.

Siemsen DW. The role of the institution. J Optom Ed 1992;17(4):117–8.

Sparks BI. Military externships: recruitment friend and foe? J Am Optom Assoc 1990;61(6):471–3.

Stein G. HMO—Here's what it's all about. J Am Optom Assoc 1976;47(2):136–41.

U.S. Department of Health, Education, and Welfare, Health Services and Mental Health Administration. Health Maintenance Organizations: The Concept of Structure. Washington, DC: Department of Health, Education, and Welfare, 1972.

Part II
Starting a Private Practice

Chapter 5

Principles of Negotiation

Lawrence S. Thal

We arg'ed the thing at breakfast, we arg'ed the thing at tea,
And the more we arg'ed the question, the more we didn't agree.

—William Carleton
Farm Ballads

While many authorities believe that good negotiators are born that way or that negotiation is a skill best learned through experience, successful negotiators are almost always those individuals who are best prepared—best prepared with information regarding their own position as well as the position of the persons with whom they are negotiating. This chapter discusses the process of negotiation to help optometrists prepare for a successful negotiating experience, whether it be for a lease, associateship or partnership, purchase of a practice, purchase or sale of equipment, or other opportunity.

Negotiation is a process in which two or more participants attempt to reach a joint decision on matters of common concern in situations where they are in actual or potential disagreement or conflict. The quality of a negotiated agreement is measured by the extent to which it meets the interests of all parties concerned. Inherent in this process is the need to determine accurately what those interests are, for both parties. It often has been proved that the negotiation that provides a clear winner in the short run provides no winners in the long run. The early "winner" often ends up a loser because the other party has realized that the agreement is unfair. Conversely, in a "win-win" negotiation, both parties are motivated to abide by their agreements, thereby avoiding conflicts and problems. Negotiation is primarily an exercise in problem solving, an exercise in which the process identifies and exploits opportunities for joint gain.

Competitive tactics, such as threats or demands, undermine a negotiator's credibility and prevent reaching a mutually beneficial outcome. Cooperative tactics, on the other hand, include reasonable offers, fair and just arguments, and concessions designed to encourage reciprocity. The use of cooperative tactics is based on the premise that behavior that is fair, reasonable, and accommodating is more likely to encourage a similar response. While the rationale for using cooperative tactics is an expectation that the other party will reciprocate, the weakness of this strategy is its vulnerability to exploitation by a negotiator who does not match a cooperative negotiator's concessions. Cooperative tactics also require an exchange of information between the negotiators and a responsiveness by the negotiators to each other's interests and needs. Each negotiator must assess the willingness of the other to be cooperative; if this willingness is not present, the offering of concessions or compromise must be curtailed.

Negotiations should follow these steps:

- Fact-finding
- Planning and preparation
- Establishment of an initial relationship with the other side

- Initial proposals
- Exchange of information
- Narrowing of differences
- Closure and implementation

Each of these steps is described briefly, as applied to negotiation by optometrists.

FACT-FINDING

The optometrist seeking to negotiate an agreement should attempt to obtain useful information regarding the other negotiator. Does this person enjoy a good reputation? Does the person have a past history of legal conflicts or problems? If there were problems, what was their nature and outcome? If the person is an optometrist, what have previous relationships with other optometrists been like? What do other associates (present and past) or other tenants have to say about the person? This type of fact-finding is aimed at determining whether the individual is someone with whom one can negotiate at all.

If this is a lease negotiation, what are the market rents? What are other tenants paying, and what are the terms of their leases? What do other tenants say about the landlord's willingness to honor the terms of the lease? What is the vacancy rate now and what has it been in the past? What mortgages exist, and what is the financial condition of the owner?

If this is a partnership, what has been the negotiator's relationship with other partners, employers, or associates? What are the revenues of the practice now, and what does a pro forma analysis reveal for the future?

If this is the sale of a practice, have there been other attempts to sell it? What was the outcome of those negotiations? What are the seller's plans: to remain in the area or to move away after the sale? What is the seller's reputation in the community? Is the practice growing? Is it economically sound? The answers to these questions, as well as to questions considering the future economic prospects of the practice, will dictate whether negotiation should be undertaken.

The negotiator with the greater knowledge of the subject matter to be negotiated is in the more advantageous position by far. Fact-finding, however, is not limited to the period before the negotiations

begin. Fact-finding continues throughout the negotiations because, to the extent that one side learns of the other side's needs and concerns, it becomes more likely that a compromise can be structured creatively to satisfy everyone's goals.

In Chapter 28, the preparation of pro forma economic analysis is discussed. Such an analysis is essential in determining a "bottom line" in the negotiation process. Too often leases are entered into because the negotiator rationalizes, "It was the best I could find," or "All the leases are that rate," regardless of what the economic projection might have shown.

Part of the fact-finding process should be devoted to considering what sources of influence, leverage, or power one party holds over the other. Each party's alternatives to a negotiated agreement and their relative needs to reach an agreement are the most important factors in determining bargaining power.

PLANNING AND PREPARATION

This part of the negotiation process involves preparing a strategy, developing goals, and anticipating arguments from the other negotiator. It involves the preparation of arguments and demonstrations (e.g., graphs, charts, economic projections) that justify an offer or show why concessions requested by the other negotiator can or cannot be met.

The willingness to show why certain positions are taken and others are rejected further contributes to a cooperative approach and helps to avoid antagonism and mistrust. Anticipating the other negotiator's position and arguments helps improve preparation and may even reveal areas where more fact-finding is necessary. This part of the process must determine—at a minimum—the specific goals, terms, and conditions necessary for the negotiation to be a success.

ESTABLISHING AN INITIAL RELATIONSHIP WITH THE OTHER SIDE

In using a cooperative strategy to achieve an agreement that is fair and just to both parties, it is necessary to develop a relationship with the other negotiator that is characterized by goodwill and trust. The first phase of negotiation sets the initial tone of the relationship between the parties and may in fact establish the character of the relationship for the remainder of the negotiation. This phase of the negotiation process may include information gathering and disclosure and exchange of initial proposals, and, to some degree, it sets the foundation for later phases.

It is usually advantageous to be the first to present an initial draft agreement or written offer. That act often establishes the first position, from which offers of compromise will be made. When a draft agreement is offered, it should be possible to determine which issues are contentious. Sometimes it is best to negotiate the least contentious issues first to build rapport and trust between the parties before tackling the most difficult topics. On the other hand, should the parties get through the most contentious issues first, it is unlikely that negotiations will break down over less disputatious provisions, thereby jeopardizing the agreements already reached. However, negotiators should avoid the tendency to allow animosity resulting from contentious bargaining on major issues to overflow into negotiations on issues that are less important.

Some negotiators believe that there is a decided advantage to negotiate on one's own premises or in one's own surroundings, and in fact, some empirical research seems to confirm that negotiators who bargain on their own territory are likely to increase both their assertiveness and the chances of a favorable negotiation outcome. However, "home" advantage means only as much as the negotiator permits it to mean. Negotiations, like sporting events, cannot always take place in the negotiator's own surroundings, and neutral sites (as diplomats often seek in Geneva or Helsinki) are not always practical. Even if a negotiator feels more comfortable and less likely to lose confidence in familiar surroundings, that seeming advantage may be offset by other factors. For example, if documents are needed to refute a certain contention, one is expected to access them immediately when negotiating in his or her own office. The documents would not necessarily be available in the other negotiator's office; this delay can allow more time for preparation.

In this phase of the negotiation process it is desirable to create an atmosphere in which negotiators attempt to maximize joint gains by first creating a psychological state characterized by mutual trust, a shared desire to achieve joint gains, and open and honest communication.

INITIAL PROPOSALS

The first proposal in a negotiation, if credible and convincing, usually becomes the focal point from which further bargaining proceeds. It should be thoughtfully and carefully considered before presentation. Justification for this initial proposal should be presented to validate its credibility and to limit the extent of further negotiation.

It is a mistake, when presenting an offer, to imply that it is the final offer or that the other side must "take it or leave it." Such an attitude destroys the negotiation process, is rarely credible, and demonstrates an attitude completely unfavorable to maximizing joint gains.

An initial proposal should be moderate enough to communicate to the other party that the negotiator is trying to be reasonable in establishing a cooperative bargaining relationship. On the other hand, the initial proposal must contain enough of a cushion to allow the negotiator to make concessions so that he or she does not appear intractable in later phases of the negotiation. Early cooperation facilitates the development of trust and a mutually beneficial, amicable relationship.

EXCHANGE OF INFORMATION

No other aspect of negotiation is as important as the exchange of information between negotiators. Negotiation can be viewed as a process in which each negotiator learns enough about what the other party needs and wants to propose an agreement that is acceptable to both sides. A full and accurate exchange of information allows both parties to participate in the creation of compromises and solutions. While providing information to the other negotiator can be risky to one's bargaining position, it dramatically enhances the ability of the negotiator to reach a fair and just compromise. The expectation is that both parties will exchange concessions in the same spirit that they trade information.

Any information that assists in determining the other side's requirements, abilities, or expectations is useful. For example, when leasing an office it is valuable to learn the terms and conditions of the lease agreements held by other tenants. Knowledge regarding the building owner's costs, renewal rates, vacancy history, financial condition, and related matters can be obtained independently, before negotiations begin. This information can be expanded during the negotiations themselves.

The most effective way to gather information is to ask questions. Even the most direct question ("What will it take to resolve this issue?") can be helpful. Less direct and open-ended questions often yield more information. Different forms of questioning should be attempted to determine which will elicit the most information. Specific questions work best, however, when the questioner's information needs are well defined.

Silence is an overlooked information-gathering technique. Obviously, it is difficult to gain information when one is doing all the talking. However, there are ethical and legal considerations involved with failing to disclose material facts. Such concealment could be fraudulent. It is important to be truthful in responses, because the other negotiator relies on the information provided as a basis for agreements.

NARROWING OF DIFFERENCES

This phase involves the bargaining or "haggling" part of the negotiation process. Even while narrowing down the differences in their positions, negotiators continue to gather information. Awarding concessions is an affirmative step. It is taken to elicit cooperation and to receive concessions in return; it is not an indication that the negotiator is losing. Human nature is such that individuals tend to cooperate with those who cooperate in return. Therefore, the willingness to offer concessions should not be viewed as a weakness in the negotiation process. Sometimes it is best to indicate flexibility on an issue before offering a specific concession, for once a concession is offered, it usually cannot be withdrawn easily.

If fatigue, irritability, or anger during this phase of negotiations threatens the success of the negotiation process, it is advisable to take a recess and resume negotiations at a later time. Often a break will allow one side or the other to develop a compromise. For example, if a lease agreement hinges on the insistence of the owner that the prospective tenant pay $2,300 per month for 7 years, when, during the first 2 years, the prospective tenant can only pay $1,600, an impasse is obviously reached. During a break in the negotiations, the prospective tenant can calculate a counter offer (based on his or her knowledge or with assistance from someone who has that knowledge) that would provide the owner exactly the same total rent in today's dollars and yet meet the prospective tenant's financial expectations. Such a counter offer might entail the use of graduated payments over the 7 years, starting with $1,600 per month in the first year and increasing each year so that over the 7-year period a $2,300 per month average is obtained.

Occasionally it may appear that negotiations are breaking down entirely. It is better to allow this to happen than to enter into a completely unfavorable agreement. Sometimes a more creative approach may be able to salvage the negotiations. The use of expert advice or of a mediator might help. Options are limited only by the creativity of the negotiator.

CLOSURE AND IMPLEMENTATION

When it appears that the parties have reached an agreement, all the elements agreed on should be repeated in summary form to ensure that there has been mutual understanding and that a "meeting of the minds" has resulted on each issue. It may be advisable to reduce the agreement to a written summary at this time. At a minimum, a letter summarizing the terms agreed on should be prepared the next day. This summary or letter can be used as the basis for a formal written contract.

Typically, one of the negotiators volunteers to have an attorney draft the written agreement. It is often to one's advantage to have one's own attorney do this, rather than the other negotiator's; the language used will not be necessarily the same from attorney to attorney. Additionally, minor details not specifically negotiated are often identified in this first draft. It is important that each party review the written contract carefully to ensure that it clearly and correctly describes each and every point. Each party will expect the other side to abide by the contract's provisions, and the contract will be used to settle any disagreements or questions arising after it has been signed.

CONCLUSION

Negotiation is a vital skill that every optometrist will be required to demonstrate periodically during a professional career. The most important phase of the negotiation process is the gathering of information, which is used to prepare for negotiations and to justify the offering of compromise positions when negotiations have reached an impasse. The underlying principle that should guide negotiators is one of fairness, which is usually attained through compromise by both parties. If an agreement is not fair, it usually will fail—with the complications and difficulties that are attendant to such failure. Therefore, negotiators should enter into discussions having obtained the necessary information, with "win-win" alternatives prepared for presentation. They should be willing to propose compromises that will obtain a successful result for both parties.

BIBLIOGRAPHY

Gifford DG. Legal Negotiation, Theory and Applications. St. Paul, MN: West Publishing, 1989;110.

Gulliver PH. Disputes and Negotiations: A Cross-Cultural Perspective. New York: Academic, 1979.

Martindale DA. Territorial dominance behavior in dyadic verbal interaction. Proceedings of the 79th Annual Convention of the American Psychological Association, 1971;6(1):305–6.

Rubin J, Brown B. The Social Psychology of Bargaining and Negotiation. New York: Academic, 1964;263–4.

Thal L. The practice sale: getting to the bottom line. Optom Manage 1986;10(6):66–7.

Chapter 6

Deciding Where To Practice

David L. Park, James Albright, and Craig Hisaka

> *Alice: I just wanted to ask you, which way I ought to go?*
>
> *Cheshire Cat: Well, that depends on where you want to get to.*
>
> *Alice: Oh, it really doesn't matter, as long as I...*
>
> *Cheshire Cat: Then it really doesn't matter which way you go.*
>
> —Lewis Carroll
> *Alice in Wonderland*

How does an optometrist decide where to practice? Many choices and options exist, in terms of the type of practice and its location. Is a private group practice specializing in contact lenses in the downtown of a major city preferable, or would a solo, small-town family practice in the rural countryside be more appealing? Would the practice of low vision hospital-based optometry be rewarding, or would a teaching career in a pediatric clinic be of more interest?

Practice opportunities exist from Guam to Alaska, from Saudi Arabia to Japan. With so many areas of the world available in which to live and work, the decision on where to locate requires serious thought and study. It also requires goal setting. If an optometrist cannot identify the type of practice and community that he or she prefers, attempting to determine a location will be an exercise in frustration. In choosing a place to practice, individual values and lifestyle, the part of the country in which one has lived, and the personal and professional goals of the person are all factors that affect the decision.

This chapter provides guidance intended to focus the optometry student's thoughts and study on selecting the ideal community. The aim is to help students (and graduates) determine what they desire in terms of the livability of a community, to assess the practice potential of the area, and to decide if the economy of the area can support the type of practice desired. The study of these questions makes up the components of a community and market analysis. This chapter helps students develop their own community and market analysis.

FINDING "VALUE" IN A LOCATION

The assessment of "value" in determining livability will be the most significant issue in deciding where to practice. Is it important that there be local access to hunting, boating, five-star restaurants, live theater, mountain climbing, golf, professional sports, or symphony performances? Would the slower pace of a rural community be preferable? Is it critical that family members live close by? Is the presence of crowds, air pollution, crime, and traffic jams bothersome?

If a practitioner loves the community in which he or she works, this attitude will be reflected to patients and staff. Similarly, if a practitioner enjoys living in a locale, the practitioner will want to become an integral part of local society and will give to the community more than just optometric care. Most patients enjoy seeing their doctor participate in local and civic activities.

Today, so much information is available that with an investment of time and effort a community can be thoroughly evaluated for livability. There are numerous books and magazines that address the livability of communities. For example, *Places Rated Almanac* (New York: Prentice-Hall) is a guide to finding the best places to live in America. The book ranks and compares 329 metropolitan areas for climate, housing, health, crime, transportation, education, the arts, recreation, and economic outlook. *Money* magazine has an annual issue that rates 300 communities in terms of health, crime, economy, housing, education, transportation, weather, leisure, and arts. A visit to the local bookstore or library will provide access to many other references that examine livability factors for communities.

If an optometrist has selected a particular state, information should be sought that has been published specific to that state. For example, if an optometrist is interested in California, it will be helpful to review the book *California, Where to Work, Where to Live* (New York: Prima Publications and Communications). The book provides essential information on such topics as affordable housing, ratings of schools, climate, cultural information, and fastest growing job areas.

The local chamber of commerce can be a helpful source of information. A letter requesting information regarding livability is usually answered with many pamphlets, flyers, and general information about the benefits of living and working in the community. A letter to a chamber of commerce is easy to write and requires little time (Figure 6.1). The addresses of chambers of commerce can be found in the *World Chamber of Commerce Directory* (Loveland, CO: Worldwide Chamber of Commerce Directory, Inc.). Optometrists should be cautious about the literature that is received, however, since each chamber of commerce is in the business of promoting its own community. The advertising that is received may be biased.

Once the decision has been narrowed to three to six communities, it is highly advisable to plan a trip to each community. These trips will inevitably include communities that appeared great on paper but may not accommodate the optometrist's priorities. On a first visit to a community, an initial impression of the city and area will be formed. If the optometrist experiences a poor first impression, he or she should continue to the next community. The optometrist should plan to spend at least one full day in those communities that give a positive first impression.

Figure 6.2 provides a necessary guideline to assist in the proper assessment of a community. The optometrist should begin by thinking about what he or she values in a community. The directions for the exercise are printed at the top of the form. The form should be filled in as directed with an H, M, or L to indicate if the item is of high, moderate, or low importance. The figure helps determine what is of priority to an individual optometrist in a community. The "high importance" elements should be used as a reference and guide when analyzing communities. The spouse or other significant advisor should also perform this exercise, so that all persons affected by the decision can analyze and discuss answers among themselves.

ASSESSING THE PAST AND PRESENT ECONOMIC PICTURES OF A COMMUNITY

When most new businesses begin (or if a business expands), an economic study is performed to determine if the community can support the business. For example, if a national chain decided to place a restaurant in a new city, the area involved would be critically and analytically studied with respect to population, employment statistics, retail sales, and many other factors. An optometrist's practice plans likewise should include an economic study, to help ensure that the community can support another practice.

To perform such an evaluation, a market study needs to be performed. Information must be collected regarding population, growth rate, new building permits, per capita income, median

Date_____

Chamber of Commerce
Main Street
Anytown, US

To Whom it May Concern:

Would you please send me information about _____?
I am interested in the economic profile, housing, weather, education, and
recreation. Helpful information would include major employers, population statistics for 1980 and 1990, ethnic breakdown, and income levels
(per capita, median household).

I would also like information about the current eye care providers in
your city. If possible, please send me a photocopy of the Yellow Pages
that list optometrists, ophthalmologists, and opticians for the area.

Thank you very much for your help. If you have any questions, please let
me know.

Sincerely,

Figure 6.1. Sample letter to a chamber of commerce requesting information about a community's economy, livability, and optometric practice potential.

household income, eye care providers, ethnic
analysis, and age analysis (Figure 6.3).

A thorough comparison of communities regarding demographic and economic characteristics will
be of great assistance in selecting a practice location. Economic characteristics include such factors
as population changes, number of households, educational attainment, income and poverty, civilian
labor force, housing units, new building permits,
municipal financial revenues, and expenditures. An
excellent source of information for statistics related to an area's economy can be found in the
*Rand McNally Commercial Atlas and Marketing
Guide* (Skokie, IL: Rand McNally). It is one of the
best resources for economic data, population demographics and estimates, and city ratings. The
atlas is an excellent reference for statistics and in-

terpretation of business data. It includes many categories, such as:

- Buying power index
- Drug store sales
- Effective buying income
- Estimated population
- Food store sales
- Per capita income
- Shopping goods sales
- Zip code sectional areas

Another source of information is the *Census
Catalog and Guide* (Washington, DC: U.S. Department of Commerce). This book, published by
the Bureau of the Census, is a resource for reports, computer tapes, maps, microfiche, online

WHAT YOU WANT A COMMUNITY TO OFFER

DIRECTIONS: For each item below, think about its relative importance or value to you. Place an (H) for high importance, (M) for moderate importance, or (L) for low importance next to each item.

_____ Clean water
_____ Low crime rate
_____ Many doctors
_____ Availability of hospitals
_____ Strong state government
_____ Cost of medical care
_____ Low income taxes
_____ Low property taxes
_____ Housing appreciation
_____ Recession insulation
_____ Inexpensive cost of living
_____ Strong local income growth
_____ Future job growth
_____ Low sales tax
_____ Cheap car insurance
_____ Good public schools
_____ Conservationists' rating
_____ Civic involvement
_____ Near lakes, oceans
_____ Close to colleges
_____ Potential state tax rise
_____ Small chance of radon gas

_____ Commuting time
_____ Low unemployment rate
_____ Local amusements
_____ Proximity to a big airport
_____ Near places of worship
_____ National forests or parks
_____ Chance of natural disasters
_____ Sunny weather
_____ Close to relatives
_____ Quality restaurants
_____ Near a big city
_____ Low housing prices
_____ Public transportation
_____ Museums nearby
_____ Major league sports teams
_____ Local symphony orchestras
_____ Major zoos or aquariums
_____ Amtrak service
_____ Skiing close by
_____ Minor league sports teams
_____ Near golf courses

Figure 6.2. Rating scale to determine the personal "value" of a community.

MARKET ANALYSIS FOR _____
CITY, STATE

CITY POPULATION   1980 _____   1990 _____

COUNTY POPULATION 1980 _____   1990 _____

CITY POPULATION FORECAST FOR 2000 _____

CITY GROWTH RATE _____% COUNTY GROWTH RATE _____%

NEW BUILDING PERMITS _____

****

PER CAPITA INCOME _____ MEDIAN HOUSEHOLD INCOME _____

PERSONS IN POVERTY _____ TOTAL HOUSEHOLDS _____

****

THREE MAJOR EMPLOYERS:

    1. _____ EMPLOYING _____

    2. _____ EMPLOYING _____

    3. _____ EMPLOYING _____

UNEMPLOYMENT RATE: _____

****

OPTOMETRISTS IN CITY _____ OPHTHALMOLOGISTS IN CITY _____

OPTICIANS IN CITY _____ OPTICAL CHAINS IN CITY _____

****

ETHNIC ANALYSIS: ASIAN/PAC. ISLAND _____ BLACK _____

AMER. INDIAN _____ HISPANIC _____ SPANISH ORIGIN _____

WHITE _____

AGE ANALYSIS

<6 _____	6–17 _____
18–64 _____	>64 _____

Figure 6.3. Research form for information collected during a marketing study.

access, and floppy disks. The information available is in areas of business, construction, housing, manufacturing, population, transportation, and related subjects.

If new major national stores have recently moved into an area, it is likely that they have conducted significant economic studies. One predominant new business can greatly impact a community's population, tax base, housing, and business climate. Conversely, the loss of a vital business can have a deleterious effect on a community.

DETERMINING THE OPTOMETRIC PRACTICE POTENTIAL FOR AN AREA

One key aspect of the study of an area is to determine if there is a need for additional optometrists. Opening a practice in an area highly saturated with eye care providers may lead to slow practice growth and development. Table 6.1 provides a current evaluation of the distribution of optometrists, including areas that are saturated and areas that need additional optometrists. A thorough study of an area's current eye care providers, the types of services provided, and the vision care needs of the population will enable the optometrist to make an intelligent assessment. Key questions to ask during this assessment include:

- Can the community support another eye care provider?
- Does the community makeup support practice goals?
- What are the referral patterns of professionals in the area?
- Does the state law allow adequate use of therapeutic pharmaceutical agents?

To find answers to these questions, the optometrist needs to analyze the practice potential of a community. A key consideration is the optometrist-to-population ratio in a community. These ratios serve as guidelines to estimate the economic viability of an area. When individual communities are studied, it may be found that a community with 10,000 people has five optometrists. However, the community may be able to support an additional optometrist who offers a particular specialty. Furthermore, the

community may have a true drawing population of 80,000 people.

Conversely, a community of 48,000 people may have only one or two eye care providers. The statistics suggest that the community could easily support an additional optometrist. However, the community may have a per capita income so low, with so many people below poverty level, that an additional optometrist would have a difficult time supporting a practice.

The rule of thumb for optometrist-to-population ratio varies from 1:5,000 to 1:8,000 in urban areas to 1:25,000 to 1:45,000 in rural areas (see Chapter 3). Optometrist-to-population ratios should be used as a guide only, and too much weight should not be given to these ratios when reaching a decision. If the buying population of the community can be accurately determined, the ratios may be more applicable. If city populations alone are used as a guide, without considering drawing areas, it may be difficult to find a community that needs an optometrist.

How does a researcher find out how many active optometrists are practicing in an area? The best way is to review the listings in the Yellow Pages of the local telephone book. Because of the high cost of Yellow Pages advertising, most optometrists who have retired or relocated will not continue a listing. A copy of the Yellow Pages for a community may be obtained from the local telephone company. It is also important to review the listings of ophthalmologists and opticians. (In addition, the Yellow Pages will be of help when calling for information regarding schools, religious institutions, real estate, shopping areas, and similar community resources.)

The *Blue Book of Optometrists* (Chicago: Professional Press/Butterworth) provides a comprehensive list of optometrists by city and state throughout the United States, Canada, and Puerto Rico. The *Blue Book* also lists retired optometrists and optometrists who are in education or research, in active military service, and in health maintenance organizations. These optometrists should not be figured into practice potential ratios. A companion reference may be found in the *Red Book of Ophthalmologists* (Stoneham, MA: Butterworth).

A second rule of thumb that has been applied over the years is to have one optometrist to every three dentists. The reason for this ratio is that, in most cases, people visit a dentist about three times

Table 6.1. Optometrist Ratios— U.S. Total and by Region, Division, and State, 1995

Area	Licensed Optometrists per 100,000 Persons	Area	Licensed Optometrists per 100,000 Persons
Total	12.3	Georgia	8.9
Northeast region	12.9	Maryland	6.4
New England division	14.7	North Carolina	10.5
Connecticut	13.1	South Carolina	8.7
Maine	13.6	Virginia	10.1
Massachusetts	16.1	West Virginia	12.8
New Hampshire	12.6	East South Central division	10.5
Rhode Island	16.9	Alabama	9.8
Vermont	11.2	Kentucky	10.0
Middle Atlantic division	12.3	Mississippi	8.4
New Jersey	12.5	Tennessee	12.5
New York	11.4	West South Central division	10.4
Pennsylvania	13.4	Arkansas	11.4
Midwest region	13.8	Louisiana	8.3
East North Central division	13.7	Oklahoma	15.7
Illinois	14.1	Texas	9.8
Indiana	16.8	**West region**	13.6
Michigan	11.4	Mountain division	12.1
Ohio	13.4	Arizona	10.0
Wisconsin	14.0	Colorado	14.1
West North Central division	14.0	Idaho	12.7
Iowa	15.1	Montana	18.2
Kansas	14.8	Nevada	11.1
Minnesota	12.3	New Mexico	11.6
Missouri	13.0	Utah	9.6
Nebraska	13.4	Wyoming	18.1
North Dakota	21.9	Pacific division	14.1
South Dakota	19.1	Alaska	9.8
South region	10.1	California	14.2
South Atlantic division	9.8	Hawaii	8.7
Delaware	9.3	Oregon	15.5
District of Columbia	6.5	Washington	13.4
Florida	11.2		

Sources: Optometrist data compiled from state licensing boards. Population data from the Area Resource File.

for every one visit to an optometrist. A third rule of thumb suggests that there should be one optometrist for every three to four physicians in a community.

Another fact to explore in relation to practice potential is the vision care needs of the population. It should be determined if the community primarily consists of senior citizens, who would require treatment for pathology and low vision services, or if it has more of a young adult population with children, who would require contact lens and pediatric services. A community profile that analyzes age categories will provide helpful information regarding the vision care needs of the population. The

local chamber of commerce usually has available census information that lists age, sex, income, and ethnic categories.

Practice potential information can be obtained through local optical laboratories. Laboratory representatives cover particular geographic areas and can serve as excellent sources of information for practice opportunities. Many laboratories have 800 numbers that would permit calls for information to be made without charge.

Opportunities for practice potential can be found through state and national placement efforts. The membership services department of the American

Optometric Association (AOA) can be contacted for placement information. The AOA Practice Resource Network is a computerized service established to help AOA member doctors of optometry and fourth-year optometry student members find mutually satisfying practice opportunities. This service provides a national listing of optometrists seeking employees, partners, and purchasers. In many states there are also placement services offered by the state optometric association.

When a selected community is visited, it is important to try to talk with as many professionals as possible about the need for optometric services, the economy of the area, and its livability. It is also useful to talk with other health care providers, (e.g., school nurses, pharmacists, physicians) about the community.

When assessing a community, local optometrists should be contacted by mail or telephone regarding potential practice opportunities. A well-written letter expressing interest in the community and asking about practice opportunities may be favorably received by an optometrist looking for an associate or potential buyer. Office visits to optometrists are usually well worth the effort; an associateship, partnership, or purchase option may develop from the encounter.

LOCATING AN OFFICE

Once a community has been chosen, the next step is to determine the location of the office. Of course, if a practice is being purchased, the location is part of the overall evaluation of the proposed sale. For a graduate looking to begin a practice, though, the location of the office is an important consideration. In fact, it is a key part of achieving financial success.

The same sources that were consulted when deciding on a community can be used to evaluate potential locations for a practice. The U.S. Economic Census for an area can be found at a city's chamber of commerce. City records can provide information of new developments in business and residential areas. Future trends about a community and patterns of population can be obtained from real estate associations, utility companies, public libraries, planning boards, school district administrators, and marketing departments of colleges. These data will be essential in guiding the deci-

sion-making process. A beginning optometrist should discuss future plans with representatives from all the foregoing organizations. The *Rand McNally Commercial Atlas and Marketing Guide* (Skokie, IL: Rand McNally) should be consulted for demographic information. A personal diary should be kept of important contacts and events during the information gathering process.

The most important consideration in selecting an office site is visibility. Visibility to the public has a positive effect on patient flow. In some communities, it may be preferable to locate in a medical complex with other health care providers. In this situation, the presence of patients in the building (and, one hopes, the referral of some of these patients by other tenants) will assist in building a patient base. In some high-visibility locations, such as malls and shopping areas, the cost of office space is high. Financial projections need to be carefully made to ensure that such a location is economically viable.

If an office is to be built or remodeled, a contractor will be needed. Determining the right person to do the job is essential. Discussions should be held with tenants, builders, and developers to obtain answers to the following questions:

- Who are the best commercial builders?
- Why is a particular builder considered to be preferable?
- Has the builder experienced legal difficulties or conflicts with clients?
- How long has the builder been in business?
- Where are some of the builder's offices located?

There should be a consistent pattern of behavior and usually a consensus of opinion about the better individuals in the building industry, especially in smaller communities.

Because practices are often open in the evenings to accommodate the schedules of working families, a well-lighted and safe location is an important priority. It is also an advantage to be near a major thoroughfare and recognizable buildings, especially when a staff member has to give patients directions to the office. Accessibility is a very important consideration when choosing an office location, and adequate parking is a key part of ensuring accessibility.

COMMUNITY ANALYSIS					
COMMUNITY	1	2	3	4	5
PRACTICE POTENTIAL INDEX					
O.D./population ratio	☐	☐	☐	☐	☐
Vision care needs	☐	☐	☐	☐	☐
Types of practices	☐	☐	☐	☐	☐
Attitude of professionals in the community	☐	☐	☐	☐	☐
Number of physicians	☐	☐	☐	☐	☐
Opinions of optical labs	☐	☐	☐	☐	☐
TOTAL					
ECONOMIC INDEX					
Employment statistics	☐	☐	☐	☐	☐
Retail sales	☐	☐	☐	☐	☐
Population growth rate	☐	☐	☐	☐	☐
Community buying power	☐	☐	☐	☐	☐
Amount of new building	☐	☐	☐	☐	☐
Rate of bank deposit	☐	☐	☐	☐	☐
Business starts	☐	☐	☐	☐	☐
TOTAL					
LIVABILITY INDEX					
Housing and neighborhood	☐	☐	☐	☐	☐
Schools	☐	☐	☐	☐	☐
Churches	☐	☐	☐	☐	☐
Cultural and recreational opportunities	☐	☐	☐	☐	☐
Shopping areas	☐	☐	☐	☐	☐
Community organizations	☐	☐	☐	☐	☐
Climate	☐	☐	☐	☐	☐
Your impression of the area	☐	☐	☐	☐	☐
TOTAL					
GRAND TOTAL					

INSTRUCTIONS: Use a scale of 1 point for the lowest value to 5 points for the highest value for each of the factors listed above. When completed, the total points for each index can be added together to determine the most desirable community.

Figure 6.4. Worksheet to rate and analyze different communities.

In most cases, the selection of an office location will be based on the input received from the business people in the community. In particular, dentists seem to understand the economics and business aspects of their profession and community. Initially, the new optometrist has to rely on and trust the opinion of others. If adequate effort has been placed on the collection of information from knowledgeable sources, the choice of location will be a good one.

PUTTING IT ALL TOGETHER

To begin the process of determining a practice location, practice goals must be established. To evaluate potential practice locations, information should be requested from different communities. A determination of what the individual optometrist values in a community should be made. A market analysis should be completed for each community that is being considered. The most promising communities should then be rated for practice potential, economics, and livability (Figure 6.4).

Finding the ideal community in which to practice is an exciting yet demanding endeavor. Planning, travel, and analysis are necessary. To find the time needed to perform an adequate assessment, the process should begin in optometry school. School holidays and summer vacations are the ideal times to plan community and practice visitations. The earlier the process can be initiated, the better the assessment that can be performed and the better the outcome realized.

BIBLIOGRAPHY

American Automobile Association. AAA Tourbook. Heathrow, FL: American Automobile Association, 1996.

American Business Directories. Optometrists, the 1993 Directory. Omaha, NE: American Business Directories, 1993.

Barreto H. California, Where to Live and Work. New York: Prima Publications and Communications, 1989.

Blue Book of Optometrists (43rd ed). Chicago: Professional Press/Butterworth, 1995.

Boyer R, Savageau D. Places Rated Almanac: Your Guide to Finding the Best Places to Live in America. New York: Prentice-Hall, 1993.

Census Catalog and Guide. Washington, DC: U.S. Department of Commerce, U.S. Bureau of the Census, 1985.

Commercial Atlas and Marketing Guide (126th ed). Skokie, IL: Rand McNally, 1995.

Statistical Abstract of the United States: The National Data Book (115th ed). Washington, DC: U.S. Department of Commerce, Bureau of the Census, 1995.

U.S. Small Business Administration. Learning about Your Market. Washington, DC: U.S. Small Business Administration, 1985.

U.S. Small Business Administration. Marketing Checklist for Small Retailers. Washington, DC: U.S. Small Business Administration, 1985.

Worldwide Chamber of Commerce Directory. Loveland, CO: Worldwide Chamber of Commerce Directory, 1988.

Chapter 7

Practice Financing

David L. Park, Craig Hisaka, and Gary Moss

Neither a borrower nor a lender be.

—William Shakespeare
Hamlet

Proper financing is an important component of success in an optometric practice. An understanding of basic financial principles is necessary to start and run an office. Many financial undertakings with great potential have failed because they were undercapitalized. It would be devastating and a personal setback for a graduate to have to close an office after a few months of operation due to the lack of a few thousand dollars and no access to capital. This chapter concentrates on key aspects of practice financing and discusses basic financial situations, types of loans, sources of financial assistance, credit worthiness, seller financing, collateral, loan restrictions and limitations, and standards of evaluation for applicants.

A written financial plan or business plan forms the basis for the success of an optometric office. The business plan is used to design business goals, make financial projections, organize the office, identify markets, and obtain financing. A business plan will need to address the basic questions posed by the potential creditor (Table 7.1).

BASIC FINANCIAL SITUATIONS

Different types of situations will require various amounts of capital to get started. For new of-

fices, space and equipment must be purchased or leased, inventory obtained, and sufficient funds left over to run the office until the practice becomes self-supporting. Buying an existing practice usually requires a sizable down payment—typically 10–25% of the purchase price—and enough money to run the office and make payments to the seller. Operating funds and payments to the seller need to be supported in the monthly operating budget.

It is necessary to determine accurately the amount of money that will be needed from a creditor. If funds are inadequate, the creditor may not be willing to extend the amount borrowed or to modify the terms of the loan. To fortify insufficient start-up capital, most optometrists incur long-term debt rather than sell equity in the practice. Long-term debt is paid with interest, usually over a period greater than 5 years; it gives the creditor neither ownership interest nor control over the practice.

Increased expenses, a slowdown in patient visits or payments, or rapid office expansion may create a shortage of working capital. The classic resolution is the use of medium- to long-term credit. However, new or additional debt should be obtained only if cash flow projections show that the loan will generate sufficient profits to pay the debt.

Table 7.1. Sample Questions That Need to be Answered in a Written Business Plan

1. Have all aspects of the desired business—including location, demographics, patient base, rent, laboratory expenses, office overhead, and so forth—been thoroughly considered?
2. How are projected expenses best estimated?
3. Is the business plan realistic and practical to implement? Has the business plan been discussed with others?
4. Has a marketing plan been thoroughly considered? Is there sufficient capital to fund the marketing program?
5. Is the borrower's credit history favorable for loan consideration?
6. What sources are available for backup or emergency funds?
7. How much of a loan does the borrower need? Does the borrower have funds to inject into the practice?
8. Does the borrower have a guarantor available if needed?

TYPES OF LOANS

The different types of financing available to optometrists are generally classified as follows:

1. *Long-term capital*: An arrangement in which repayment extends over more than 5 years. Long-term loans are repaid from earnings. This type of loan is usually required when purchasing a practice or when a practice is unable to meet the obligations of an intermediate-term loan.

2. *Intermediate-term capital*: An arrangement in which repayment must be made over a period of 1–5 years. These loans are also repaid from earnings. Most conventional bank loans permit repayment in 5 or fewer years.

3. *Short-term capital*: An arrangement in which repayment must be made within 1 year of the loan. Short-term loans are repaid from the liquidation of current assets or of inventory that the loan has financed. An example of a short-term loan is the financed purchase of a large quantity of new frames, with the repayment coming from the sale of the frames at a profit.

Banks loan funds based on the borrower's reputation and may, thereby, provide either an unsecured or a secured loan. An unsecured loan is often used for short-term situations. Collateral is not required because the bank counts on the borrower's credit standing. Credit cards and lines of credit are examples of unsecured loans. A secured loan requires the borrower to possess an asset (the collateral) that can be taken or sold by the bank if the borrower cannot repay the loan. The bank requires the collateral as protec-

tion for its depositors against the risk that the loan will fail.

Many factors are involved in the loan process, and the borrower has no control over some of these factors. Recessionary times, the fluctuating cost of credit, and changes in banking regulations can interfere with an optometrist's ability to obtain financing.

SOURCES OF FINANCING FOR OPTOMETRISTS

Three facts should be understood when facing the formidable task of obtaining funds from a borrower:

1. An established office (typically, 10 years or more in business) with a good record of operations has a better chance of obtaining a loan than a new office.
2. Some personal capital investment in an office is almost a requirement to obtain any type of creditor support.
3. The more collateral or security the borrower is willing to give, the easier it will be to obtain a loan.

Financing is available from a variety of sources, including both commercial and government lenders. These sources include the following:

1. *Banks*. Full-service banks are the most visible lenders and make the greatest number and variety of loans. Bankers look for borrowers with experience in the business, excellent credit records, and good ability to repay the loan.

2. *Commercial financial companies*. These companies are similar to banks and many offer the same

Table 7.2. Sources for Funds When Financing is Needed to Start an Optometric Practice

---

Loans from relatives or friends
Loans from equipment dealers
Trade credit (e.g., credit given by laboratories)
Personal resources from savings or inheritance
Bank loans
Small Business Administration loans
Mortgage loans
Small business investment company loans
Partners
Spouse
Retirement accounts

---

types of loans and terms as banks. Commercial financial companies often provide loans based on the borrower's collateral rather than on the office's track record. Finance company loans sometimes exceed the net worth of the borrower, a situation that is undesirable to most banks.

3. *Life insurance companies.* A whole life insurance policy can work as business cash when the owner borrows on the policy. Repayment to most insurance companies is made with interest, in the same manner as standard loans from banks.

4. *Consumer finance companies.* These companies are high-risk lenders that charge higher interest rates than banks for similar types of loans. They typically supply personal loans for any personal need, including money for a small business.

5. *Savings institutions.* These businesses specialize in real estate financing. They often make loans on commercial, industrial, and personal residences.

6. *Small Business Administration (SBA).* The SBA guarantees bank loans (up to 90% of the amount borrowed) to small businesses and makes a limited number of direct loans to small businesses.

7. *Small business investment companies.* These companies are privately owned venture capital firms eligible for federal loans that are used to invest in or lend to small businesses.

8. *Minority enterprise small business investment companies.* These companies serve small businesses that are at least 51% owned by socially or economically disadvantaged Americans.

9. *Farmers Home Administration (FHA).* The FHA guarantees bank loans to nonfarming businesses in rural areas. It does not make direct loans

but will guarantee up to 90% of a bank loan to a qualifying applicant.

Additional suggestions for sources of loans are listed in Table 7.2.

When looking for a creditor, the borrower may have to search many avenues. Some lenders base loans on debt ratio, whereas other lenders look at collateral. A loan proposal requires the expenditure of significant work and energy (see Chapter 8). However, with persistence, motivation, and entrepreneurial enthusiasm, an optometry school graduate should be able to obtain funding for an optometric practice.

CREDIT WORTHINESS

When applying for a loan, there are two major questions that will be asked by the creditor. The first question is: "Can the borrower repay the debt?" To answer this question, the creditor will analyze the borrower's profit and loss statement, balance sheet, and cash flow summary. Loan institutions often request all data about both business and personal income, including expenses and equity. For start-up offices, industry data must be consulted for income and expense projection purposes. If the borrower is purchasing a practice, financial information from the existing practice will be requested as part of the loan proposal.

The creditor's second question is: "What is the borrower's credit history and credit data (TRW report)?" To answer this question, the creditor will investigate the borrower's past ability to repay debt. The borrower's prior payment records will be obtained and scrutinized by the lending agency. Any late payments, even from years earlier, will require proper explanation to the lending company. A poor credit repayment history will severely affect the borrower's ability to obtain funds. An excellent credit rating will not guarantee a loan but will help significantly in the total process of obtaining funds.

Before a lending agency will advance money, the institution must be satisfied with the answers to the questions listed in Table 7.3.

To determine if a borrower's business is credit worthy, satisfactory financial data will be necessary. Loan institutions want to make loans to businesses that are solvent, earning profits, and expanding. The two fundamental financial documents used to ascertain those positions are the in-

Table 7.3. Questions a Lending Institution Will Ask the Borrower

1.	What type of individual is the borrower? Most often personal qualities come first. What is the borrower's ability to manage an office?
2.	What is the purpose of the loan? The answer will determine if a short- or long-term loan is being obtained. Money to be used for inventory may require faster repayment terms than money used to buy equipment.
3.	Do income and expense projections allow the borrower to pay the loan back and afford ample income for all projected living expenses?
4.	Is there a cushion in the loan to make allowances for unforeseen developments?
5.	What is the outlook for optometry in general and for the proposed office in particular?

come statement and the balance sheet. The income statement is a primary measure of profits and losses, and the balance sheet is a fundamental gauge for assets and liabilities. The bank usually will request the profit and loss statements and balance sheets of an office for at least the 5 years preceding the loan. If these documents are not available, tax returns are substituted. A consecutive sequence of these two statements over a period of time is the primary means for measuring financial balance and development capacity.

In reviewing loan documents, the banker will be particularly interested in the following:

1. *Fixed assets.* What is the fair market value of the major equipment and furnishings? What are the depreciation values? Fair market value appraisals by qualified appraisers for banks often will need to be obtained. Qualified appraisers for ophthalmic equipment can often be hired from companies involved in selling ophthalmic equipment. The loan institution will inform the borrower of its requirements for an appraisal.

A second type of appraisal involves the calculation of book value. The book value for equipment is determined by taking the original cost of the equipment and subtracting from it the amount of depreciation claimed. Depreciation tables often will be needed to determine an item's book value.

2. *Accounts receivable.* Are accounts receivable part of the sale and value of the practice? Are the accounts receivable poor because many patients are behind in payments? What is the percentage of accounts receivable that are collected? The lending institution must be asked to state its policy on loans that include accounts receivable. If funds are not available for the payment of accounts receivable, the purchase agreement must be negotiated with the

seller so that the accounts receivable are not part of the sale.

3. *Inventory.* Are frames and supplies current? Is a large part of the inventory on consignment? Is the inventory turnover similar to other offices? Many lending institutions prefer not to support a portion of a loan that is backed with inventory as collateral. The reason is that inventory used as collateral is difficult to liquidate by a creditor in case of foreclosure.

4. *Customary information.* Are the books and records up-to-date? What are the salaries? Have the taxes been paid? What is the number of employees? Is insurance provided by the office? These and similar questions will customarily be posed by the creditor.

AMOUNT OF FINANCING

The quantity of funds needed by a borrower depends on the objectives for use of the capital. Determining the amount of money required for equipment, furnishings, supplies, construction, expansion, or buy-out is easy. Equipment companies, architects, and builders will eagerly supply cost calculations. On the other hand, the amount of working capital that is needed depends on the projection of income and expenses.

In general, most lending agencies will provide loans that can be secured by collateral. However, it can be difficult to obtain a loan for working capital (which involves no collateral). To obtain money needed for operating expenses, the borrower will need to contact lending agencies regarding a line of credit. A line of credit is an agreement by a creditor to supply funds—up to a certain stated maximum— for use by the borrower. After the line of credit is es-

Table 7.4. Initial Start-up Expenses*

Purchase or lease of ophthalmic equipment
Purchase or lease of office equipment
Leasehold improvements or remodeling
Ophthalmic inventory
Printing expenses
Accounting, legal, and license fees
Initial marketing program
Rental (first month's, last month's, security deposit)
Projected living expenses (e.g., rent, food, utilities, insurance) for 6 months
Miscellaneous (for unforeseen expenses)
Total

*The calculations for each item help the borrower determine the cash needed to start up an office.

tablished, the borrower can draw against it as needed. No obligation to repay is incurred until money is actually withdrawn. Often such an arrangement can be used to serve as a source of working capital.

The amount of money needed to start an optometric practice can be roughly calculated by using Table 7.4.

COLLATERAL

Collateral is the offering of a form of security or guarantee that a loan will be repaid. If a loan cannot be justified by financial statements, a pledge of security may enable the borrower to secure the loan. If the borrower defaults, the collateral can be used by the creditor to offset the borrower's lack of payment. A borrower may offer the bank collateral in many different forms. Each lending institution has certain collateral that it will accept. Some of the common types of collateral are listed in Table 7.5.

RESTRICTIONS AND LIMITATIONS

In general, a financially sound practice will incur few limitations on a loan. A new practice started "cold" or a practitioner who is a poor credit risk can expect to incur greater restrictions and limitations in the loan agreement. Limitations include requirements intended to protect the creditor's investment and usually involve:

- Type of collateral
- Repayment terms (length of time and interest amount)
- Periodic reporting (required reporting by the borrower)

Restrictions are found in a loan agreement in the section known as covenants; these obligations can be either positive or negative. Negative covenants are things the borrower cannot do without approval from the lender. An example of a negative covenant is the inability of the borrower to take on additional debt without the lender's approval. Positive covenants include things the borrower must do—for example, the maintenance, by the borrower, of a minimum net working capital and the borrower's repayment of the loan according to the stated terms.

A borrower should keep in mind that all terms are negotiable, and being prepared to negotiate various terms is an important part of the loan process. A borrower should not be afraid to fight to protect personal interests. For this reason, it is a good practice to obtain the loan documents in advance before closing.

STANDARDS OF EVALUATION

After a borrower has furnished the required data, the next phase in the borrowing process is the evaluation of the application. Most lending agencies consider similar factors when determining whether to award or decline a loan. In most instances, the evaluator looks for the following:

- The borrower's prior debt-paying record
- The ratio of the borrower's debt to net worth
- Past performance of the practice
- The value and condition of collateral

SELLER FINANCING

One popular method for transferring the ownership of a practice in recent years has been the use of financing by the selling optometrist. Seller financing can be both primary or secondary and can involve the use of mortgages. A mortgage is the purchase of property in which the buyer is given the title to the property, even though the

Table 7.5. Different Types of Collateral That May Be Offered When Applying for a Loan

1. Borrower's signature: such as a line of credit or a signature loan.
2. Endorsers: other people sign the note as endorsers to improve the borrower's credit. The endorsers are liable for the loan if the borrower fails to make payments.
3. Chattel mortgages: if equipment such as a visual field instrument is purchased, the bank is given a security interest in the equipment (and may sell the equipment to satisfy the loan if the borrower fails to make payments).
4. Real estate: an excellent and preferred type of collateral. If the borrower is willing to take a risk by putting real estate up as collateral, the bank usually becomes more willing to provide a loan.
5. Accounts receivable: can sometimes be used as collateral. Banks count on patients paying their bills, and a good report of the borrower's accounts receivable performance is necessary to use this aspect as collateral. It may be possible to borrow up to 50% of current (<30 days) receivables.
6. Savings accounts: can be assigned to the bank to act as collateral.
7. Life insurance: cash value in a life insurance policy can serve as collateral. The policy is assigned to the bank.
8. Stocks and bonds: serve as collateral if they are marketable. Up to 75% of the value of the stocks and bonds may be eligible to be borrowed.

purchase is financed by a loan from a creditor. The creditor may proceed to take title to the property, however, if the buyer does not repay the loan. The creditor may also sell the property to obtain the amount due.

An example of primary seller financing may be found in the following practice sale agreement. The buyer agrees to purchase the practice for $150,000 and makes a 20% down payment ($30,000) to the seller. The seller is willing to finance the balance of $120,000 and is given a mortgage by the buyer for that amount.

An example of secondary seller financing may be found in the following example. The buyer agrees to buy the practice for $150,000 and borrows $50,000 from a bank for a down payment. The remaining balance of $100,000 is financed by the seller, who is given a second mortgage for that amount. In this arrangement, the bank holds the first mortgage of $50,000, and the seller holds the second mortgage for the remaining balance.

In the first case, although the seller obtained a smaller down payment, the interest is more secure because the seller holds a first mortgage. In the second case, the seller obtains more money as a down payment, but the position is less secure because, in the event the buyer is unable to pay, the seller's

mortgage can only be satisfied after the bank's mortgage. The bank holds first mortgage and thus may sell the practice equipment and other collateral to obtain payment for the amount due. The seller can attempt to obtain payment only after the bank's first mortgage is satisfied. There are advantages to both buyer and seller in this arrangement, and some disadvantages as well (Table 7.6).

Due to the difficulty of obtaining financing, creative methods for the transfer of practice ownership have been devised. In the situation where a prospective buyer is unable to obtain the full financing necessary to purchase a practice, the seller's willingness to finance part of the purchase price will often enable the transfer of ownership to take place.

CONCLUSION

The information in this chapter provides an introduction to the basic fundamentals of financing an optometric practice. In Chapter 8, the details of business loans are discussed, and an example of a loan proposal is presented. This proposal includes a projected profit and loss statement, a projected income statement, and a sample business plan.

Table 7.6. Advantages and Disadvantages of Seller Financing

Advantages

To the Buyer:

1. The buyer usually needs to provide less money to purchase the practice:
   - The buyer often saves money, with minimal closing costs and no points.
   - The buyer may be able to negotiate a lower down payment to the seller than the payment required by a bank (typically 20%).
   - The buyer has more control over costs such as appraisals, inspections, and reports.
2. Financing keeps a selling practitioner more active in the practice (to keep the practitioner's investment secure). The selling practitioner has a vested interest in the success of the new owner and wants the new practitioner to succeed.
3. The buyer may be able to negotiate a lower interest rate than through a commercial loan.
4. Seller financing may be the only means to purchase a practice if banks are unwilling to provide capital to a new practitioner who has high debt and minimal collateral.

To the Seller:

1. Since there will be principal and interest paid over a period of time on a monthly basis, this money will add to the seller's retirement living expenses.
2. The tax consequences will be lessened if the practice is purchased over time, due to a reduction in capital gains.

Disadvantages

To the Buyer:

1. This method of financing may entail more years of monthly payments than other methods, and thus would ultimately cost more.

To the Seller:

1. The seller does not receive a large sum of money as a down payment that can be invested.

BIBLIOGRAPHY

American Optometric Association. Focus on Your Future. St. Louis: American Optometric Association, 1988.

Bank of America. Financing Small Business, SBR-104. San Francisco: Bank of America, 1985.

Bank of America. Loan Preparation Guide, AD-1016. San Francisco: Bank of America, 1985.

California Optometric Credit Union. Optometric Practice Loan Application Requirements. Sacramento, CA: California Optometric Credit Union, 1985.

U.S. Small Business Administration. The ABC's of Borrowing. Management Aid 1001. Washington, DC: Office of Business Development, U.S. Small Business Administration, 1985.

U.S. Small Business Administration. Business Basics for the Growing Optometric Practice, publication 88-1062. Washington, DC: U.S. Small Business Administration, Office of Business Development, 1988.

Chapter 8

Obtaining a Business Loan

John G. Classé

Hold fast to dreams
For if dreams die
Life is a broken winged bird
That cannot fly.

—Langston Hughes
The World Tomorrow

The traditional means of delivering optometric services—sole proprietorship—requires offices to be equipped with an array of up-to-date instruments, inventories of frames and contact lenses, and tasteful fixtures and furnishings. This obligation places a heavy financial burden on practitioners seeking to practice in the time-honored way. In addition, there are operating costs that must be met (e.g., rent, taxes, utilities, and salaries). That means that the graduate seeking entry into private practice must obtain financing in order to afford the start-up costs of private practice.

Usually, financing must be acquired for both capital assets and operating expenses. Thus, the creditor may be required to lend more money than there will be collateral to serve as security. This possibility necessitates careful planning and meticulous preparation on the part of the borrower, because the creditor will have to be convinced that there is minimal risk in making such a partially unsecured loan. To ensure that the risk is low, the creditor will dictate the terms of the agreement and will protect the interest in the collateral. This chapter discusses the conventional devices used by creditors to secure loans and to protect collateral in the event of default on the part of the borrower. It also describes the preparation of a loan proposal intended to secure the necessary financing.

FUNDAMENTALS OF FINANCING

The usual source of loans for the initiation of a practice is a full-service bank. The most basic aspects of bank financing involve the method of repayment and the type of interest. Borrowing money involves not only the act of obtaining the loan but also the repayment of principal and interest. Although there are a number of methods used for the repayment of loans and for the computation of interest, this discussion will be limited to the usual techniques employed by banks.

Banks rely on two principal methods for the repayment of loans:

1. *Renewable short-term notes*. These instruments acknowledge the lending of money for relatively brief periods (usually 90 days) with provisions for renewal at the option of the lender. At the close of any 90-day period, the lender can demand payment in full of the balance due.
2. *Installment notes*. These instruments provide for the periodic repayment of a stated sum at regular intervals, such as monthly payments, usually over a period of 3–5 years.

Either of two interest rates—simple or add-on—may be applied to short-term loans:

Table 8.1. Sample Simple Interest Loan

If $10,000 is borrowed at 10% simple interest on a renewable 90-day note, what would be the interest payable at the end of 90 days?	
Amount borrowed	$10,000
Interest rate	× 10%
Total interest if the note was held for a year	$1,000
Interest for one-fourth of a year	$250
If the note is due in 90 days without renewal, the total amount that has to be repaid is $10,250.	

Source: Reprinted from JG Classé. Legal Aspects of Optometry. Stoneham, MA: Butterworth, 1989.

Table 8.2. Sample Add-On Interest Loan

If $10,000 was borrowed at 10% add-on interest for a period of 3 years, what would be the total cost to the borrower?	
Multiply $10,000	$10,000
By 10%	× .10
Yearly interest	$ 1,000
Multiply by 3 years	× 3
Finance charge	$ 3,000
Add principal	+10,000
Total amount financed	$13,000
Divide by 36 months	÷ 36
Monthly payments	$ 361.11

Source: Reprinted from JG Classé. Legal Aspects of Optometry. Stoneham, MA: Butterworth, 1989.

Table 8.3. Calculation of Interest Under the "Rule of 78"

How is $1,000 in interest computed over a 12-month period under the "Rule of 78?"
The 12-month period is summed as follows:
    $12 + 11 + 10 + 9 + 8 + 7 + 6 + 5 + 4 + 3 + 2 + 1 = 78$
The interest is computed as follows:

First month	12/78 =	$153.84
Second month	11/78 =	$141.02
Third month	10/78 =	$128.20
Fourth month	9/78 =	$115.38
Fifth month	8/78 =	$102.56
Sixth month	7/78 =	$ 89.74
Total		$730.74

Therefore, 73% of the interest due is paid in the first 6 months, leaving $270 of interest to be paid in the last 6 months.

Source: Reprinted from JG Classé. Legal Aspects of Optometry. Stoneham, MA: Butterworth, 1989.

1. *Simple interest.* This rate applies a fixed percentage rate to the amount borrowed for a stated period of time. An example will illustrate how the interest is computed (Table 8.1). Simple interest is one of the most advantageous ways to borrow money. Should the borrower decide to pay off the loan early, there is no prepayment penalty, because the interest is prorated for the actual number of days that the money has been borrowed. However, renewable 90-day notes are subject to fluctuating interest rates based on the prime lending rate during any 90-day period. Rates may be set at the start of the 90-day period or they may change each time the prime rate goes up or down. In the latter case, the rate may change many times over the course of the life of the note. Simple interest short-term bank loans are the preferred means of borrowing money to purchase equipment and start a practice.

2. *Add-on interest.* This method of determining interest is the more costly of the two rates. It is called add-on because the interest is computed on the amount borrowed, without proration, and added to the principal. This total is then repaid in installments over the course of the loan—usually 3, 4, or 5 years. An example will illustrate the method of determining repayment (Table 8.2). Add-on interest is commonly encountered in installment loans, such as are used for the purchase of automobiles and boats. If a borrower decides to prepay an installment loan (i.e., pay before maturity), the interest is short-rated rather than prorated. Short-rating means that if the borrower pays off the loan early, the lender will charge a fee for administrative expenses and profit. Normally this fee is governed by the Rule of 78, which is a standard formula for figuring the interest due (Table 8.3). If the borrower believes there is a possibility that the loan could be repaid early, before borrowing money he or she should always inquire into the short-rate charge with add-on interest. Early repayment of an add-on loan is usually not advantageous if the interest is short-rated. The reason is that the interest charge is heavily weighed toward the start of the loan (Table 8.4).

The usual banking custom is to use simple interest notes for relatively small amounts and for short periods of time, if based on the borrower's signature. Although an unsecured simple interest

Table 8.4. Short-Rated Interest Under the "Rule of 78"

3-Year Note	4-Year Note	5-Year Note
50% of interest in first year	43% of interest in first year	36% of interest in first year
33% of interest in second year	29% of interest in second year	28% of interest in second year
17% of interest in third year	18% of interest in third year	18% of interest in third year
	9% of interest in fourth year	2% of interest in fourth year
		6% of interest in fifth year

Source: Reprinted from JG Classé. Legal Aspects of Optometry. Stoneham, MA: Butterworth, 1989.

note can often be obtained for various personal needs, the financing of equipment and the start-up of a practice will necessitate the use of the equipment (and other collateral) to provide security for the loan.

Add-on interest is used for longer-term financing, involving periodic payments, and is normally secured by the automobile, equipment, or other collateral that is financed. Of course, the personal endorsement of the borrower is also obtained.

The burden is on the borrower to determine the type of financing that is being offered and whether the rate and terms of the loan are favorable and competitive for the market.

BASIC PROVISIONS OF A BANK LOAN AGREEMENT

Although individual bank agreements may differ somewhat in their terms, there is a commonality to these contracts that permits some generalizations to be made. The basic provisions of loan agreements invariably include the amount to be borrowed and the terms of the loan, the interest type and rate, the collateral requirements, the limitations on additional indebtedness, the repayment provisions, and an acceleration clause.

AMOUNT AND TERMS

Any creditor will have loan limits that will not be exceeded without good cause. The creditor will have established loan repayment terms that vary with the purpose of the loan and the amount borrowed. For example, most automobile loans are for 3–4 years; most practice loans are for 5–7 years. There will be an upper limit on the amount

lent that can be utilized for nontangible items. The more conservative the bank, the lower the amount allowed for these expenses (e.g., working capital).

INTEREST RATE

If the loan is for simple interest, it is likely that the agreement will specify a short-term renewable note. In this event, the interest charge probably will fluctuate in accordance with changes in the prime interest rate; the only variable will be the frequency with which the rate changes. Most banks specify a floating rate that changes whenever the prime rate rises or falls, but some may set the rate at the renewal of the note (e.g., quarterly).

If the loan is for add-on interest, the rate is usually set at the start of the loan and does not change thereafter. (Add-on rates are customarily found on installment notes.) If add-on interest is used in conjunction with a renewable short-term note, the rate can be changed at each renewal.

COLLATERAL REQUIREMENTS

There are two customary collateral requirements in practice loans: a purchase money security interest in the equipment (and other tangibles) and a life insurance policy that is assigned to the bank.

A security interest is created when the borrower and creditor follow certain procedures:

1. The creditor and the borrower must agree, in writing, to the formation of the security interest. This is done through the execution of a security agreement.
2. The creditor must make the loan, and the borrower must acquire the property.

3. The creditor must file a financing statement, a document putting the public on notice that the creditor has a financial interest in the property.

The filing requirement is necessary to protect the creditor from subsequent creditors. If the borrower fails to repay the loan, the creditors will have to fight among themselves for whatever assets remain, and the creditor who has filed the earliest security interest will prevail over the others. For this reason, there is considerable emphasis placed on security interests by creditors.

The bank usually requires the borrower to assign to the bank a life insurance policy that will sufficiently cover the loan balance in the event of the borrower's death. An assignment is a transfer of a contractual right or benefit that operates to extinguish the right for the one making the transfer and establish the right exclusively for the benefit of the one to whom it is transferred. Many banks will require the borrower to assign the rights to a life insurance policy to the bank, placing the bank before any other beneficiary in terms of payment if the borrower dies before the loan is repaid.

The borrower will be asked to execute an assignment agreement and will have to surrender the policy to the bank, which will hold it as long as the loan is outstanding. When the loan is repaid, the assignment will be extinguished and the policy will be returned to the borrower.

In addition to the life insurance policy, the bank may require the borrower to maintain other types of insurance coverage. These requirements obligate the practitioner to purchase property and professional liability insurance sufficient to indemnify the bank in the event of the loss of the collateral. Of course, the bank may require additional collateral, a co-signer, or other such items as it deems necessary to protect its security adequately.

LIMITATION ON ADDITIONAL INDEBTEDNESS

To prevent borrowers from overextending themselves, some banks limit the ability of borrowers to obtain additional loans from other creditors. The limitation is usually expressed as a cash limit, not to be exceeded without the prior approval of the bank. These limits do not apply to consumer purchases or to debts incurred during the course of everyday practice activities.

REPAYMENT PROVISIONS

Repayment provisions vary widely from bank to bank and with the type of note and interest charged. Installment notes specify a payment each month for the period of the note. The monthly payment does not change during the repayment period, which is usually for 3–5 years but may be longer. Short-term renewable notes offer the bank more options. These loans are described as being for a period of years (usually 4–5) but are actually renewable at the option of the bank—at stated intervals that are specified in the loan agreement. Renewable periods may be as brief as 90 days or may be for as long as a term of years. Notes retain a degree of flexibility that enables the bank to adjust the repayment schedule as necessary to accommodate the borrower's ability to pay. Some notes specify interest repayment only during the first year of the loan, then amortize the principal and interest over a period of several years thereafter. Other notes will allow the borrower to pay less during the first years of the repayment period.

Regardless of the type of note or repayment schedule, the bank will require the borrower to submit periodic financial statements so that the status of the borrower's practice can be assessed.

ACCELERATION CLAUSE

Any note will contain a so-called acceleration clause, which permits the bank to demand the full amount of the loan due and payable in the event the borrower fails to comply with the provisions of the agreement. This provision affords the bank some protection in the event the borrower cannot make the required payments, because it allows the bank to claim its collateral and proceed as necessary to collect the full outstanding amount. These clauses are a standard aspect of any financial agreement and can only be enforced by the creditor if there is some default on the part of the borrower.

Loan agreements are complex and comprehensive documents that typically involve the transfer of large sums of money. A potential borrower who is not knowledgeable in financial affairs would be well advised to secure professional counsel before entering into any long-term financial arrangements with a creditor.

LOAN PROPOSAL

The loan proposal, which is used to secure funding for the operation of the practice, is a key element of the practice plan (Figure 8.1). To start a practice, buy a practice, or acquire a partnership interest in a practice requires financial investment. The amount of money needed can be many thousands. A creditor is often required to provide financial support. Part of the amount borrowed will be unsecured—unprotected by assets that a creditor can sell if the borrower fails—which motivates the creditor to review the borrower's status meticulously. The loan proposal is used to create confidence in the borrower's financial acumen, to justify the amount being borrowed, and to provide monetary projections against which the borrower's progress can be measured. It requires a considerable amount of time to prepare. Usually, there are three phases of the proposal process: research, drafting the proposal, and presentation.

Research

Research is the key component of preparing a loan proposal. The value of the proposal is directly related to the accuracy of the information it contains. Reliable figures should be used for calculations. For example, repayment of educational loans is a financial burden that most new graduates must consider. The amount of each monthly payment and when payments will begin can be accurately determined, as can the cost of leasing an office, purchasing insurance, or paying for water, gas, and electricity. The effort taken to secure accurate information will pay for itself many times, for the value of the loan proposal as a true measuring rod for financial success will be far greater if reliable information is used. The creditor may also doubt the validity of the proposal if many projections are obviously inaccurate. The biggest fault of insufficient research is that the predictive value of the

proposal is lost and it serves only as a justification for funding. Ideally, the loan proposal should continue to be useful after funding has been secured and the practice plan initiated, as part of the effort to measure success toward financial goals. It should be constantly updated and revised to reflect the evolving situation in the practice. In such a role, it fulfills the short-term goal orientation that is so necessary to a successful outcome.

Drafting the Proposal

The loan proposal requires a stepwise approach. First, all items that are to be purchased—equipment, furniture, real estate, computer, inventory of frames—need to be valued. Second, other key expenditures, such as loans, taxes, leases, utilities, and so forth, need to be determined. Third, projections need to be calculated on a month-by-month basis for the first year and annually thereafter for each year of the loan repayment period (which generally is 4–7 years). Fourth, practice income projections need to be calculated. Fifth, the "bottom line"—the profit or loss to be realized—needs to be determined, month by month for the first year and annually for all subsequent years.

Step 1: Valuing Purchases

The fair market value should be determined for all items that must be purchased. The cost of a phoropter, a sofa, a computer, or any other item can be reasonably ascertained. If an inventory of frames is needed, its value will have been negotiated. For all items of purchase, an accurate determination of value should be obtained.

Step 2: Valuing Key Expenditures

One important goal of the loan proposal is comprehensiveness. It should seek to include all costs that can reasonably be expected to arise during the projected period of years. Key expenditures that should be considered include the projected cost of:

- Repaying educational loans
- Repaying the loan proposal
- An office lease
- Modifications or improvements to an office

<h2 style="text-align:center">LOAN PROPOSAL</h2>

Purpose
To acquire capital to establish an optometric practice in southeast Townsville.

Proposal
The location of the practice will be in southeast Townsville on Vision Ease Road. At present the ratio of optometrists to population in the Townsville area is 1:16,000. The preferred ratio for an optometrist in a similar area is 1:5,000 to 1:8,000. Enclosed is a map of the Townsville city school system with the vision care providers marked in. Although there are numerous dentists and pharmacies in the southeast area, there is no vision care provider at present. The closest provider is at least 8 miles away from the proposed site. As the southeast area is an affluent and rapidly growing area of Townsville that will need vision care services, I feel that with adequate capital I can provide the vision care needed.

Office Lease
I have negotiated an office lease at the proposed location. The lease is for 5 years with an option to renew for another 5 years. A copy of the lease is enclosed.

Insurance Coverage
I have been approved to purchase a term life insurance policy in the amount of $40,000 to pay off the loan from the bank should I die before the loan is repaid. In addition, I have acquired an umbrella liability policy to cover malpractice, other types of liability claims, and property loss by fire or other casualty. A list of these policies, the insurers, and the premium costs is enclosed.

Financial Status
A financial statement is enclosed. At present, my only significant debts are an educational loan, which totals $28,366, and automobile loans with this bank, (in my name and my spouse's name), which total $17,322.
I have also enclosed our federal income tax return for the past year.

Capital Needed
I need a loan of $40,000 to establish my practice. Of this amount, $3,700 will be unsecured. The remainder will be used to purchase equipment for which a purchase money security interest may be obtained by the bank.

Financial Summary
A year-by-year summary of my projected income and expenses for the 6 years needed to repay the loan is enclosed. My spouse has been offered employment in Townsville. My spouse's income is included in the projections for each year.

Year	Projected income	Projected expenses
1[a]	$98,200	$137,200
2[b]	121,500	117,262
3	146,000	141,656
4	171,750	168,274
5	198,750	196,566
6	227,000	223,775

[a] For year 1, projected income and expenses are itemized in Schedule A, projected professional and personal expenses are itemized in Schedule C, and a spreadsheet of monthly projected income and expenses is outlined in Schedule D.
[b] For years 2–6, projected income and expenses are itemized in Schedule B.

Alternative Plan for Financial Supplementation
If practice revenues do not meet projections, it may become necessary to supplement practice income with outside employment. I have investigated the opportunities available to me in the Townsville area for part-time employment outside the practice. I anticipate that these opportunities will be available in the first year after I open my practice. There are three potential sources at this time:
• Employment with an ophthalmologist in northwest Townsville. I would provide low vision services.
• Instructor at Townsville State Community College. I would teach biology, which was my undergraduate major.
• Eye care provider at Bigtime Correctional Facility, which is located 30 miles from Townsville.

Summary
The projections of income and expenses used in this proposal are based on conservative national estimates. They represent reasonable goals for overhead and generated income. Based on these projections, the practice begins to generate a profit after 6 months and for the entire year incurs a loss of only $1,470. Profit in the second year should be sufficient to permit income use for practice improvements, anticipated increases in the cost of living, and for a greater doctor's draw. After the sixth year, the loan will be retired.

Schedule A: Projected Income and Expenses for Year 1
Expenses

Purchase of equipment and modification of office	$44,155
Operating expenses for office (see Schedule C)	58,050
Loan cost	-0-
Taxes (income, Social Security)	2,041
Doctor's draw	35,000
Total	$137,200

Assets and income

Cash on hand	-0-
Projected practice income	
(250 days at $150 gross per approximately	
1.54 patients per day)	$56,200
Spouse's income	42,000
Total	$98,200
Net	-40,000
Loan amount needed	$40,000

Figure 8.1. Sample loan proposal.

Schedule B: Projected Income and Expenses for Years 2 through 6

Year 2	
Expenses	
Operating expenses for office	$61,062
Bank loan repayment	11,400
Taxes	4,800
Doctor's draw	35,000
Practice improvement	5,000
Total	$117,262
Assets and income	
Projected practice income	
(250 days at $155 gross per approximately	
2.0 patients per day)	$77,500
Spouse's income	44,000
Total	$121,500
Net	$4,238

Year 3	
Expenses	
Operating expenses for office	$71,256
Bank loan repayment	11,400
Taxes	9,000
Doctor's draw	40,000
Practice improvement	10,000
Total	$141,656
Assets and income	
Projected practice income	
250 days at $160 gross per approximately	
2.5 patients per day)	$100,000
Spouse's income	46,000
Total	$146,000
Net	$4,344

Year 4	
Expenses	
Operating expenses for office	$80,874
Bank loan repayment	11,400
Taxes	16,000
Doctor's draw	45,000
Practice improvement	15,000
Total	$168,274
Assets and income	
Projected practice income	
(250 days at $165 gross per approximately	
3.0 patients per day)	$123,750
Spouse's income	48,000
Total	$171,750
Net	$3,476

Year 5	
Expenses	
Operating expenses for office	$91,166
Bank loan repayment	11,400
Taxes	24,000
Doctor's draw	50,000
Practice improvement	20,000
Total	$198,566
Assets and income	
Projected practice income	
(250 days st $170 gross per approximately	
3.5 patients per day)	$148,750
Spouse's income	50,000
Total	$198,750
Net	$2,184

Year 6	
Expenses	
Operating expenses for office	$101,375
Bank loan repayment	11,400
Taxes	31,000
Doctor's draw	60,000
Practice improvement	20,000
Total	$223,775
Assets and income	
Projected practice income	
(250 days at $175 gross per approximately	
4.0 patients per day)	$175,000
Spouse's income	52,000
Total	$227,000
Net	$3,225

Figure 8.1 (continued)

- Salaries for office staff
- Social Security payments and unemployment compensation taxes for office staff
- Utilities for the office (telephone, electricity, water, gas)
- Premium costs for insurance coverage—life, disability, personal property, and professional liability
- Laboratory bills
- Inventories of frames, lenses, and supplies
- Income for the practitioner
- Taxes on the practitioner's income

The more complete the list, the more accurate the determination of the total cost to operate the practice. These expenditures should be calculated for each month of the first year of practice and for each year thereafter, until the loan repayment has been satisfied. These expenditures, taken with the cost of purchases, constitute the "overhead" of the practice. It is important that, for a new practice, the overhead not be too high. The higher the overhead, the larger the number of patients that must be seen to break even or show a profit. If the overhead is so high that the loan proposal projects

Schedule C: Projections of Professional and Personal Expenses for Year 1

Operating Expenses for the Practice		Personal Living Expenses	
Office lease	$10,800	Apartment rent	$7,400
Laboratory costs	16,860	Automobile loans (2 cars)	6,064
Employee salary and benefits	15,000	Educational loans	3,600
Utilities	2,700	Automobile insurance (2 cars)	1,276
Telephone and facsimile costs	1,200	Health insurance (paid by spouse's employer)	-0-
Computer	1,690	Utilities (electricity, water, telephone)	2,160
Drugs, supplies, and postage	1,200	Subsistence	6,800
Repairs to office and equipment	500	Clothing allowance	1,200
Automobile expenses	600	Automobile operating expenses	700
Continuing education, professional dues, and licenses	2,000	Miscellaneous personal expenses	2,000
Umbrella liability insurance coverage	1,000		
Life insurance (decreasing term policy)	700		
Employee taxes	1,450		
Self-employment tax	-0-		
Legal and accounting fees	1,000		
Announcement for opening of office	550		
Total	$58,050	**Total**	$30,000

Schedule D: Projected Income and Expenses for First Year in Practice

Month	1	2	3	4	5	6	7	8	9	10	11	12	
Patients per day	1.0	1.1	1.2	1.3	1.4	1.5	1.6	1.7	1.8	1.9	2.0	2.1	
Income													
Income per patient	$150	$150	$150	$150	$150	$150	$150	$150	$150	$150	$150	$150	
TOTAL	$3000	$3300	$3600	$3900	$4200	$4500	$4800	$5100	$5400	$5700	$6100	$6500	$56200
Expenses													
Laboratory costs	$900	$990	$1080	$1170	$1260	$1350	$1440	$1530	$1620	$1710	$1860	$1950	$16860
Office lease	$900	$900	$900	$900	$900	$900	$900	$900	$900	$900	$900	$900	$10800
Employee salary and taxes	$1370	$1370	$1370	$1370	$1370	$1370	$1370	$1370	$1370	$1370	$1370	$1370	$16450
Utilities	$325	$325	$325	$325	$325	$325	$325	$325	$325	$325	$325	$325	$3900
Insurance	$141	$141	$141	$141	$141	$141	$141	$141	$141	$141	$141	$141	$1700
Other	$695	$695	$695	$695	$695	$695	$695	$695	$695	$695	$695	$695	$8340
TOTAL	$4331	$4421	$4511	$4601	$4691	$4781	$4871	$4961	$5051	$5141	$5231	$5321	$58050
Net Income													
Net loss or profit	-$1331	-$1121	-$911	-$701	-$491	-$281	$71	$139	$349	$559	$869	$1179	
Cumulative loss or profit	-$1331	-$2252	-$3163	-$3864	-$4355	-$4636	-$4565	-$4426	-$4077	-$3518	-$2649	-$1470	

Figure 8.1 (continued)

that the practice will operate at a deficit for years before patient flow can generate a profit, it is likely that the loan proposal will be rejected. Therefore, overhead should always be kept at a reasonable level, and extravagant expenditures should be discarded. Expensive items, such as an automated perimeter or an edging laboratory, may not be feasible for a plan to start a practice "cold." The bottom line should be carefully scrutinized. Creditors do not like to fund operations when it appears that it will take a long time to generate a profit.

Step 3: Drafting Projections

Once all information on expenditures has been compiled, it is organized in a spreadsheet format. The first-year projections are arranged month by month; for the subsequent years a total figure is used. Projecting overhead costs for these subsequent years is an art; cost of living increases should be added to each year to approximate the rise in costs that can be anticipated.

Step 4: Projecting Income

Perhaps the most difficult aspect of creating a loan proposal is to project expected income, especially for a new practice. If there are other practitioners who have recently opened a practice, it may be possible to obtain information about their experience. If there is no source of recent information, it may be useful to provide projections so that they specify the number of patients needed to pay the overhead or to generate a certain profit level. For the first-year projections, the number of patients seen daily should be determined with a specific gross income attributed to each. Local practitioners can be consulted to determine the amount of income that can be expected per type of patient. Eye health examinations generate different amounts of income than contact lens assessments or binocular vision evaluations. The number of expected patients for each service, and the projected income for each, must be calculated. If a practice has been purchased, it is much easier to make income projections. It should be remembered, however, that some loss of patient base—approximately

10–20%—can be expected during the first year. The number of new patients needed to eliminate this potential deficit should be determined and used as a goal.

Step 5: Calculating the "Bottom Line"

The income and overhead for each month of the first year are used to determine if there will be a profit or loss. For a new practice, it is not unusual for the first several months to produce a deficit rather than a profit. However, the anticipated income should be such that, within the year, a monthly profit can be reasonably expected. The "bottom line" calculations are the goals against which the practice's actual performance is to be measured. If the calculations are inaccurate, they can be adjusted to reflect the actual financial circumstances of the practice and a new set of goals can be created.

Once the loan proposal has been calculated, it must be reduced to writing and supporting documents must be added. The proposal should begin with a statement of purpose, which summarizes the financial goals of the borrower. Documents that may be attached to the loan proposal include:

- A personal financial statement
- The income tax return for the past year
- A copy of the office lease (if available)
- An insurance list describing policies and premium costs

Presentation of the Proposal

The presentation of the proposal to the creditor should be planned, and answers to anticipated questions should be rehearsed. Professional attire should be worn for the occasion. If accepted, the usual means of financing is a line of credit, against which the borrower may draw as the need for money arises. Since creditors do not like to extend lines of credit beyond those originally agreed on, the amount of credit secured should be adequate for the practice's financial obligations. Of course, interest is charged on the amount actually withdrawn for use.

CONCLUSION

The loan proposal is the financial heart of the practice plan. To make the plan viable, the loan proposal must contain accurate information, attainable goals, and reasonable projections, and must be capable of modification to meet the changing circumstances that are an inevitable part of practice.

BIBLIOGRAPHY

Gregg J. The Business of Optometric Practice. White Plains, NY: Advisory Enterprises, 1984.
Runninger J. Your new wellspring of ready credit. Optom Manage 1981;17(2):27–31.

Chapter 9

Understanding Office Leases

Lawrence S. Thal and Harry Kaplan

Why so large cost, having so short a lease,
Dost thou upon thy fading mansion spend?

—William Shakespeare
Sonnets

The signing of a lease can represent the largest financial transaction ever made by a prospective tenant. The lease agreement is legally binding and can be enforced on the parties involved. While a lease should be reviewed by competent advisors or legal counsel, it is unusual for counsel to actively negotiate its terms; that burden inevitably falls on the prospective tenant. For this reason, a prospective tenant should be aware of the common terms and the usual pitfalls associated with leases. This chapter reviews many of the problems that are encountered when attempting to negotiate a lease for a professional office.

The person who occupies property owned by another is called a lessee. Negotiation of the lease agreement with the owner—the lessor—might be limited to the presentation of a contract by the owner, accompanied by the following language: "Enclosed please find your standard lease form. You should sign where indicated, initial each page, and return at your earliest convenience."

This language can be the first introduction the tenant has to the lease, and while the term *standard* might seem to imply some degree of conformity or regularity, the only standard aspects of an individual lease are the matters that it addresses. There is not one customary way to address these matters, and they should be fully negotiated and understood by the tenant.

A lease is a contract binding its signatories to its terms, and the tenant should assume, at the inception of the relationship, that all terms are fully enforceable. There are many pitfalls for the novice tenant, and even what is perceived to be the fairest of leases might contain provisions that can lead to disastrous financial consequences. Therefore, it is important to obtain competent advice before executing a contract such as a lease.

A shrewd attorney for the tenant could write a lease allowing the tenant to delay or offset rent payments for a myriad of reasons—even reasons beyond the landlord's control. A landlord's attorney could be equally shrewd in writing a lease with complicated clauses that provide for rapid and unfair rent increases. The object of any negotiation, however, should be to reach a contract that is fair, equitable, and easily understood.

Often it is perceived that certain landlords—such as shopping center owners—are inflexible and powerful and that, as a result, all tenants sign the same lease. Prospective tenants should not overlook the fact that they are the ones with the power to sign or not sign a lease. Printed lease forms are sometimes meant to epitomize inflexibility or to emphasize the power of the landlord. Tenants should not be fooled by how impressively worded the lease is, or by how large the law firm is that supposedly drafted the lease. Concessions can still be awarded by the landlord.

NEGOTIATING FOR CONCESSIONS

It is usually 2–3 months after the lease agreement has been signed before the first patient walks through the door. During this period, without the benefit of patient income, the optometrist will be paying for alterations, instruments, office furniture, and similar items. To offset these expenditures, the practitioner should not be afraid to ask the landlord for help in the form of concessions. Possible concessions in the lease agreement include:

- Out-and-out reduction in the rent for the full term of the lease (if the rent is out of line for the space and location)
- A few months of free rent to help the optometrist reduce overhead expenditures while alterations are being performed on the premises or equipment is being delivered and installed
- Payment by the landlord for all or part of the alterations to the office
- A step-up lease (the rent is paid at a reduced rate for the first 6–12 months and increases to the full rate over time)

In some cases, the landlord might refuse to make any concessions. If the office space is highly desirable and the market for office space is very limited, the prospective tenant might have to be comforted by the knowledge that previous tenants have worked successfully under such leases. In such a case, it is appropriate to check with the other tenants. If the landlord has dealt reasonably and fairly with them, there is a reasonable likelihood that the prospective tenant will not encounter any extraordinary difficulties. The landlord has a reputation to protect, and if tenants have been treated unfairly in the past, it will suffer. In addition, a high turnover rate will drive up the landlord's costs of doing business.

SELECTING COMPETENT COUNSEL

The tenant should solicit recommendations for real estate attorneys from other health care professionals in the area. Successful professionals are likely to have identified and hired the best attorneys and accountants because physicians, dentists, and other health care providers demand good advice and are willing to pay for it. The prospective tenant should not hesitate to schedule an interview with an attorney to obtain information about the attorney's background, philosophy of practice, fees, and experience with real estate. There is normally no charge for this initial interview. The attorney will value the opportunity to discuss matters of mutual interest with a prospective long-term client.

LOCATION

The same type of investigation of local demographic information should be conducted to determine the best locations in which to seek an office. Real estate agents, the staff of the local planning commission, or the office of the Chamber of Commerce can provide demographic data. Practice sites should be prominent and readily visible to the public. In addition, the office location should be easily accessible—near public transportation and with adequate parking available.

If an office is highly visible (e.g., next to a bank, across from the post office), the practice will become known immediately. Being in the local "professional building" or in an area with other professional offices is excellent. It is worth some extra cost to obtain a good, visible location; the additional expenditure will be returned many times over. It is also important to obtain adequate space. The consistent rise in net income due to such a practice site will usually compensate for the higher cost of the lease.

SPECIFIC CONTRACT CLAUSES

Several specific clauses of the lease agreement are of particular importance. These clauses include identification of the parties, property description, term, rent, tenant mix, assignment, disaster escape, maintenance, warning before eviction, leasehold improvements, costs of alterations, broker's fee, exculpation, warranty to practice, and security deposits.

Parties

The parties to the contract must be identified; these are the parties who will be expected to comply with the lease's terms and conditions.

Property Description

The lease should clearly define the property to be rented. If the property is free-standing it is relatively easy to describe the premises for which maintenance will be performed, taxes assessed, and insurance provided. This description is not as clear when the premises are part of an office complex or shopping center that includes parking facilities, elevators, and other common areas. In these cases, tenants will normally pay a percentage of the taxes, insurance, or maintenance that is assessed on the whole building. The percentage to be paid should be negotiated based on the square footage occupied, rent amount, anticipated use of parking and other common areas, and type of business conducted.

Term

For a credit-worthy tenant, successful in a business endeavor, a long lease term can be beneficial to both the tenant and the landlord. Conversely, a long-term lease can be disastrous for the optometrist who is less successful. While adequate investigation, planning, and market research should minimize that risk, it is always possible for unexpected events to adversely affect anticipated revenues.

Many landlords will not be anxious to lease to an optometrist who wants only a 3-year term. A 5-year term can be more acceptable, even for a new practice. For an already established practice with anticipated revenue based on historical performance, a 10-year lease can be more reasonable. In any case, the optometrist should negotiate for renewal options to be included in the lease. These options are exercised at the discretion of the tenant, and they extend the lease period for a stated number of years. The rent to be paid during the new term should be calculated on a pre-agreed basis.

Whatever the term of the lease, the tenant should request a provision that allows the tenant to stay month-to-month at the prevailing rental charge when the lease expires. Another useful provision is one that provides for possible practice growth by requesting first refusal on adjoining or other space in the building if it becomes available.

Rent

Leases are often characterized as being either "net leases" or "gross leases." A net lease implies that the tenant will pay the landlord rent that includes the "net" cost of all taxes, insurance, or maintenance expenses (i.e., the tenant pays these in addition to rent). A gross lease implies that the landlord pays the expenses for taxes, insurance, and maintenance out of the rent proceeds. A fully negotiated lease should be a compromise between these extremes.

While some practitioners live in communities that have experimented with various artificial methods of controlling residential rents, those that advocate such foolishness live in a fantasy world—one where new buildings will be constructed and improved with no regard to profit and where conventional lenders will provide construction loans solely because of their sense of social responsibility. Conversely—and realistically—a fair rent should be determined from the marketplace, which is to say by demand and availability. It is a mistake, however, for the optometrist to use market factors as the only determinant of rent. A pro forma analysis (see Chapter 28) will indicate the maximum rent that will not unreasonably drain the resources of a practice. A landlord should have the motivation, as well, to ensure that rents are fair and affordable to tenants. A contract to the contrary is an invitation to early vacancy, cessation of rents, and possible litigation.

Most net leases establish a base or fixed rent (often called minimum rent); additional amounts are added to reimburse the building owner for operating costs, which can include taxes, insurance, or common area maintenance (e.g., landscaping, janitorial services, elevator maintenance, parking lot resurfacing, common area lighting). In shopping centers a percentage rent can be used; this provides a bonus to the owners of the shopping center based on the tenant's success.

The tenant should attempt to negotiate "caps"—maximums on the reimbursement of operating costs—or, at a minimum, the tenant should expect a guarantee that the total expenses reimbursed to the landlord by all tenants will not exceed 100% of the actual costs incurred. Optometrists who do not wish landlords to perform advertising on their behalf should exclude assessments for advertising. Where advertising is to be performed by the landlord, copies of the advertisements should be submitted to the optometrist for approval and to ensure that they conform to applicable state laws.

While percentage rents provide some protection to landlords from inflation, a rent based on the number of examinations performed or eyeglasses dispensed might be disagreeable to the optometrist. The negotiation of rents is a business matter, but many optometrists have difficulty reaching business decisions without some regard to practice morals or professional ethics. The decision to pay percentage rents is an individual one, and, if it is agreed to, the amount to be paid should be negotiated based on the rents paid by other tenants. A percentage rent requires that monthly accounts of income or profit and loss statements be provided to the landlord. It can be preferable to pay a higher base or fixed rent instead of such an arrangement.

When and if percentage rents are paid, a fair percentage must be considered in relation to the total amount that the optometrist can budget for rent. A pro forma analysis should identify the maximum available rent the optometrist can pay. Even a 2% percentage rent could increase payment over a fixed rent amount by many thousands of dollars. For example, the tenant would have to pay $4,000 if the percentage rent applied to all of a $200,000 gross income, but would only pay $2,000 if it was limited to gross income in excess of $100,000.

There are other factors that should also be considered, including rental per square foot per year, automatic rent increases, and steps-up in rent.

Rental per Square Foot per Year

The tenant should determine if the "per square foot" cost is in line with what is being charged for comparable offices in the vicinity. The tenant should attempt to have the cost-per-square-foot figure applied only to the office's actual floor space and should try to avoid payment of a prorated share of the building's common footage, such as halls and lobbies. Economic surveys of established practices that have been performed by the American Opto-

metric Association have indicated that rent cost usually equals 5–7% of gross earnings. This percentage is similar to that found in other professions.

Automatic Increases

Many leases permit a landlord to raise the rent to allow for rises in property taxes, maintenance costs, or the cost-of-living index. If such a clause must be accepted, the tenant should attempt to limit the annual increment to a maximum fixed percentage. Late charges should be clearly stated. If a landlord expects to recover a penalty for any rent payments made late, the amount of the penalty and the date by which the penalty would be incurred need to be carefully described.

Step-Up Rents

When negotiating rents, it can be advantageous to start off a lease term with a low rent that increases over time—hopefully, as income also increases. Most accountants should be able to determine an equitable rent structure. For example, if a landlord is asking for $1,000 a month for a 4-year term, the tenant can offer $700 a month for the first year, $900 a month for the second year, and $1,230 a month for the last 2 years. (Assuming a 6% interest rate, this proposal nets the landlord exactly the same amount as $1,000 a month over the 4 years.)

The attractiveness of many community shopping centers as lease premises lies in the presence of a nationally known anchor tenant: a large department store or supermarket that attracts consumers. Should one of these tenants vacate the shopping center, the optometrist could experience a dramatic loss in revenue, making monthly rent payments a hardship. Thus, it would certainly be fair to negotiate a clause that allows for reduced rental payments during the period such major tenant vacancies persist.

It is also reasonable to restrict landlords so they may not offer leases or subleases to competitors (other optometrists or opticians) within the part of the facility that is under the landlord's control.

What should a tenant do if the landlord wants to raise the rent by a tremendous amount at the termination of the current lease? It is difficult to protect against this event except through automatic renewal options that can be asserted by the tenant at stipulated periods. In the absence of such an option, it is probably best to open negotiations for a new lease early (e.g., 4–6 months before the lease expires) to prevent this from happening. Another strategy is to ask other tenants about the past history of the landlord before signing the original lease. Has the landlord been reasonable? Have the rent increases been reasonable?

Tenant Mix

Landlords can claim that they entered into a lease with individuals who met specific criteria or with careful consideration of tenant mix. While some restrictions are appropriate to protect the landlord against the assignment of leases to undesirable tenants, absolute restrictions are unfair. Absolute restrictions on assignment might even prohibit an optometrist from selling the practice to another tenant.

Assignment

Although many leases prohibit a tenant from assigning or subletting a lease, a prospective tenant needs to weigh these provisions carefully. Without such a right, an optometrist or the optometrist's heirs might be responsible for lease payments even in the case of death, disability, or lack of economic success. In planning for such an event, the optometrist will want to ensure that the lease could be assigned to another party, or perhaps be terminated altogether. In the case of death or disability, it should be possible to terminate the lease when the appropriate notice is given. (e.g., 90 days).

The landlord can insist that approval be obtained if the tenant wishes to move before the conclusion of the lease term and to turn the premises over to another tenant. If the landlord insists on reserving the right to veto any proposed subtenant, the following compromise should be suggested: "The tenant shall not sublet without the landlord's consent, which consent shall not be withheld unreasonably." Another proposal is for the optometrist to ask for an automatic end to the lease within 90 days (or within another reasonable period) after a disabling accident

or illness has been suffered, the optometrist has been called for military duty, or the optometrist has died. A clause should also be sought that guarantees that a practitioner who buys the practice has the right to continue under the terms of the lease.

It should also be clear what the tenant's rights are when title to the property being leased reverts to the owner of a mortgage. The lease should clearly state that the rights of a tenant are not subordinated to the interests of a mortgage lender (called a mortgagee). This clause would prevent a lender from evicting tenants in the case of a mortgage foreclosure, a situation in which a transfer of ownership is effected from the original landlord to a mortgage lender.

Both parties to a lease should have the right to terminate or cancel the lease should the other significantly default on lease provisions. A reasonable period of time in which to remedy such a default should be provided.

Some leases obligate a tenant to keep paying rent for the full term even if the building is severely damaged by fire or other casualty or if an essential facility like air conditioning breaks down and the landlord fails to repair it. The lease should allow the tenant to terminate the agreement under such circumstances without penalty or, at most, by paying a fixed maximum rent charge (e.g., 3 months' rent).

Maintenance

Typically, the landlord would like to repair nothing, while the tenant would like the landlord to repair everything. Absent other concessions, a fair agreement is somewhere in between these two extremes. A possible fair agreement would have the building owner liable for all repairs to the building exterior, including roof and exterior glass, as well as mechanical systems such as central heating and air conditioning, while the tenant would be responsible for repairs to plumbing, the electrical system, interior painting, carpeting, and so forth. Maintenance provisions are subject to negotiation, and results can vary considerably, depending on the amount of rent paid and the length of the lease term.

Insurance on the building is normally carried by the owner; it is required by the building's mortgagee. The owner, likewise, should have the burden of rebuilding in the case of destruction by fire or other casualty. The tenant should be properly insured for the replacement of interior leasehold improvements, furniture, equipment, and supplies.

Maintenance of the exterior affects building appearance; thus, standards for exterior signage should be established. A professional tenant like an optometrist should be protected from the garish signs of a retail store or amusement area next door. In fact, the optometrist can request protection from such a tenant being allowed in the same building. Examples of such restrictions include prohibitions on pawn shops, massage parlors, sex paraphernalia shops, or exotic dancing.

Responsibility for exterior painting and for maintenance of sidewalks or parking areas should be covered in the lease. A tenant might be compensated for maintenance violations by a landlord through fair rent reductions, providing that the tenant has appropriately notified the owner of the violation and that adequate time has been given for the defaults to be cured.

Warning Before Eviction

A tenant should ensure that eviction will not result the first time a house rule (e.g., "objectionable conduct") is broken. The tenant should ask to be given written notice when in violation of a rule and to be allowed an opportunity to correct the error. A flat "no" should be given to any clause that says breaking a rule renders the tenant not only liable to be evicted but also responsible for the payment of the rent for the balance of the lease. If these clauses cannot be stricken from the lease in their entirety, then "objectionable conduct" (or other terms) must be clearly defined.

Leasehold Improvements

Seldom will office space vacated by one tenant be acceptable to another without renovation. The payment of office renovation costs needs to be negotiated, not only in terms of how the costs are to be borne, the extent of the renovations, and the period of time involved for them to be performed, but also in terms of the effect of the costs on the rent to be paid by the tenant during the lease term. Options for payment should be considered.

Where an owner is highly dependent on full occupancy or where office space has had a long vacancy, a prospective tenant might be able to negotiate for the landlord to pay the renovation costs or—if the tenant pays the costs—for the landlord to provide a period of free rent or of reduced rent. When office space is in high demand and rents are fair, it might be unreasonable to expect concessions of this type.

It can be strategically advantageous for a tenant to offer a higher rent than requested if, in return, the owner agrees to absorb the cost of renovations. When owners agree to perform renovations for a tenant there should also be provisions in the lease for monetary damages resulting from construction delays.

The landlord might agree to follow a tenant's specifications at the landlord's expense if the office needs painting, partitioning, or structural changes to suit the tenant's practice. If not, the tenant can suggest that an improvement allowance be rewarded as a rent rebate.

Alterations and repairs usually should not be initiated until the term of the lease begins. If the office is vacant, written permission should be obtained to start the modifications immediately. Customarily, the tenant is obligated to pay for services (e.g., electricity, water, gas) once alterations have begun. The tenant should try not to accept any clause requiring the premises to be restored to their original condition. The cost of recreating a bare rectangle can be high. Also, improvements are assets to the landlord and should not have to be removed.

Broker's Fee

A broker's fee is usually due in leasing transactions and is generally payable by the landlord. In a sublease situation, the existing tenant will pay the fee. The lease should identify any brokers involved and should clearly establish who is responsible for the broker's fee.

Exculpation

An exculpation clause limits the liability of a landlord to the interest in the property itself. The clause frees the landlord from legal responsibility for certain acts—committed by the tenant—that cause injury to persons on the property. It is not unusual for an owner to attempt to limit personal liability in this way.

Warranty to Practice

The tenant should be sure to include a clause stating that if local zoning laws forbid the practice of optometry on the premises or the operation of a business, the lease is null and void.

Security Deposit

The prepayment of 1–2 months' rent will earn the landlord money as long as the deposit is held. Unless local law so requires, the landlord will not offer to pay interest on the deposit. The tenant can ask for payment of the interest on the deposit held by the landlord.

Other Terms

In shopping plazas, the leases often state that all tenants must maintain the same hours (e.g., 9:00 AM–9:00 PM 6 days per week). A professional tenant can usually have this provision changed, and the change should be written into the lease.

The parking privileges available to staff and patients should be specified. The lease agreement should be examined to determine if there are any additional costs for parking. The rules and regulations of the landlord should be checked for availability of parking during the hours the practice is to be open. Ideally, there should be seven to eight parking spaces for each professional in a building. If the practitioner and the staff do not use the spaces, a minimum of four to five spaces might be adequate.

The tenant should be sure that there are specific rights to erect customary signs—both inside and outside the building—and that these rights are in the lease.

CONCLUSION

When considering the rental of office space, other tenants should always be consulted to determine the integrity of a landlord. The law of supply and demand governs a tenant's bargaining position. That bargaining strength depends on how badly the tenant wants the space and how much the tenant is willing to pay for it. If there are two or three other prospective locations and time is not of the essence, a tenant is in a better position to bargain.

In the low-to-moderate rental field, the demand for space usually exceeds the supply. In more expensive areas, the reverse is true. Being a professional is in a tenant's favor when bargaining. Landlords would prefer to have a professional as a tenant, and a young professional should not be afraid to ask the landlord for changes and concessions.

Lease provisions can be looked at this way: A tenant is unlikely to get every clause requested in every instance. However, a prospective tenant can be sure that provisions favoring the tenant won't appear in the landlord's standard contract and that the landlord will not bring up such provisions unless asked to do so. How much compromise a landlord allows will depend on how desirable the space seems and how likely it is that a prospective tenant can find other suitable space in the locality.

From the landlord's viewpoint, professionals are good tenants. They usually pay their rent on time and do not often cause problems; they add prestige to the building and typically sign long-term contracts. These facts should not be forgotten by a young optometrist seeking to negotiate even that very first lease arrangement.

BIBLIOGRAPHY

Classé JG. Legal Aspects of Optometry. Stoneham, MA: Butterworth, 1989.

Cotton H. Medical Practice Management. Oradell, NJ: Medical Economics, 1977.

Dean M, Nicholas F, Caplan R. Commercial Real Property Lease Practice. Berkeley, CA: California Continuing Education of the Bar, 1976.

Dean M, Turner W. Commercial Real Property Lease Practice (update). Berkeley, CA: Continuing Education of the Bar, 1992.

Elmstron G. Advanced Management for Optometrists. Chicago: Professional Press, 1974.

Sachs L. The Professional Practice Problem Solver. Englewood Cliffs, NJ: Prentice-Hall, 1991.

Chapter 10

Office Design

Neil B. Gailmard and John Rumpakis

*Let us see these handsome houses where the wealthy
nobles dwell.*

—Alfred, Lord Tennyson
Locksley Hall

The general public forms an impression of a professional office by the physical appearance of the exterior, and, as patients visit the office, their perception of the whole practice can be strongly influenced by the interior decor. These impressions can exert a significant effect on future visits and on referrals of new patients. For this reason, it is important for the practitioner to become knowledgeable in the areas of office design, decoration, and some aspects of remodeling and construction.

The goal of this chapter is to stimulate ideas about office design, based on how optometric practices function. The chapter provides a description of the "ideal" office design; it is not expected that new practitioners will be able to incorporate all the ideas presented into a beginning practice. Rather, the descriptions are intended to serve as a model, toward which a beginning practitioner could aspire.

Obviously, an optometrist will need the services of qualified professionals in the building trade, and finding the right people can be the biggest challenge. Architects, designers, contractors, and decorators should be chosen in the same manner as any advisor—by reputation in the community and by a trusted referral if possible. An interview to discuss the scope of the project and the cost and time involved should assist in the effort to make an intelligent selection. It is always wise to check with previous clients of building professionals. Specific questions to ask include: "Was the cost estimate on

target?" "Was the work completed on time?" "Was the client satisfied with the work?"

The location of a practice adds to the image it projects to the public. For the same reason, the design and appearance of the office should follow a theme. If the professional philosophy is one of excellence in medical care, a professional and clinical look would be desired. If the emphasis is on optical dispensing, then a retail or boutique theme would be appropriate. In some cases, both elements can be achieved with separate entrances.

The exterior of the office depends on the type of building in which the practice will be located (Figure 10.1). In the case of a freestanding building, much can be done to positively influence the exterior, including the use of extensive landscaping, signage, and lighting. When the practice is located in a professional building or medical center, these options might not be under the optometrist's direct control. However, design options might be influenced at the time a lease is negotiated. Other possible office locations include downtown storefront locations, strip shopping centers, and large enclosed malls.

It is important to develop an efficient floor plan so that practitioners, staff, and patients can all work effectively and logically. The best time to consider the floor plan is when selecting a new office location. Sometimes a practitioner might be the first tenant in an open space and can have the luxury of constructing interior walls to suit the needs of the practice. In other cases,

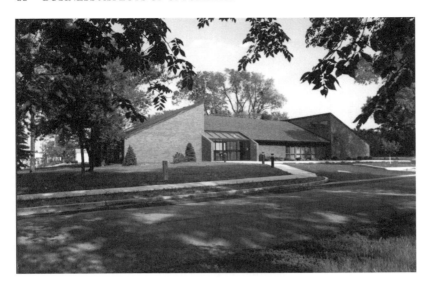

Figure 10.1. Building exterior, Gailmard Eye Center. (Courtesy of Gailmard Eye Center, Munster, Indiana.)

interior walls could already be in place and might have to be used "as is" for economical reasons. An established practitioner might wish to remove walls and add new walls to improve the floor plan and office flow.

It is extremely valuable to visit as many practices as possible before designing a new office or making major revisions. Photographs should be taken, if allowed, along with plenty of notes and a sketch of the floor plan. Actual measurements of existing rooms can give a better understanding of space requirements than any floor plan. Many eye care management journals feature photographs of and stories about office designs, and these can stimulate ideas.

DESIGN OF THE OPTOMETRIC OFFICE

A designer or contractor should be consulted when functional considerations for individual rooms within the office are being decided. Since this is a specialized field and the special needs of optometric offices are not generally known, this chapter covers key ideas to consider on a room-by-room basis. Obviously, not every office will have all the rooms listed, but this list should stimulate ideas for present needs and for future planning.

VESTIBULE OR LOBBY

A pleasant first impression is created when the front entrance to a building opens into a lobby or even a small vestibule. This area generally serves as a weather buffer to prevent shocks of cold or heat or rain from entering the reception area of the office (Figure 10.2). Lobby space can also serve as a convenient area for a patient who is waiting for transportation. Tile makes an excellent floor covering for this space, and replaceable rug mats provide a surface to absorb dirt and moisture.

RECEPTION AREA

The reception area is also known as the waiting room, but calling it a reception area provides a more welcoming tone (Figure 10.3A). The reception area should immediately welcome visitors in comfort. Unlike the examination area, this is a space that patients will identify with, since it consists of items with which the public is familiar, such as sofas, chairs, carpeting, and wall coverings. This reception room should be kept very clean and should be remodeled at least every 5 years.

The size of the reception area will be dictated by the size of the practice and the number of patients who will be asked to wait. Because pupillary dilation is now a standard procedure, a larger reception area might be needed. A secondary, inner waiting room can also serve as a "holding" area, reducing the number of people who must be seated in the reception room and therefore decreasing the size of the area needed. The reception area must also accommodate the family members or friends who

Figure 10.2. Entrance lobby to professional office. (Courtesy of Gailmard Eye Center, Munster, Indiana.)

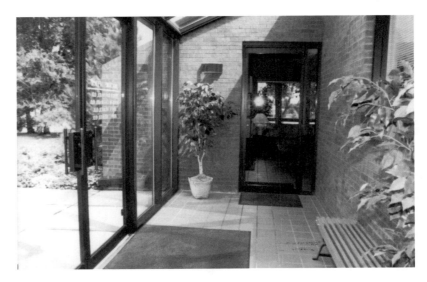

might accompany the patient. The seating in the reception area should be visible to the receptionist from the business office desk or counter. In small offices, the receptionist can have a desk, rather than a built-in counter, within the reception area. In large clinics, the reception area can be a common area for the patients of many practitioners.

Anything that can make the reception room unique and special is desirable, if it is done in good taste. Considerations such as an aquarium, well cared for plants, unusual windows with attractive exterior views, or a fireplace can set the practice apart from others and can become a form of internal marketing. Other unique ideas that can be incorporated into a reception room include bookcases with large print and regular print reading materials, a TV and VCR with cable news and weather or videotapes on eye care topics or children's cartoons, a display of antique eyewear, or a refreshment bar that might offer coffee, tea, or soft drinks. It is desirable to have a restroom available for patients immediately adjacent to the reception area so that the office staff does not have to be interrupted by patients seeking toilet facilities.

The choice of seating is a very important consideration and must provide durability while offering comfort and safety for handicapped and elderly patients. Single seating is preferable to couches, since strangers do not like to sit together. Lighting should be adequate for comfortable reading and should remind patients of the important relation-

ship between good lighting and sharp acuity. A coat rack or closet is a nice addition and should be located within view of the receptionist. A bulletin board for announcements to patients is a useful accessory. A special corner or other built-in environment can be reserved for children, with a table and chairs as well as toys and children's reading materials (Figure 10.3B). This area demonstrates that the practice cares for children's eyes. The reception room should provide a clear path from the front entrance doors to the receptionist's desk. Tile or vinyl floor coverings make a practical walkway to the front desk, while the rest of the reception area can be carpeted.

BUSINESS OFFICE

The business area will serve to provide an office for the receptionist and business office staff (Figure 10.4). This area should be easily accessible to patients and should give the image of being open and available. An adjacent door to the reception room can provide for security and privacy. It works well if patients can be seen at an inner office counter to make payments and appointment arrangements, rather than having to return to the reception room where others will overhear. This inner area could be simply a widened hallway. Care should be given to the location of telephones so the receptionist can view the reception room

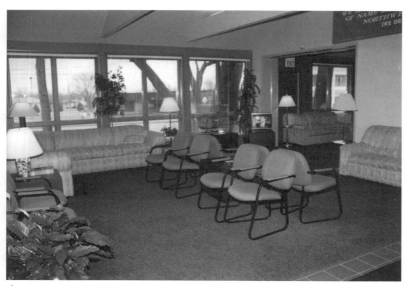

Figure 10.3. A. Reception area. (Courtesy of Gailmard Eye Center, Munster, Indiana.) B. Children's playhouse, located adjacent to reception area. (Courtesy of Drs. Bob Baldwin, Bobby Christensen, and Russell Laverty, Midwest City, Oklahoma)

A

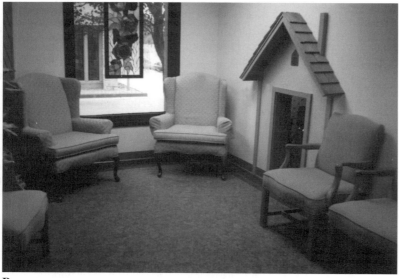

B

and still have some privacy for phone calls (including outgoing calls) that can be of a more sensitive nature.

The business office usually contains file cabinets or shelving units to maintain current patient files. It might be necessary to install an additional remote filing area when the number of files exceeds the front office capacity. A system to purge older files must be devised for patients who have

not returned in a certain number of years. Countertops and cabinets should be provided to allow for storage of office supplies.

The typical office equipment located in the business area can include the telephone, the typewriter, the computer system and printer, a fax machine, credit card impression devices, and a photocopier. Wall-mounted shelving units can provide an excellent visual display of contact lens solutions and

Figure 10.4. Business area, showing moveable filing cabinets. (Courtesy of Alderwood Vision Clinic, Lynnwood, Washington.)

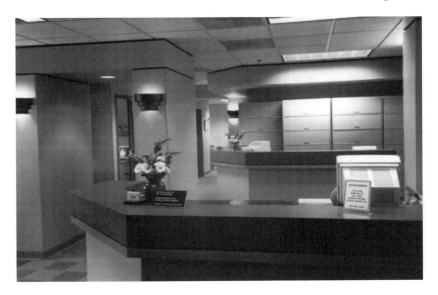

other eye care supplies. Having this visually available at the time of final billing will result in convenience purchases. The telephone system can generally incorporate an intercom to the other rooms in the office and can even be used as a light signaling system. An additional light signal panel can be mounted in the business area to show which examination rooms are occupied by individual staff members. In smaller offices, it is convenient if the business office permits a view of the examination rooms. This method can be more efficient than light signaling systems, because the receptionist can simply look to see if doors are open or closed to determine when the next patient can be brought into the inner office.

This area, along with most of the office, will typically be carpeted and will have a suspended ceiling; both factors help absorb sound and provide a nicer working environment. A short-weave, commercial-grade carpet is best, to allow for ease of cleaning and to permit office chairs and stools to roll easily. A color and texture should be chosen that will not show traffic patterns and soil. Fluorescent lighting, within the suspended ceiling, is most often used in offices because it is cool and inexpensive. Various grid covers or lenses are available for fluorescent fixtures. The use of incandescent can spotlighting provides additional light where needed for emphasis and adds some style to the office.

ADMINISTRATIVE AREA

It might be desirable in larger office spaces to have an additional business area that is not accessible or visible to patients. This area allows behind-the-scenes work by office staff—including the numerous billing and mailing activities that are part of a successful practice. Such activities can include billing statements, recall notices, service agreement reminders, and other direct mail pieces. Additionally, this room can be used for receiving deliveries and mail and can provide a private area for the telephone activities of the staff, including calls to patients about past due accounts and the use of telephone marketing techniques. This room can have a conference table as well as an additional computer, telephone, postage meter, and photocopier.

DATA COLLECTION ROOM

The data collection room is used for preliminary testing, usually by an optometric technician (Figure 10.5). In some practices, it can be used as a special procedures room for procedures such as visual fields and retinal photography. A smaller examination room with a minimum size of 10 × 12 feet could serve this purpose. It can be desirable to have more than one data collection room, since the use of many instruments in one room

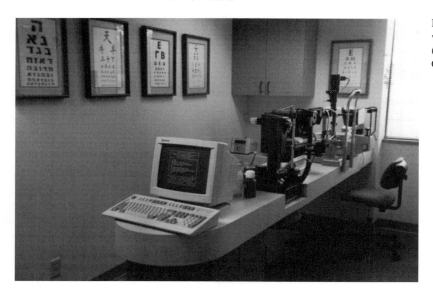

Figure 10.5. Pretesting area with computerized data entry. (Courtesy of Alderwood Vision Clinic, Lynnwood, Washington.)

Table 10.1. Procedures for Data Collection Rooms

1. Case history
2. Visual acuity (far and near)
3. Noncontact tonometry
4. Autorefraction
5. Keratometry
6. Lensometry
7. Telebinocular visual skills
8. Visual field testing
9. Retinal photography
10. Color vision
11. Stereopsis
12. Blood pressure measurement
13. Corneal topography

will require testing for significant periods of time. It is not likely that a practice will duplicate some of the computerized automated instruments that can be found in data collection rooms, so it might be preferable to conduct some of the tests in the first room and then move the patient to the second room. This opens the first room for the next patient. A sink is useful here so that technicians can wash their hands and contact lenses can be removed and reinserted. There are various instrument delivery tables, ranging from automated rotating tables to individually adjusted tables for each instrument.

Thought should be given to the techniques that will be performed in this room so that room size and other aspects of design can be planned. For example, light switches should be easily turned on or off by a technician seated at the instrument. If this room is to be used for visual acuity, the placement of mirrors or other devices to measure acuity should be considered. Table 10.1 lists several procedures that could be performed in a data collection room.

EXAMINATION ROOM

Multiple examination rooms should be considered for all but the smallest practices. Various methods for making the examination room more efficient include the refractive duo concept, in which the patient end of the room is wider and the far end of the room is narrower. Often, two rooms can be designed so that they are adjacent to one another. Mirrored examination rooms have become very popular, however, and provide a nicer look than long, narrow lanes.

A room as small as 8 × 12 feet can be made acceptable for refractive distances of 20 feet with the use of refractive mirrors. These mirrors can be set up in a very effective manner and should not be regarded as too difficult or too confusing. If space permits, an ideal examination room might be 10

Figure 10.6. Examination room. (Courtesy of Drs. Terry Hawks and Gregory Besler, Overland Park, Kansas.)

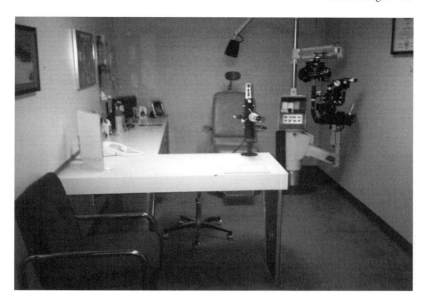

feet wide and 20 feet long. These dimensions provide the refractive characteristics needed along with a large, open feeling, and plenty of room is available for chairside technicians and visitors who might accompany the patient. It should be noted, however, that the examination chair will be at least 2 feet from the back wall of the room and that the refractive distance will be close to 18 feet. The acuity chart can be adjusted to compensate for this test distance.

Examination rooms should be designed specifically for use by a right-handed or left-handed practitioner, and individual preferences should be taken into consideration (Figure 10.6). It is important to have a sink near the examination chair so that hands can be washed and solutions and contact lenses can be handled. An excellent concept is the use of the refraction desk, which will serve as a writing surface and storage area near the sink and vanity. Handheld diagnostic instruments are placed in recharging wells within this refraction desk, and an inclined drawer stores the trial lens tray. Placement of a manual chart projector on the refraction desk allows easy operation by the practitioner, especially if a small rearview mirror is incorporated so the practitioner does not have to turn around to see the chart. Remote-control devices allow the projector to be mounted virtually anywhere in the room. The refraction desk can be

electrically wired to control wall outlets so that various instruments can be controlled at the refraction desk. The room lights can be dimmed or turned off by controls on the refraction desk if they are prewired. It is somewhat complex to use a dimmer on fluorescent light fixtures, so it might be more practical to turn them off and use the reading light on the instrument stand as the only light for low illumination.

A clean, professional look is desirable for examination and treatment rooms, although some decoration is needed to prevent a too-sterile look. Subdued and textured wall coverings, tasteful art work, or a display of professional certificates are some decorating possibilities. Windows are not desirable in the examination room because of the need for lighting control, but if they already exist in the room, they can be covered with blinds or drapes. Some practitioners use windows as an adjunct to trial frame testing at a far distance.

CONTACT LENS ROOM

A special area reserved for contact lenses is a must for most practices (Figure 10.7). The contact lens area can serve as a laboratory and an inventory room that is only accessible to staff members, or it can also include a dispensing and

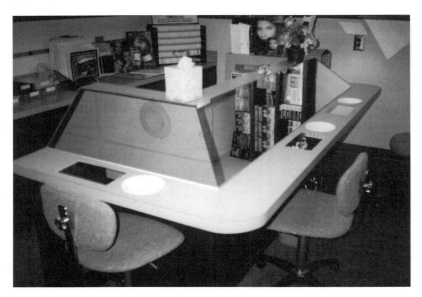

Figure 10.7. Contact lens training center. (Courtesy of Drs. Bob Baldwin, Bobby Christensen, and Russell Laverty, Midwest City, Oklahoma.)

patient education room that would be used to instruct patients in contact lens use. As a laboratory, this room should have counters with convenient electrical outlets for instruments such as a radiuscope, lensometer, shadowscope, or microscope. A modification unit and sink should also be located in this room. With increased use of disposable contact lenses, larger areas are needed to store larger inventories. Having most lenses in stock is regarded by some practitioners as a significant practice asset, although the trend toward doctor-directed shipment from the manufacturer may reduce this need.

Special dispensing counters with built-in sinks, tissue dispensers, and individual mirrors create an excellent environment for multiple or single patient training by the technician. Other considerations for this room include a dedicated video recorder and television, for educational tapes about contact lenses, and storage for educational brochures and fitting agreement forms.

OPTICAL DISPENSARY

A large area within the office should be devoted to frame displays and optical dispensing since this area usually produces a large portion of a practice's gross income (Figure 10.8A). A small dispensary is 200 square feet or smaller; a medium to large traditional dispensary is 500–1,000 square feet; and a superoptical size dispensary runs from 2,000–3,000 square feet. Wall space is typically used to mount frame display units or glass shelves for frames. Windows are desirable if sunlight can be controlled and if they leave some wall space. Professional designers can be of great help in this more retail-like area. The companies that manufacture and sell optical display furnishings can be of assistance with the overall look of the dispensary.

A lens design center can be a good concept to include as a central theme in the dispensary. This center directs attention to ophthalmic lenses and optional lens features before frames are selected. A video frame viewing center is another concept that can be included. A special area or individual booths for delivering and adjusting finished glasses should be considered because they provide some privacy and reserve the use of dispensing tables for frame selection purposes. Special sections showcasing frames for men, women, and children are fairly standard, but special areas for sports eyewear and brand name sunglasses are more unique (Figure 10.8B). An optical laboratory adjacent to the dispensary is recommended, possibly with large windows to show off lens fabrication operations.

Figure 10.8. A. Optical dispensary. (Courtesy of Gailmard Eye Center, Munster, Indiana.) B. Sunwear display area. (Courtesy of Drs. Terry Hawks and Gregory Besler, Overland Park, Kansas.)

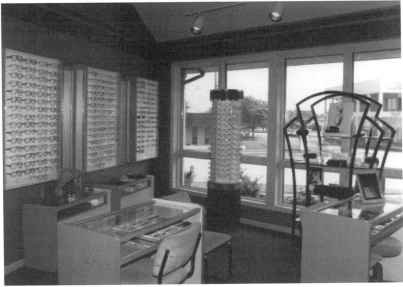

A

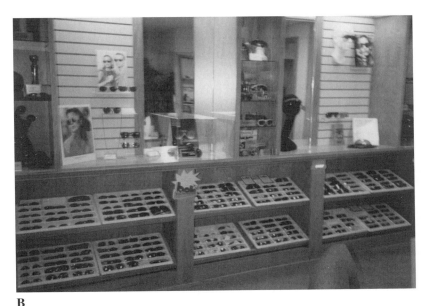

B

Lighting deserves special planning to highlight merchandise displays and to make skin tones most attractive. Track lights work well for dramatic highlights but might need to be supplemented with fluorescent light and daylight. Indirect lighting—reflected off ceilings or walls—can be quite pleasing. Skylights are a popular architectural detail.

Many practices provide an entrance to the optical dispensary that is separate from the entrance to the professional practice. This feature allows a separate identity for the dispensary and allows more aggressive marketing than a practitioner might be comfortable with if it were strictly part of the practice. A separate entrance can prove quite functional for patients stopping in to pick up eyewear or to receive adjustments.

OPTICAL LABORATORY

The optical laboratory can range from a small repair center to a full-service laboratory with finishing and surfacing equipment (Figure 10.9A). Square footage can range from a minimal 60–80 square feet up to 1,000 squre feet for a very large laboratory.

Attention should be given to the special requirements of water supply and waste drains, electrical outlets and voltage supply, and excellent lighting and sound control.

The logical flow of equipment based on function will dictate how the laboratory should be designed. Ample counters at a 36-inch height for standing are needed, and equipment must be placed in a manner so that each job can flow from beginning to end. Base cabinets and wall cabinets provide important storage (Figure 10.9B). If certain tasks require seating, the use of a bar stool is effective, but an opening must be left between cabinets as a knee/leg hole. Certain tasks, such as computerized lens design, might need a special section of the counter to be placed at the desk height of 30 inches.

Special care must be taken in the tinting area to provide for excellent air ventilation, such as the installation of an exhaust hood (similar to those found above a household stove). The walls and floor of this area will have dye splashed on them and, for that reason, can warrant special protection.

PRACTITIONER'S PRIVATE OFFICE

It is recommended that practitioners have a private office that can be used for conducting the business aspects of managing a practice (Figure 10.10). It must be remembered that practice administration is a vital component to successful operation, and that not all of the optometrist's time is spent examining patients. As the owner of a small business, the practitioner must have a space to perform paperwork and meet with staff members and business associates. If space is limited, an area within an examina-

tion room can have a desk and chairs and double as the private office.

CONFERENCE ROOM

A luxury in most offices is the use of a dedicated conference room (Figure 10.11). This room can have a long conference table at which all staff members could be seated. The room can include an area for a slide projector or overhead projector, as well as special felt tip marker boards. The inclusion of a conference room will encourage regular and more productive staff meetings.

STAFF LOUNGE

If space permits, a staff lounge or lunch room is a nice addition to the office. This room can provide a lunch table, sink, refrigerator, microwave oven, telephone, and perhaps a television.

STORAGE ROOMS

Most practitioners, like homeowners, will agree that one can never have too much storage. Unfortunately, with the high cost of commercial real estate, revenue-producing activities must take precedence over storage. In planning an office, practitioners should consider the need for convenient storage of office records and invoices, contact lens solution inventory, extra displays for the dispensary, office stationery, cleaning supplies, and maintenance tools.

OFFICE SIZE

The space requirements needed for an office will depend on numerous factors, but, in general, a small office will require less than 1,000 square feet (Table 10.2), a moderate-sized office will need less than 2,500 square feet (Table 10.3), and a large office could demand as much as 6,000 or more square feet (Table 10.4). Obviously, individual designs can produce requirements that require more or less space, but these figures provide approximate indications

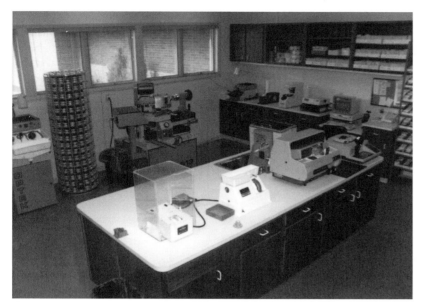

A

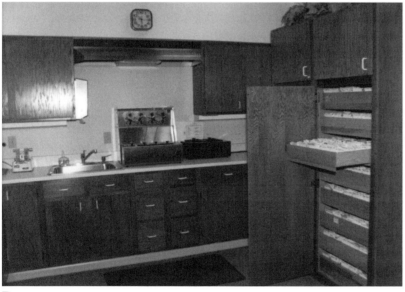

B

Figure 10.9. A. Lens fabrication laboratory. (Courtesy of Gailmard Eye Center, Munster, Indiana.) B. Uncut lens storage cabinets. (Courtesy of Gailmard Eye Center, Munster, Indiana.)

of the space needed for small, moderate, and large practices.

BUILDING AND REMODELING

It is strongly recommended that the practitioner meet with an architect or designer as early as possible to plan adequately for any remodeling or new office construction. Most towns and cities have building codes and zoning ordinances, and it is best to check with the town's building inspectors before performing any construction, no matter how minor. This precaution should be taken even if the construction involves the placement of new exterior signs.

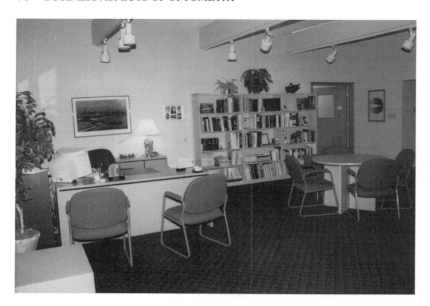

Figure 10.10. Doctor's private office. (Courtesy of Gailmard Eye Center, Munster, Indiana.)

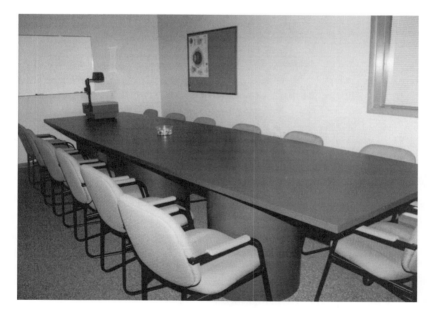

Figure 10.11. Conference room. (Courtesy of Gailmard Eye Center, Munster, Indiana.)

Parking plays a vitally important part in how an office is perceived by the public. Businesses that have easy parking will have a better chance of reaching a high level of success. One must anticipate growth in the planning of any office, and that includes more parking. Doctors' offices typically have the greatest requirement for parking by town ordinance, usually based on square footage such as 1 space per 100 square feet.

Special considerations for wiring exist when remodeling or planning new construction. Planning must be instituted for burglar alarm systems, telephone systems, computer systems, light signal systems, stereo music systems, and intercoms. When working with architects and designers, the best way to approach planning meetings is with a written list of the special needs of the office. Designers can help recommend some aspects of construction, such

Table 10.2. Room Requirements for a Small Office

1. Reception room: $12 \times 15 = 180$ square feet
2. Business office: $10 \times 12 = 120$ square feet
3. Exam room: $10 \times 12 = 120$ square feet
4. Laboratory: $6 \times 12 = 72$ square feet
5. Dispensary: $10 \times 20 = 200$ square feet
6. Hallway and bathroom: 100 square feet

Total = 792 square feet

Table 10.3. Room Requirements for a Moderate Office

1. Reception room: $10 \times 20 = 200$ square feet
2. Business office: $10 \times 15 = 150$ square feet
3. Data collection room: $10 \times 12 = 120$ square feet
4. Exam room: $10 \times 14 = 140$ square feet
5. Exam room: $10 \times 14 = 140$ square feet
6. Contact lens room: $10 \times 18 = 180$ square feet
7. Finishing laboratory: $14 \times 18 = 252$ square feet
8. Dispensary: $20 \times 30 = 600$ square feet
9. Private office: $12 \times 12 = 144$ square feet
10. Hallways, storage, and 2 bathrooms: 300 square feet

Total = 2,226 square feet

Table 10.4. Room Requirements for a Large Office

1. Lobby: $6 \times 12 = 72$ square feet
2. Reception room: $20 \times 25 = 500$ square feet
3. Business office: $15 \times 20 = 300$ square feet
4. Administrative area: $12 \times 14 = 168$ square feet
5. Office manager's office: $10 \times 12 = 120$ square feet
6. 2 data collection rooms: $10 \times 12 = 120 \times 2 = 240$ square feet
7. 4 exam rooms: $10 \times 20 = 200 \times 4 = 800$ square feet; or 6 exam rooms: $10 \times 14 = 140 \times 6 = 840$ square feet
8. Contact lens laboratory: $8 \times 20 = 160$ square feet
9. Patient education room: $12 \times 16 = 192$ square feet
10. Dispensary: $30 \times 60 = 1,800$ square feet
11. Finishing lab: $20 \times 20 = 400$ square feet
12. Private office: $10 \times 20 = 200$ square feet
13. Staff lounge: $10 \times 20 = 200$ square feet
14. Storage, hallways, and 3 bathrooms: 600 square feet

Total = 5,752–5,792 square feet

as size requirements, lighting, heating and air conditioning needs, plumbing and electrical needs, and so on, but they must know individual needs, which are very specific to optometry.

It is customary, after plans are drawn, to accept bids by contractors. An architect can serve as a construction manager—a person who generally serves as an advisor—and can eliminate the need for a general contractor. With the use of a construction manager, subcontracts to individual specialty contractors such as plumbers and electricians can be made directly, possibly saving some of the administrative costs that would be built in by a general contractor. With this arrangement, the practitioner is the general contractor. It should be noted, however, that a general contractor can be quite necessary for a busy practitioner who might not have time to coordinate and supervise all of the contract work. Many general contractors also serve as designers and can provide a complete turnkey job.

Regardless of the specific approach taken, it should be expected that construction will take longer and cost more than the amount originally anticipated.

BIBLIOGRAPHY

Baldwin BL, Christensen B, Melton T. Rx for Success. Midwest City, OK: Vision Publications, 1983;33–58.

Bennett I. Management for the Eye Care Practitioner. Boston: Butterworth-Heinemann, 1993;6–15.

Blackwood F. Design do's and don'ts. Eyecare Bus 1993;8(6):72–4.

Blackwood F. Shedding light on lighting. Eyecare Bus 1991;6(7):51.

Bostick DB. Dispensary relocation: creating separate retail and clinical environments. Optom Today 1993;1(4):19.

Chase C. Don't fall into these office design traps. Optom Manage 1993;28(5):25–8, 30.

D'Addono B. Five offices where form meets function. Here's what designers like to see when they work on an office. Rev Optom 1994;131(10):45–6, 48.

D'Addono B. How to get what you want from an office designer. Rev Optom 1995;132(9):37–40.

D'Addono B. Keep your patients out of each other's space. Rev Optom 1995;132(3):37–8,43–4.

D'Addono B. The waiting room from hell: nine ways to avoid it. Rev Optom 1995;132(6):47–52.

Del Pizzo N. Blueprints: success by design. 20/20 1994;21(9):59–60, 62.

Gailmard NB. Office design: Gailmard Eye Center. J Am Optom Assoc 1987;58(8):680–3.

Gailmard NB. When your practice screams for an extra exam room. Rev Optom 1993;130(3):115–16.

Goldberg DW. Seeing your interior as patients see it. Eyecare Bus 1988;3(7):64, 67.

Hanks AJ. A "purpose built" practice. Optom Econ 1996;6(1):38–40.

Herrick T. Blueprints for success: Doctors Blackman, Lentz and Murphy. 20/20 1991;18(8):56.

Herrin S. Make your office larger than life. Optom Manage 1993;28(3):33–4.

Lee G. Office renovations. Optom Econ 1992;2(11):11–4.

Lee J. How to prevent parking problems. Optom Manage 1992;27(12):27–9.

Persico J. What does your reception area say about you? Optom Manage 1992;27(7):33–8.

Sachs L. Limited office space (Here are 17 ways to maximize it). Optom Econ 1992;2(2):33–4.

Schwartz CA. How safe are your habits? Optom Econ 1992;2(3):12–19.

Stoltzfus JH. Blueprint for a successful office conversion. Optom Manage 1994;29(2):28–31.

Thumann C. Make your new look solve your old problems. Rev Optom 1993;130(7):37–40.

Winslow C. These steps can avoid an inefficient office. Rev Optom 1991;128(9):48–53.

Wrench J. Practice design in today's market place. Optom Today 1995;35(4):38, 40.

Wright BL. Ophthalmic Office Design Guide. Los Angeles: Wright Design Group, 1991.

Chapter 11

Instrumentation and Equipment

Neil B. Gailmard and John G. Classé

It is the Age of Machinery, in every outward and inward sense of the word.

—Thomas Carlyle
Critical and Miscellaneous Essays

Optometry is a profession that requires the use of sophisticated (and often expensive) instrumentation and equipment. The use of this technology involves all aspects of care, from diagnostic evaluation of patients to fabrication of eyewear to billing for services. Involvement in the purchase of instruments and equipment is an inevitable part of the practice of optometry, and one of the most costly in terms of financial investment.

For optometry school graduates, purchasing decisions are important steps in the process of beginning a practice. The selection of instrumentation and equipment is a major consideration in opening a new practice that must be completely equipped. When purchasing a practice, existing instrumentation and equipment often need to be replaced. The selection of equipment is, in fact, a large, never-ending task, for even well-established practitioners find it necessary periodically to replace or update clinical instruments, office furnishings, and business equipment. Choosing the right supplier is a crucial part of making this investment successfully. As in selecting any professional advisor, referrals from trusted sources (such as fellow optometrists) are an excellent guide. The purchaser should always allow time to compare prices and service among sellers. An excellent way to compare different brands of instruments, and the dealers who sell and service them, is by attending the exhibit hall at major eye care seminars and conventions. Because

the purchase of equipment is an expensive investment, one with significant legal ramifications, potential legal issues should be understood before entering into a purchase agreement.

LEGAL CONSIDERATIONS WHEN PURCHASING INSTRUMENTS AND EQUIPMENT

There is a tendency on the part of new graduates to assume a rather cavalier attitude toward the agreements used for the purchase of equipment. This is due, in part, to the circumstances of the usual purchase. The buyer places an order, which the seller promises to deliver at a time that is often several weeks or months in the future; the buyer signs what is not much more than a list of agreed-on items; and no money actually changes hands. Although equipment purchase agreements would not seem to be in the same category as practice purchase agreements— which require lawyers, accountants, a bank loan, and usually a period of bargaining—nothing could be farther from the truth. As with agreements to purchase a practice, equipment purchase agreements are contracts that are formal, binding, and enforceable.

These agreements cannot be voided merely because of some unforeseen circumstance, such as the disability of the buyer or the failure of the buyer to obtain an optometry license as expected. Under these circumstances, the buyer will have to pay damages to the seller or try to sell the equipment to another buyer. The damages incurred by the seller can be relatively small if another buyer is quickly found, or they can be rather consequential if the equipment must be warehoused, transported, and resold at a loss. In either event, the buyer's breach of the agreement creates liability for the expenses incurred.

The only way to void a purchase agreement is to place a clause within the agreement that specifies that the contract will not be binding should a certain described event occur. An example circumstance would be failure to obtain an optometry license. Although a clause stating that the purchase agreement would be void if the buyer failed to receive a license would be legal and enforceable, it is unlikely that the seller would agree to it. Contingency clauses are not in a seller's best interest, and they are not customarily included in equipment purchase agreements for that reason.

There are issues other than the contract that are important when purchasing instrumentation and equipment, such as budgeting for instrument purchases, financing, the use of leasing rather than buying, tax considerations, and selecting the appropriate equipment.

BUDGETING FOR PURCHASES

A budget should be determined for the capital investment of a practice since it is very easy to add excessively to the list of needed instruments. A rule of thumb, if opening a new practice, is to buy only what is needed to provide competent professional care. When the practice is economically sound, it is a wise strategy to reinvest income into the practice in the form of additional and more automated instrumentation. Another rule of thumb is to allocate 2–5% of net income every year to this fund. Each practitioner should develop a list for instruments, identifying and prioritizing the items needed in the practice. As funds are available, the desired items can be purchased.

There is a market for used equipment when it functions well and looks good. Buying directly from another practitioner or a reliable equipment dealer will allow substantial savings when compared to the cost of new equipment. An equipment vendor gives the advantage of cleaning, servicing,

recalibrating, and possibly even applying a new paint finish to instruments. It is always wise to inquire about warranties, which might not be offered with some used equipment. Instruments with advanced electronics can be very difficult and expensive to service. Equipment maintenance should be performed on a regular basis according to the manufacturer's guidelines. This maintenance might simply involve regular cleaning, which is important for accurate operation. Staff members should be trained to clean instruments daily, since lenses and mirrors can be damaged if cleaned improperly, and instruments can be broken if mishandled.

FINANCING THE PURCHASE

Buying new professional instruments often involves financing. There are several options available to the purchaser, but the usual choices made by optometrists are bank loans or financing through the equipment dealer. Another option is leasing rather than buying. In many cases, the time savings achieved by the use of the new instrumentation or the additional fees generated by use of the instrumentation can offset its cost. For example, an autoperimeter with threshold capability is an expensive device costing several thousands of dollars. If an optometrist's practice requires the frequent use of autoperimetry—for the management of glaucoma patients—the income generated by the device could more than pay for the cost of its purchase. When contemplating the purchase of equipment, thought should be given to the capacity of the device to add to services and to generate income. This consideration is particularly important for optometry school graduates seeking to start a new practice. For new practices, it is essential to keep overhead expenses—the fixed expenses that must be paid every month—as low as possible.

Another important issue related to equipment purchased with a loan is that the equipment serves as collateral for the loan. In such cases, the creditor retains a security interest in the equipment. In the event that the borrower defaults on the loan (cannot pay the creditor), the security interest allows the creditor to take possession of the collateral and sell it in an attempt to minimize financial loss. If the collateral cannot be sold for the amount that is owed, the creditor might be able to have other as-

Table 11.1. Leasing of Ophthalmic Instruments and Equipment

Advantages

100% financing of the equipment.

No down payment.

100% of the lease cost may be deducted.

After the term of the lease, the equipment does not have to be purchased; instead, a new lease for new equipment can be entered into.

The financing charge for the lease period does not change, so fluctuating interest rates do not affect the amount due.

Disadvantages

Most new practices do not earn enough income to justify the tax advantages of the full lease deduction.

The cost of a lease is greater than the cost of purchasing the same equipment; at the end of the lease period a payment will have to be made (usually 10–15% of the equipment's fair market value) to obtain the title to it.

The depreciation deduction is claimed by the leasing company.

The equipment must be kept for the full term of the lease. The only exception is if the equipment is upgraded or if equipment of greater value is obtained. If the equipment is returned because of a default in payments, it can be sold and any deficit in what is owed can be collected from the defaulting practitioner.

The lease agreement will probably require the practitioner to pay for insurance on the equipment; the practitioner may also be required to pay for all repairs (although this will depend on the warranty received from the equipment seller or manufacturer).

sets of the creditor seized and sold in an attempt to collect the difference. If, even worse, the creditor becomes insolvent, those to whom the creditor is indebted might be able to sell the equipment themselves. This unlikely event can occur if the security interest signed by the buyer is not actually with the seller but, rather, with the creditor of the seller.

To avoid misfortune, new graduates should negotiate with dealers who have acquired a good reputation over a period of time and not fall prey to impulses or succumb to the allure of cut-rate prices. Buyers should always obtain competent legal advice before entering into any contract that involves the expenditure of a considerable amount of money or requires years of obligation to repay.

LEASING OPHTHALMIC EQUIPMENT

When considering the acquisition of ophthalmic equipment, the buyer should consider whether it is more advantageous to lease the equipment than to buy it (Table 11.1). Although leasing is usually more expensive than financing through a bank (or purchasing equipment outright), the use of leasing can allow a practitioner to use savings for the purchase of another asset (such as a home). While it is not technically the same as financing, there is a built-in interest rate in a lease (which usually

does not fluctuate over the period of the lease). This financing cost is generally higher with leases than with bank loans. The main advantage of leasing is that a lease does not usually require a down payment or affect a line of credit that might be established at a bank. Leases from different companies should be examined and compared in detail. The term (length) of the lease is for a period of years and is very difficult to change after the lease has begun.

At the end of the lease term the equipment can be returned to the leasing company or purchased for an agreed-on amount. The amount paid will depend on the lease agreement, but it is usually the used market value of the equipment or 10–15% of the equipment's fair market value. The purchase option will affect the amount of the monthly lease payment. There are several tax issues that must be understood before entering into a lease agreement. A certified public accountant or tax attorney should be consulted to clarify individual provisions of lease agreements (Table 11.2).

TAX CONSIDERATIONS OF BUYING VERSUS LEASING

For tax purposes, an equipment lease must be managed differently than a bank loan used for the pur-

Table 11.2. Common Provisions of Equipment Lease Agreements

Identification of the parties
If the lease is to be taken out by a professional association or corporation or by a partnership, the lease agreement should be signed accordingly.

Description of the lease property
The practitioner will select the equipment that is to be purchased and the leasing company will provide the funds to purchase it. The lease agreement needs to describe the equipment with specificity so that there is no mistake or question about the items subject to the lease.

Term of the lease
The lease period may vary from 1 to 7 years; some companies may permit even longer periods.

Option to purchase
At the conclusion of the lease period, the practitioner will have the right to purchase the equipment. The price can be set at the onset of the arrangement or may be expressed as a percentage that cannot be exceeded. If the practitioner does not wish to purchase the equipment, it is returned to the leasing company at the end of the lease term.

Cost of the lease
The interest, though higher than that charged by a bank, will be stable throughout the lease term. (However, if interest rates should go up significantly during the lease term, the interest rate charged by the leasing company may actually fall below the rate charged by a bank.) A monthly payment is established for the term of the lease, which does not change from month to month. (Some leasing companies offer a graduated payment schedule, whereby the lease payments are lower in the first years and gradually escalate over the later years of the lease term.)

Responsibility for repairs
The leasing company does not provide repairs; the practitioner will have to find an equipment dealer to perform repairs, and the practitioner will have to pay for them. (However, the equipment manufacturer will provide maintenance and repairs during the warranty period.)

Insurance
The practitioner will probably be required to purchase insurance sufficient to indemnify the leasing company in the event the equipment is lost in a fire or other casualty.

Right of exchange
The practitioner may wish to exchange certain equipment before the lease term is concluded, to obtain a newer model or a different piece of equipment altogether. The lease may recognize the right to perform exchanges (with proper adjustments in the cost of the lease).

Failure to make timely payment
The lease will provide certain remedies to the leasing company should the practitioner fail to make the lease payments as provided in the agreement. Among the remedies typically available to the leasing company are the acceleration of payments, increased charges for late payments, and seizure and sale of the equipment. The penalties for late payment should be clearly understood by the practitioner.

chase of equipment. When money is borrowed from a bank, both principal and interest must be repaid. Only the interest, however, can be deducted. When an equipment lease is entered into, each monthly repayment is tax deductible. Therefore, 100% of the lease amount can be deducted.

Some consideration must be given to whether the lease deduction is advantageous for a given practice. It is often not particularly advantageous for a beginning practice, but for an established practice a lease arrangement might offer some tax benefits. Again, professional advice should be solicited before entering into an agreement.

MAKING THE APPROPRIATE CHOICES

There is a practice-building and promotional aspect to having excellent instruments. Patients will judge the quality of the examination based on an impression of how up-to-date instruments are. Even if instruments are not new, they should look new. Automated and computerized instruments provide accuracy of measurement, state-of-the-art technology, public relations benefits, and savings of time because their use is delegated to support personnel. Informing patients about the special diagnostic instruments used in the practice is an excellent means

Table 11.3. Equipment Checklist
for the Data Collection Room

Basic
1. Keratometer
2. Telebinocular
3. Color vision plates
4. Stereopsis test
5. Sphygmomanometer and stethoscope
6. Lensometer
7. Patient chair and examiner stool

Advanced (substitute or add to above)
1. Autorefractor
2. Noncontact tonometer
3. Autokeratometer
4. Autolensometer
5. Autoperimeter
6. Retinal camera
7. Rotating instrument table
8. Power patient chair

Table 11.4. Equipment Checklist
for the Examination Room

Basic
A. Refraction
    1. Examination chair
    2. Instrument stand
    3. Phoropter
    4. Keratometer
    5. Chart projector and screen or chart display terminal
    6. Trial lens set and frame
    7. Retinoscope
    8. Examiner's stool
B. Ocular disease management
    1. Slit lamp biomicroscope
    2. Goldmann tonometer
    3. Binocular indirect ophthalmoscope
    4. Direct ophthalmoscope
    5. Various hand-held devices for emergency and primary care
C. Additional
    1. Corneal topography analyzer
    2. Electrodiagnostic instrumentation
    3. Pachometer
    4. Slit lamp 35-mm camera
    5. Slit lamp video system
    6. Low vision diagnostic aids
    7. Binocular vision testing and/or training equipment

of providing internal marketing, which can result in more word-of-mouth referrals. For that reason, new instrumentation is a great topic for newsletters, recall reminders, and office brochures.

The determination of the appropriate instruments and equipment for a practice is one of the most important tasks a practitioner faces. As has been described, it is particularly important for beginning practitioners to be selective and to purchase only the equipment essential to start a practice, adding on when necessary as the patient base and income grow.

Tables 11.3 through 11.6 summarize the pieces of equipment to be considered for a practice, organized by the rooms in which they are typically used. A large range of costs and features are usually found for each instrument and, of course, some items are necessities while others are luxuries.

BIBLIOGRAPHY

Aldridge C. How to choose the right payment option: is it better to buy, lease or finance your new instrument? Optom Manage 1994;29(1):22–4.

Table 11.5. Equipment Checklist
for the Laboratory

A. Optical
    1. Automatic diamond lens edger
    2. Hand edger
    3. Lensometer
    4. Layout marker and blocker
    5. Rimless grooving machine
    6. Edge polishing machine
    7. Lens tinting machine
    8. Chemical hardener
    9. Heat-tempering oven
   10. Frame warmer
   11. Various dispensing tools
B. Contact lens
    1. Contact lens modification unit and tools
    2. Radiuscope
    3. Shadowscope or dissecting microscope

Table 11.6. Equipment Checklist
for the Business Office

1. Typewriter
2. Telephone system
3. Calculator
4. Photocopier
5. Answering machine
6. File cabinets
7. Postage meter
8. Dictation equipment
9. Computer system and printer
10. Fax machine
11. Light signal system (interoffice communication)

Allergan, Inc. Pathways in Optometry. Irvine, CA: Allergan, 1992:63–75.

Arkin J. Time to replace your old equipment? Using these calculations, you may find it's costing you more than buying new. Eyecare Bus 1988;3(12):61–2.

Baldwin BL, Christensen B, Melton T. Rx for Success. Midwest City, OK: Vision Publications, 1982;59–63.

Barnett D. Are your instruments in tune with your practice? Rev Optom 1992;129(8):19.

Bayusik L. The fine-tuning of an instruments market. Eyecare Bus 1989; 4(3):41,44–5, 48.

Classé JG. Legal Aspects of Optometry. Stoneham, MA: Butterworth, 1989;607–11.

Cleinman AH. Remove risk from technology investments. Optom Manage 1994;29(2):21.

Coady C. To lease or not to lease. Eyecare Bus 1995; 10(10):53.

Coleman DL. Your new ophthalmic equipment (First decide which is better for you. Then make sure you know the rules). Optom Econ 1992;2(4):30–3.

Donoghue SK. The paperless practice: the future is now. Eyecare Tech 1993;3(2):13–16, 26.

Gailmard NB. The consultant's corner: are your investments secret information? Rev Optom 1992;129(6):25.

Gailmard NB. Guide to diagnostic instruments and equipment. Rev Optom 1993;130(3):111–28.

Gailmard NB. When your practice screams for an extra exam room. Rev Optom 1993;130(3):115–6.

Goldsborough R. Five ways to ease the strain of opening cold. Rev Optom 1987;124(5):97–103.

Goldsborough R, Gailmard NB. Pick your exam room. Rev Optom 1987;124(9):48–56.

Gorin SB. Equipment purchases: to lease or buy? Optom Econ 1993;3(7):47–8.

Harris L. Build a testing room for the '90s. Optom Manage 1994;29(3):55–6.

Hayes J. How much to spend on new instruments. Optom Manage 1993;28(4):15.

Kirkner R. Instruments for the sake of patient care [editorial]. Rev Optom 1992;129(8):19.

Kreda SH. Enter the office of the future. Optom Manage 1995;30(4):31–2.

Legerton JA. Sound purchasing decisions (analyzing the what, when, why and how of purchasing ophthalmic equipment). Optom Econ 1992;2(10):34–8.

Perry P. Look before you lease. Eyecare Bus 1993; 8(4):90–91.

Ramsay WK. Miniaturizing equipment: small and portable instruments for optometrists today. Optom Today 1995;3(3):37,39.

Schwartz CA. Capitalizing on high-tech equipment. Optom Econ 1993;3(5):28–31.

Chapter 12

Use of Computers

Stuart Rothman and Michael Usdan

The computer is no better than its program.

—Elting Elmore Morison
Men, Machines and Modern Times

Recent surveys indicate that the vast majority of modern optometric offices are using computer systems. The range of uses for these systems can be as limited as word processing on a single personal computer and as extensive as the paperless office on a multiuser system.

This chapter describes the various roles and functions of personal computers in contemporary optometric practice. Specific patient management, business management, inventory management, and time management applications are discussed.

USE OF THE PERSONAL COMPUTER

The personal computer has revolutionized optometric office management in the same way it has revolutionized all small businesses. Computers save time by performing many of the functions that used to be performed by hand, and they also have expanded the capabilities of the optometric office to manage data.

Patient information, such as name, address, telephone number, birth date, and recall date, has been expanded by computerization to include diagnoses, insurance information, spectacle prescription, and contact lens information. A noncomputerized office has to create and maintain a separate file for each patient; when information is needed, it has to be retrieved by hand. The computerized office can store, obtain, and analyze information with the stroke of a few keys, which greatly expands the practice's ability to retrieve and sort the information collected.

Communication between practitioner and patients, prospective patients, and potential referral sources is enhanced with computers. The merger of word processing with stored data allows a computerized office to send personalized letters to all these sources, permitting the office to market itself in ways that a noncomputerized office either cannot offer or can offer only with the expenditure of significant time and expense.

Financial management has been enhanced in the computerized office, from simple tracking of accounts receivable, to accurate up-to-date summaries of the financial health of the practice, to projections of future practice growth with changes in fees, addition of equipment, or use of ancillary personnel.

Computerized inventory management includes the tracking of ophthalmic materials such as frames and contact lenses, which allows for more efficient purchasing of these items by the practice. With the advent of frequent replacement and disposable contact lens wear programs, inventory management has become increasingly more important. The use of laser scanners and bar codes on these items by the optical industry makes inventory control even easier.

Computers can also be used for the management of patients. Equipment such as automated refractors, corneal topography units, automated lensometers, and visual field analyzers can be linked to personal computers to store pertinent data and to assist in the interpretation of this data, creating a "paperless" office environment. The use of computers in such areas as contact lens design, low vision care, and visual therapy has allowed optometrists to provide better, more efficient care to patients. Optometrists who are online have access to discussion groups and thus can acquire information on patient management, developments in clinical care, and ophthalmic products.

SPECIFIC OFFICE MANAGEMENT APPLICATIONS

Applications in the optometric office include patient information, insurance use, financial information, inventory control, services information, material tracking, appointments, referrals, payroll information, and marketing.

Patient Information

Computerization allows all the pieces of information about individual patients to be stored in one place. Patients can be categorized, sorted, and identified based on any one of the pieces of information that have been collected. For example, computer storage makes it possible for practitioners to learn the demographics of a practice. A practitioner considering a move to another location might want to analyze the patient population by zip code or address so that the most geographically desirable location for the move can be identified. Another application is marketing. Practitioners can perform internal marketing through the use of newsletters or other literature sent to a computer-generated lists of patients.

Typical patient information stored on a computer might include name, address, date of birth, telephone number, insurance information, referral source, the individual responsible for payment of fees, examination date, recall date, reason for recall, diagnoses, contact lens type, contact lens service agreement information, spectacle lens information, frame information, and account information (Figure 12.1).

Any of this information can be accessed, retrieved, sorted, and reviewed through the computer. For example, the office might want to inform all patients with high myopic refractive errors about a new type of lens material. Without a computer, retrieval of this information would require considerable staff time, because individual patient files would have to be reviewed. With a personal computer, a list of the appropriate patients can easily be compiled, and mailing labels or letters can be sent to each patient, with minimal staff time and effort involved.

Insurance Information

In addition to allowing insurance information to be listed with other patient data, a computer will permit the office to more efficiently process and keep track of insurance payments. Many software programs will print standard patient insurance forms, and some will transfer information electronically (e.g., for Medicare patients). These procedures can hasten the reimbursement process and thus improve the office's cash flow. In the future, it is likely that many insurers will insist on the electronic transfer of claims as a condition for participating in managed care plans.

As more and more optometric patients obtain insurance coverage from third-party insurance plans, it will become necessary to monitor when payments are due from individual payers and to track third-party payment schedules. Medicare now allows electronic filers to tap into its computer network to determine the status of claims being processed—a development that will become the standard procedure for most insurers in the future. Computerization also allows for easier and more efficient communication with third-party payors by permitting the use of standardized letters and forms.

Financial Information

Computerized billing and tracking of accounts receivable enables a practice to more efficiently bill and collect money owed. Many software programs will allow the office to set payment schedules for patients. The computer will calculate interest charges and present the patient with preprinted receipts to return to the practice when money is due (Figure 12.2).

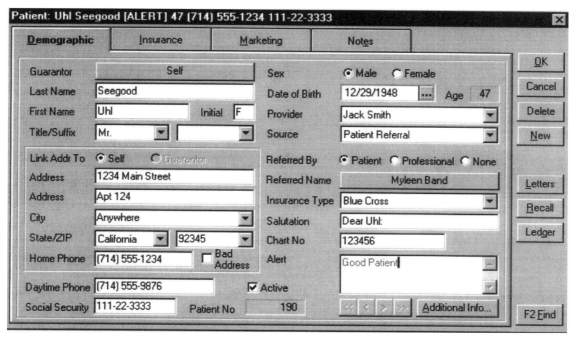

Figure 12.1. Patient information screen with information to be collected on each patient. This information can later be selectively retrieved. Patients can also be sorted by various pieces of information. (Courtesy of Officemate.)

Tracking of accounts payable is made easier through computerized programs that can act like a checkbook to record and categorize payments, write checks, and monitor accounts. These programs enable the office to obtain profit and loss statements as needed rather than having to wait for quarterly accounting reports.

The financial productivity of an office can be determined by the day, week, or year; as needed, income can be tracked for tax purposes. The financial contributions of the practitioners and staff can also be determined, an essential capacity in offices where practitioner income is divided on the basis of productivity or where bonuses are paid to staff based on performance or office productivity.

Inventory Information

Many practitioners maintain large inventories of contact lenses, on consignment, in the office so that patients can receive same-day service on replacement lenses or can be provided with lenses imme-

diately after fitting. Management of inventory can be cumbersome without computerized inventory control. The computerization of inventory also makes it possible for the receptionist or contact lens technician to immediately tell a patient calling for a replacement lens whether the lens is in stock. The growing popularity of frequent replacement and disposable contact lenses places a much greater burden on inventory control. An efficiently run inventory control system can mean a substantial income savings for the practitioner.

Inventories of contact lens supplies and solutions can also be more effectively managed by computer. Many offices stock contact lens solutions for patients, and these solutions must be monitored for turnover rates and expiration dates. Determining when and how frequently solutions and other supplies must be repurchased can allow the office to take advantage of cost savings by buying supplies when they are discounted.

Most practices invest a substantial amount of money in a frame inventory. Computerized management of frames can provide information such as

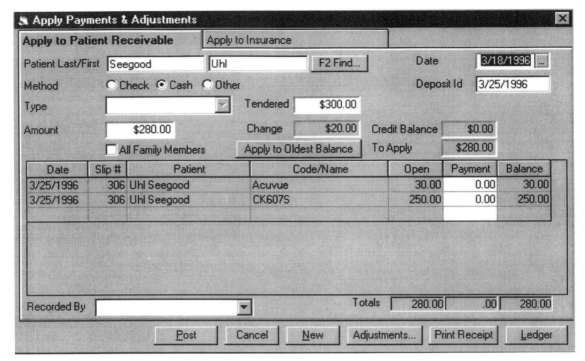

Figure 12.2. Patient receipt generated at the time of visit. This could be attached to the patient's medical insurance form for reimbursement. (Courtesy of Officemate.)

when the frame was purchased, how long it has been offered for sale, how frequently similar frames are sold, and whether similar frames are still in inventory. Reports can be generated by frame type, manufacturer, and cost. These reports can be used to make purchasing decisions for the practice (Figure 12.3).

Services Information

As patients are seen in the office, the type of services provided will be keyed into the computer. Computerization allows the office to track the services provided to any patient on any given day. It also allows the office to keep track of the number of services provided and the income received by the practice from a particular service. This information is used to print out a bill or insurance form for the patient at the time of the office visit. The information can also be used to identify sec-

ondary services or specialized procedures and their use. Financial data can be used to allocate space and money for new equipment based on the amount of income generated by each procedure or service.

Material Tracking

Patient orders for contact lenses and spectacles must be monitored for delivery time. Because patients expect prompt dispensing of ophthalmic materials, a failure on the part of the practice to provide timely service can result in loss of orders. Many ophthalmic laboratories now accept electronic transfer of information, which can eliminate the time-consuming method of messenger or postal delivery. Computerization of this aspect of optometric practice can also aid in the more efficient payment of laboratory bills by enabling credits and invoices to be followed more easily.

COMPANY	FRAME NAME	COLOR	EYE SIZE	DATE RECEIVED	DATE DISPENSED
ALRAY	G 308	ANT TORT	52	10/02/95	12/19/95
	GV 742	315	56	10/02/95	12/08/95
ALTAIR	220	BLACK	60	03/20/96	03/23/96
	710	TORT	54	12/19/94	04/12/96
AUSTRALIAN OPTICAL	AUSSIE 9 CLIP	VIOLET	48	04/29/96	04/29/96
	AUSSIE 9	VIOLET	48	04/29/96	04/29/96
AVANT GARDE	TEEN 83	GEPMUAVE	44	01/09/95	03/14/95
	402	MIDNITEJADE	47	01/09/95	03/22/95
	FRAN	SKYPINK	54	01/09/95	04/15/95
	BB 101	1006	50	01/09/95	02/22/95
	SENATOR	GEP	51	10/03/94	03/14/95
	VEGAS	LITECOPPER	50	09/30/94	03/27/95
	434	GEP BLACK	51	03/19/93	12/16/94
EASTERN STATES	2208	229	49	05/26/95	06/28/95
	1099	BK/GL	52	05/26/95	09/11/95
	7515	203B	56	05/26/95	08/01/95
	2204	848	48	05/24/95	05/24/95
FRATELLI LOZZA	IVY	RASPBERRY	51	04/24/96	04/29/96
	PLYMOUTH	BLACK	53	01/03/96	04/22/96
	SAMANTHA	BURG WEB	54	11/03/95	03/15/96
	FRASER	AMBER	56	10/28/95	03/23/96
	PLYMOUTH CLIP	PEWTER	53	06/16/95	04/22/96
KENMARK	MERYL	GREY	52	02/06/96	03/08/96
	IVY	ANT/BLUE/GREEN	51	06/27/95	11/13/95
	AGATHA SPRING	LAVENDER	53	09/28/94	10/17/95
L'AMY	INES F	PASTELS	54	02/12/96	02/21/96
	USA 50	BLACK AMBER	52	11/17/95	02/21/96
	FREEPORT	BLACK	59	07/31/95	04/27/96
	FREEPORT CLIP	BLACK	59	07/31/95	04/27/96
	LACOSTE 787F	GOLDBROWN	57	06/30/95	04/12/96
	415V	AMBERDEMI/GOLD	44	06/07/95	01/15/96
LAURA ASHLEY	ELEANOR	WINE	49	07/31/95	11/27/95
LAWRENCE	IM14	PURPLE	47	03/23/96	04/12/96
OPTIC STUDIO	P501	27	48	09/30/94	12/19/95
SAFILO	4552	BROWNMARBLE	56	01/20/96	04/16/96
	LADY ELASTA 4550	AQUAMARBLE	54	07/25/94	04/03/96
SAVVY	GB 1101	TO/AS	51	12/29/95	02/26/96
	GB 1119	TO/APTR	49	12/08/95	03/27/96
	GB 1119 CLIP	TO/APTR	49	12/08/95	03/27/96
	GB 1102	DA/YG	50	09/18/95	03/27/96
VIVA	GU252	DT	52	09/18/93	03/29/94

Figure 12.3. Report of frame inventory by manufacturer.

Referral Information

The life-blood of professional optometric practice is the referral. Whether from existing patients, other health care practitioners, or community contacts, re-ferrals keep pumping new blood into a practice. Being able to properly recognize and thank each re-ferral source will make it more likely that these sources will continue to send new patients. Most software programs will facilitate the sending of thank you notices to a referral source. Many will also monitor the numbers of patients each referral source has contributed as well as the income generated by each referral source. For referrals from other health care providers, reports can be generated to allow the referring practitioner to keep up to date on a patient's progress. Managed care plans require prompt communication between the optometrist and the primary care physician gatekeeper. This communication is essential if the optometrist is to continue to receive referrals.

Payroll Information

As the number of employees in an optometric office increases, so does the time needed to handle payroll and tax reporting information. Computerization allows the office to calculate tax withholding, determine net salaries, and even print payroll checks. This information can be summarized and sorted by employees so that payroll taxes can be calculated quarterly as required.

Information about employee salaries and tax withholding can also be printed out on a year-end statement for use when completing tax returns.

Appointment Scheduling

Many software systems designed for optometric offices have an appointment scheduler. In multipractitioner or multilocation offices, these systems can aid in more efficient use of time and can help to avoid improper scheduling. The computer can allocate the proper amount of time for a procedure, assign patients to a given practitioner, and locate available appointment dates and times. Many offices will pre-appoint patients months and even years in advance in a perpetual appointment recall system. Computerization of this system allows the office to efficiently keep track of the appointments made, confirm them in advance, and refill the time slots if patients do not respond or cancel scheduled appointments.

Marketing

A computer will make it easier to carry out all levels of a marketing plan. The first step is to identify a need or problem, such as the failure of many contact lens patients to renew their service agreements. The next step is to implement a marketing concept. For contact lens patients, a letter can be generated by the computer, reminding these patients that regular contact lens care is needed to maintain ocular health. An invitation to renew the service agreement can be included, offering an incentive if renewal is obtained by a specific date. The key element of any marketing plan is an ability to monitor the success of the marketing effort; then the return on investment can be determined. The computer is used to track those patients to whom the letter was sent and the number of patients who responded positively.

HOW TO GET STARTED COMPUTERIZING AN OFFICE

Computerizing an existing office is never an easy task. The actual procedures used can depend on the software system chosen. Certain software companies will load patient information into the system so that the office is "up and running." This process will cost more initially but can save money in the long run, because staff time will not be required to enter information into the computer system. The office will also be fully functional on the computer for standard monthly procedures like recall appointments and billing of accounts receivable. New patients will be added to the system as they come into the office.

Other software systems will allow the office staff to enter patients with outstanding balances so that billing can be computerized from date of installation. Patients to be recalled are entered into the system monthly, requiring additional staff time before recall notices can be mailed. Full data on these patients are entered as they return to the office. For new patients, data are entered at the initial visit.

Some offices will prefer to enter patients as they return for care or when they are seen for the first time. This approach can require the least amount of additional staff time, but it has the disadvantage of delaying the computerization process, because the staff has to go through both a computerized list and a noncomputerized list when sending out recalls, bills, or other patient correspondence. If the average patient visits the office once every 2 years, it will be at least that long before the office will be fully computerized.

Despite the initial disruptions to office procedure, computerization can benefit any size office. Smaller offices that seem to function quite efficiently without computers can still benefit from the additional capabilities that computerization offers. Costs of hardware and software products have regularly decreased, even while computer technology continues to expand. There is no "perfect time" to make the decision to computerize. Software will be improved periodically, and hardware can always be upgraded. Waiting until computer technology is "perfected" only means delaying the tremendous advantages of computerization.

For new offices, computers should be included as initial equipment in much the same way as a phoropter or ophthalmoscope. The use of the computer in marketing, report writing, and patient communication will aid in the development of the new practice. The cost of computerization will be spread out over the lifetime of a practice loan in the same way as other optometric equipment.

SELECTING COMPUTER SOFTWARE

For the computer novice, the use and applications of office computers can be discussed with fellow practitioners, with experts in the field, and with the office staff of colleagues. Vendors from various companies can be found at large continuing education seminars. Salespeople should be able to demonstrate the capabilities of software. Information can be obtained about the support the company offers, what is included in the price of the software, and how often upgrades are provided. Many companies will offer demonstration videotapes of their software; these allow the person who does not own a computer to get a feel for the capabilities of the software.

For the non-novice who has access to a computer, demonstration disks will give a more realistic demonstration of the ease of operation of the software. These demonstration disks will typically allow entry of a small number of patients or can be used for a specified period of time.

For the experienced computer user, testing a product in the office can be of value. Many experienced users decide to purchase a nonoptometric, commercially available database program. Such programs will usually be less expensive than optometric software but will require considerable time to program. The experienced user can use the software to customize a program that suits the particular needs of the office.

PRIORITIZING USE

Once the possible applications of software are understood, it should be determined how the computer will be used in the office. The initial investigation of a software package should reveal its strengths and weaknesses, and knowing the functions that the computer must handle, along with the priority of functions, should assist the practitioner in making the software choice. For example, a program that is strong on inventory control will offer little benefit for an optometrist in a nondispensing practice. Most independent optometrists will find that a software program strong in patient information storage, billing, patient communication, and inventory control will meet all their needs.

Planning where the computer (or computers) will be located will help determine whether patient information will be entered as the patient comes in or "batch processed" for all patients at the end of a work day. It will also help determine the functions that will take priority on the computer. For example, the office with a sole computer that is located on the receptionist's desk will find it difficult to use the computer for inventory assessment and control by staff in the dispensary. Identifying the priorities for computer use will assist in the effort to establish hardware requirements and will help to determine the location of computer workstations. Any and all hardware and software should allow for expansion if the needs of the office change.

KNOWING THE SOFTWARE COMPANY

The software system should be "user friendly." Since the office staff will be the primary users of the system, the software should be designed with simple on-screen menus and explanations. This capability eliminates the need for extensive retraining every time a new staff person is hired. It also eliminates the new staff member's need to refer to a manual when using the computer for a waiting patient.

Support for the software can be provided in various ways. Some companies will use a 900 telephone number, for which advice is billed at a per-minute rate. Other companies will offer a yearly support fee, paid in advance, that allows the user to call for assistance. Many companies will insist that the user purchase a telephone modem, which will allow support personnel to view the problem on their own computer screens and make any corrections or adjustments.

Upgrades of hardware and software systems must be considered a regular expense of doing business. As technology improves, these updates ensure that software is kept current. A company that issues regular updates stands behind its products and is investing in research for new products.

HARDWARE REQUIREMENTS

Hardware requirements will be described for currently available optometric software. Hardware can usually be purchased from the software vendor or, separately, from a local hardware vendor.

Most optometric software runs on DOS or Windows-compatible personal computers. The software will specify the processing chip needed, the suggested speed of operation, the operating system, hard disk capacity, random access memory, and floppy disk requirements. Most software vendors recommend a tape backup system. Peripheral hardware such as internal fax modems and CD-ROM drives might also be recommended. Networking requirements include software and hardware connections to allow multiple-user stations. Remote software allows access to the computer system by the practitioner from home or from a satellite office. Printers can be dot matrix, ink jet, or laser quality. The type of printer can be determined by the software system that is chosen and the type of correspondence used. Many offices will use a dot matrix printer for patient statements and insurance claim forms and use a laser printer for reports and letters.

The computer work station should be designed to provide maximum comfort and efficiency. Chairs should have proper back support and adjustable seats. Monitors should be placed slightly below eye level and should have antiglare screens. Keyboards should have wrist rests and should be adjustable so the operator can reduce strain on upper back and neck muscles. Dot matrix printers, which are more noisy than other printers, should be placed away from areas where conversations will be held with patients or telephones are located.

The time spent on the computer by staff members should be regulated if possible. If one person has specific responsibility for data entry, work periods should be of limited duration and periodic breaks provided. The work station should also be properly designed.

CLINICAL APPLICATIONS FOR COMPUTERS

Computers are beginning to have applications beyond those that provide standard office management. As technology improves, the potential for increased clinical use will expand. Some of the current software options include the following:

1. *Report writing.* This application allows the office to mail a full range of patient, referral source, and other practitioner reports by entering information from the patient examination.

2. *Dispensing.* Software availability includes a computerized display of lifestyle dispensing options; the ability to show patients their appearance with various frame shapes, sizes, and colors; and frame availability by manufacturer and distributors. New products take the computerized image of a patient's face and design an optically correct pair of spectacles with the proper eye-face-spectacle relationship.

3. *Differential diagnoses and therapy.* Software programs exist to analyze and store data for various diagnostic tests. This data can be used for determining the course of therapy or the effectiveness of therapy. Today, most visual field instruments come with statistical software packages that analyze visual field defects, determine the probabilities of such defects, and compare multiple fields on the same patient. Software also exists to transfer and compare findings on various automated devices. Instruments have been developed to obtain a computerized analysis of the optic nerve head so that minute changes, not visible to even the most experienced retinologist, can

be detected. Databases also exist to help practitioners determine the differential diagnosis of pathologic conditions. Modems and communications software hold the promise of being able to transmit patient data, findings, or images to another location for immediate consultation.

4. *Pharmacology.* Current software allows a practitioner to enter the name of ocular or systemic medication taken by a patient and to obtain a list of ocular and systemic side effects. The information can be entered from a case history and printed for the practitioner before the patient is examined. This information can also be printed and given to the patient to take home as a reminder.

5. *Vision therapy.* Computer programs offer practitioners the ability to treat various binocular, oculomotor, and visual perceptual deficits. These programs are often highly motivating for younger patients because of their resemblance to computer games. Vision therapy programs replace older instrumentation that is no longer made and allow for easier quantification of patient progress during therapy. For practices that offer in-office training, the computer therapy programs allow increased flexibility by not requiring the constant supervision of the optometrist or therapist.

6. *Contact lenses.* Computers can aid in the design of rigid contact lens parameters as well as specialty lens parameters. Corneal topography can be analyzed using photokeratography. This technique promises to allow more precise measurement of the cornea-contact lens relationship and of corneal changes occurring over time. Corneal topography software allows practitioners to determine how a particular contact lens might fit a patient's eye and can refine the lens design and fitting process, allowing for less trial and error.

7. *Low vision.* Computers can be used as low vision devices for the partially sighted and as aural word processing devices by the blind population. Various manufacturers produce computers that can be used with standard software to magnify the computer image to any level for the partially sighted; contrast and illumination can also be controlled. Talking computers are available to interface with standard software and enable the blind patient to perform word processing and database management.

CONCLUSION

Computer applications have produced dramatic advances, for both business and personal use. In the optometric office of the future, the computer will be one of the most important pieces of equipment used, for it has the potential to manage both the business and professional care aspects of the practice. Because of this versatility of use, optometrists must understand and be prepared to apply computer technology to the wide array of business and patient care needs faced in private practice.

BIBLIOGRAPHY

Anonymous. Directory of automated instruments and lab equipment. Eye Care Tech 1995(Suppl);5(3):7–34.

Baggarly BA. Who's on line? Optom Econ 1991;1(1):48–51.

Baldwin BL, Christensen B, Melton JW. Rx for Success. Midwest City, OK: Vision Publications, 1983;161–7.

Ensman RG. How do you rate on computer care? Optom Econ 1994;4(4):28–9.

Freeman DN. Recall on line. Optom Econ 1991;1(6):32–7.

Hamada K. The promise of paperless practice. Optom Econ 1994;4(5):22–4.

Maino J. How to network yourself. Optom Manage 1991;26(7):58.

Maino J. Optometric software: how 5 programs rate. Optom Manage 1992;27(7):41–4.

Maino J. A smarter way to shop for office software. Optom Manage 1992;27(3):51–2.

Maino J. Why you should buy a clone. Optom Manage 1991;26(11):55.

Maino JH, Maino DM, Davidson D. Computer Applications in Optometry. Stoneham, MA: Butterworth, 1989.

Mathe N. Computers: the key to success in the 1990's. Optom Econ 1992;2(12):10–4.

Mathe N. Software guidance counseling. Optom Manage 1991;26(1):39–40.

Mathe N, Reisner R. Optometric practice management software directory and buyers guide. Optom Manage 1991;26(1):D1–D22.

Mayo WA. Optometric software looks ahead. Optom Econ 1994;4(7):8–13.

Mortimer MD. Computerize without busting the budget. Optom Econ 1991;1(1):42–5.

Professional Enhancement Program. Monograph MN 16: Optimize Your Professional Opportunities through Business Equipment and Computers. St. Louis: American Optometric Association, 1986.

Sachs L. The right computer. Optom Econ 1991;1(12):24–7.

Chapter 13

Selecting and Using an Optical Laboratory

Donald H. Lakin

It has long been an axiom of mine that the little things are infinitely the most important.

—Sir Arthur Conan Doyle
The Adventures of Sherlock Holmes

Although most optometrists have accounts with many laboratories and frame companies, in the majority of practices one source is used for over half of the laboratory work. There are several factors that lead to the selection of a primary laboratory:

- Communication with sales representatives and laboratory managers
- Sources of frames
- Availability, service, and quality in obtaining frames
- Inventory control of frames
- Quality lens control
- Laboratory service
- Pricing of materials
- Laboratory policies and the facility to expedite laboratory work and materials

These topics constitute the subject matter of this chapter.

MEETING WITH OPTICAL SALES REPRESENTATIVES

Whether starting or buying a practice, it is necessary to establish a board of advisors (attorney, accountant, banker, financial advisor, and similar individuals with technical expertise). Another important advisor will be a trusted representative of the ophthalmic industry. To a considerable degree, financial success in practice will depend on that tangible aspect of the optometry product, the glasses dispensed. Approximately one-third of the revenues generated in an optometric practice are used directly for the payment of ophthalmic materials.

Experienced laboratory representatives are familiar with the ophthalmic marketplace and can be used for advice on subjects as diverse as the tentative location of a practice, the demographics of eye care providers in an area, how to design and furnish a dispensing area, and how to budget for an initial frame inventory. It is a representative's business to know the current trends in the eyewear field and what has been successfully received by the public.

Once a relationship with a representative has been established, the representative becomes a source for the practice's eyewear. He or she will bring to the office new products or products that the practitioner has seen advertised in journals. These representatives also become the individuals who must be contacted regarding quality of work, laboratory services, and cost of materials. As a practice grows, these representatives can provide an important service by educating staff members on the advantages to patients of specific lenses and frames. Many laboratories and suppliers will offer in-office, after-hours seminars to teach staff members how to present specific ophthalmic products to patients.

SOURCES OF SPECTACLE FRAMES

Until the late 1960s, most spectacle frames were sold through wholesale distributors or optical laboratories. These companies were referred to as "full-service laboratories" and usually supplied frames from an in-house frame inventory while providing lenses and lens services from their surfacing and finishing laboratory. In addition, these companies usually sold full lines of ophthalmic equipment. During this era it was possible to deal with one optical laboratory. If all of the frames in a practitioner's dispensary were from the same company that provided the lenses, orders for completed glasses could be phoned or mailed to the laboratory. Logistically, there is still a sizable advantage to working this way, and laboratories that maintain inventories of frames should be considered whenever they can satisfy the need for good service and price. Over the years, however, imported frames have become a bigger part of the ophthalmic market, and direct sales of frames by manufacturers have become very common. Many of these products are high-fashion frames or are provided to fill specific market niches. Imported frames have greatly expanded the frame market and have also changed the way frames are distributed. Companies selling imported frames have their own sales representatives, and these individuals call on private practitioners for orders just as they call on national chains. These companies bill practitioners directly and often offer discounts on quantity orders or provide contracts to use a specific number of frames per month, quarter, or year. Most optometrists work with a number of these direct sales manufacturers so that a wide variety of eyewear can be offered to patients. The number of representatives is usually limited to three to four individuals to increase the opportunity for greater volume discounts and decrease the time spent reviewing products.

Because of the financial advantage of ordering ophthalmic materials and contact lenses in large quantities, private practitioners have formed "buying groups." Originally these groups consisted of optometrists, opticians, or both, who pooled their buying ability to negotiate with suppliers for the purchase of materials at discounted prices that approximated those being offered to national chains or very large practices. These buying groups have been quite successful, and some have expanded to regional size, while a few have even been able to distribute their services nationally. Some are associated with optometric management consulting firms or national franchisers of ophthalmic materials. A few of the larger, more progressive "full-service" optical companies and laboratories are now negotiating with direct frame distributors to have the frames shown and sold by company representatives and billed at the lowest possible price to optometrists who order the frames through their laboratory. As single frames are needed for patients' orders, they are sent and billed to the laboratory, and the discounted cost, with a minimal handling charge, is passed on to the optometrist. The advantages of this process to optometrists is that the service is faster, there are fewer accounts to deal with, and frame materials can still be obtained at the lowest possible cost.

FRAME QUALITY, SERVICE, AND PRICE

Quality, service, and price are three principal concerns when purchasing frames for a dispensary. Since frames vary considerably with regard to material, style, and features, quality is related to the suitability of the product for the specific type of patient that it is intended to serve. For example, a child's frame used for a Medicaid patient would need to be more durable than a fashionable, rimless mounting, because eyewear for Medicaid patients must typically last for several years before it can be replaced. Since most frames are ordered to fill a patient's immediate needs, service in getting frames promptly when ordered is critical to patient satisfaction. Patients do not understand back orders, whether for initial orders, parts, or replacement frames. Most frame manufacturers provide a warranty for frames, with the minimum period being 1 year. The manufacturer's policy should be understood before putting a new frame in the dispensary. Availability of frames must be satisfactory both for the initial dispensing and for any follow-up services related to the frames.

There is a difference in the way that frames are priced by manufacturers. To maximize value to patients, maintain fees for materials at a competitive level, and still have the dispensary make a financial contribution to practice overhead and income, it is necessary to monitor what is paid for frames on a total and a per unit basis.

INVENTORY CONTROL OF FRAMES

Demographics of the practice population will dictate the makeup of the frame inventory. To obtain demographic data, both the current or projected patient base and the market area must be analyzed. Statistics on age, sex, and income provide a guide for the frame styles and price ranges that should be stocked. Optometrists (or their ophthalmic assistants) commonly make the mistake of purchasing products they like instead of what demographics tell them. Laboratory or frame representatives can help practitioners better understand the preferences and practices of a given patient population or practice area. This information and the anticipated volume of frame sales should serve as a guide to inventory control.

It is necessary to have a plan for inventory control. The plan might be to achieve the goal of an inventory that turns over four times a year, an accepted industry goal for a reasonable return on the investment made in this part of a practice. Therefore, if the practice dispenses or plans to dispense 1,200 frames a year, ideally the inventory should be held at 300 frames. This number might be too low, however, to allow presentation of a satisfactory variety of styles to patients. It can be necessary to accept a three or even two times turnover rate until the patient load increases to reach this four times turnover goal. Depending on where the practice is located, the competition from other ophthalmic providers, and the demographics of the practice, 400–700 frames might be necessary. Considering all of these factors, the inventory plan should establish the total number of frames that is appropriate for the practice.

Having established the inventory number, frames must further be divided by gender and age. If the total number of frames is to be 500 and 60% of the patients in the practice are female, 40% are male, and 15% require child-sized frames, frames should be stocked with approximately 250 women's frames, 175 men's frames, and 75 children's frames. Approximately 60% of the frames should be in the "stable" category—frames that are basic to the market, have long-range stability, and consistent turnover. "Fads"—frames that are momentarily popular—should be monitored closely. These frames are often shown and recommended by frame representatives. They are usually demanded by some patients, but for an abbreviated period of time. Fad frames can prove not to be popular in a particular practice, and therefore it is wise to inquire about return policies before purchasing them. The dispensary should offer some frames for sports and avocational use. These frames help to meet the various ophthalmic needs of the patient population, which is the primary goal of having a dispensary in the office.

The selecting and purchasing of frames is often delegated to the person responsible for the fitting and dispensing of ophthalmic materials. Selecting and purchasing frames can be best performed when a plan is in place and the person assuming the responsibility understands the plan, the goals of the dispensary, and the need for inventory control.

Most offices need to have an inventory log book or file to record the name or number of the frame, vendor, style, colors, sizes, price, and date received of all frames in stock (Figure 13.1). This log can be maintained on a rotary file and kept on or near the styling table. This type of file allows the dispenser to have frame information at hand and also to determine which frame styles and types are being used most frequently.

Maintaining a frame stock inventory by computer has proved to be successful for some practices, but there must be a commitment by all staff members handling frames to keep the information up-to-date. The use of bar codes on frames is also used in some practices. This system works best when frames are being directly dispensed from existing coded stock.

In the past, because the variety of frames, styles, and colors was often limited and the investment in frame "samples" was much less, many optometrists ordered all frames from the laboratory rather than using frames from inventory. Since changes in the "samples" were much less frequent, as these frames became shopworn they were disposed of, with the loss being considered just a cost of doing business. In today's market, which requires a large number and variety of frames in most offices, if the frame selected by the patient is the proper size and color, it is usually removed from display and dispensed to

```
MARCHON
MANUFACTOR  NAME           COLOR       SIZE    W/P     R/P
Marchon     Autoflex 1     Brown       56-18   79.95   170.00 +
Marchon     Autoflex 3     GEP         52-15   77.95   166.00 +
Marchon     Autoflex 5     Black       52-20   95.95   190.00 +
Marchon     Autoflex 7     GEP         51-14   77.95   166.00 +
Marchon     Autoflex 10    Brown       57-16   97.95   206.00 1195
Marchon     Autoflex 10    Havana      61-16   97.95   206.00 1195
Marchon     Autoflex 12    Havana      54-19   97.95   206.00 0895
Marchon     Autoflex 17    GEP         59-17   99.95   210.00 1195
Marchon     Autoflex 17    SteelGrey   55-17   99.95   210.00 1195
Marchon     Autoflex 19    GEP Nat     54-16   99.95   210.00 +
Marchon     Autoflex 22    DemiBld     44-19   89.95   190.00 0895
Marchon     Autoflex 22    Havana      48-19   89.95   190.00 0895
Marchon     Autoflex 22    Grapeberry  46-19   89.95   190.00 0895
Marchon     Autoflex 25    DBld/SGEP   52-18   94.95   200.00 +
Marchon     Autoflex 30    HvnGEP      51-18   89.95   190.00 1195
Marchon     BlueRibbon 4   BrwnCrstl   56-14   24.95    63.00 1195
Marchon     BlueRibbon 5   BrnFade     61-16   24.95    63.00 1195
Marchon     BlueRibbon 7   CrtlGrey    54-20   24.95    63.00 1195
Marchon     BlueRibbon 9   PastelPink  58-14   29.95    75.00 1195
Marchon     BlueRibbon 9   HrvstRnbow  56-14   29.95    75.00 1195
Marchon     CEO 105        LilacSilk   56-15   54.95   120.00 +
Marchon     CEO 105        EmldSilk    54-15   54.95   120.00 +
Marchon     CEO 109        Lav Silk    53-18   54.95   120.00 +
Marchon     CEO 109        Teal Silk   51-18   54.95   120.00 +
Marchon     CEO 112        Blue/Sat    52-20   54.95   120.00 0196
Marchon     CEO 112        Orchid/Sat  50-20   54.95   120.00 0196
Marchon     CFG 1 Clip     448 Pewter  55      28.95    39.55 1195
Marchon     CFG 5          62          51-18   34.95    79.00
Marchon     CFG 7          191         51-21   39.95    91.00 +
Marchon     CFG 7          190         51-21   39.95    91.00 +
Marchon     CFG 29         60          56-13   44.95    96.00
Marchon     CFG 31         168         54-18   44.95    96.00
Marchon     CFG 34         184         51-14   42.95    90.00
Marchon     CFG 34         185         53-14   42.95    90.00
Marchon     CFG 35         90          56-15   42.95    90.00
Marchon     Colours 102/103 clip Gep   50-20   24.95    35.00 0895
Marchon     Colours 108    Demi Aqua   50-19   49.95   110.00
Marchon     Colours 108    Mat Tort    52-19   49.95   110.00
Marchon     Colours 113    Mauvtique   48-21   49.95   110.00
Marchon     Colours 114    Snst Red    52-20   49.95   110.00
Marchon     Colours 115    DAbrAqBrn   51-20   49.95   110.00
Marchon     Colours 115    MtBlkAqPw   49-20   49.95   110.00
Marchon     Colours 116    DGrn/AntGrn 50-20   49.95   110.00
Marchon     Colours 123    GreyTort    52-20   49.95   110.00 1195
Marchon     Colours 124    TortBlk     52-20   49.95   110.00
Marchon     Colours 125    SAmber      50-20   44.95   100.00 0895
Marchon     Colours 125    Mediterrean 48-20   44.95   100.00 0895
Marchon     Disney 3       OP          42-16   39.95    91.00
Marchon     Disney 5       BS          42-18   39.95    91.00
Marchon     Disney 24      TacLilac    46-18   39.95    90.00
Marchon     Disney 24      Pstl Psly   46-18   39.95    90.00
Marchon     Disney 24      Confetti    44-18   39.95    90.00
Marchon     Disney 25      Tortoise    46-18   39.95    90.00
Marchon     Disney 27      Mauvtique   44-18   39.95    90.00
Marchon     Disney 27      AGepMatHvn  50-18   39.95    90.00
Marchon     Dinsey 32      Pstl Psly   44-17   42.95    96.00
Marchon     Disney 33      MatTort     46-18   39.95    90.00 0895
```

Figure 13.1. Sample frame inventory record (taken from computer) for spectacle frames. Information recorded (left to right): frame manufacturer, frame name, frame color, size, wholesale price, retail price, and date received in stock.

the patient. Dispensing from stock not only eliminates the cost of wornout samples but also allows for replacement with newer frames, thereby providing a better service to patients. In addition, there is never a delay in obtaining a frame in stock. When dispensing from stock, frames should be available to replace those being sold. This reserve of frames can be as little as 10% of the frame stock if the plan is to alternate the frames being shown. Some offices will obtain more depth in stock, particularly in the "stable" category, to replace frames removed for sale. There can be a cost advantage to buying some of these "stable" frames in quantity. If there is an in-office laboratory, a larger frame stock can also be required (see Chapter 12).

To obtain an ongoing control of inventory, it is necessary to compare what has been purchased to what has been sold. This process requires periodic review of the records of frame orders and sales. A computer makes the task easier, but it will still be necessary to take the time to make the comparison and take corrective steps as needed. A yearly count of the frame inventory certainly tells if the buying plan has been followed, but the inventory can be out of control if not checked more frequently. Plans to stock inventory are based on dispensing patterns, which can and should be reviewed at least annually. The primary goal for the dispensing function of a practice is to meet the ophthalmic needs and wants of patients. The frames bought for this purpose are a

Table 13.1. Tolerances for Single-Vision and Multifocal Lenses*

Meridian of highest absolute power	Tolerance on each meridian (A)	Tolerance on nominal value of the cylinder (B)			
		0.00 up to 0.75	>0.75 up to 4.00	>4.00 up to 6.00	>6.00
0.00 up to 3.00	±0.12	±0.09	±0.12	±0.18	±0.25
>3.00 up to 6.00	±0.12	±0.12	±0.12	±0.18	±0.25
>6.00 up to 9.00	±0.12	±0.12	±0.18	±0.18	±0.25
>9.00 up to 12.00	±0.18	±0.12	±0.18	±0.25	±0.25
>12.00 up to 20.00	±0.25	±0.18	±0.25	±0.25	±0.25
>20.00	±0.37	±0.25	±0.25	±0.37	±0.37

*The distance refractive power imbalance between a pair of lenses in each meridian shall not exceed ⅔ of the sum of the tolerances for each lens for that meridian.
Source: Adapted from American National Standards Institute. Prescription Ophthalmic Lenses—Recommendations. ANSI Z80.1-1995. Available from the American National Standards Institute, 11 West 42nd Street, New York, NY 10036. Reprinted with permission.

critical part of providing total eye care and eyewear for patients.

The following "purchasing tips" should be kept in mind when buying frames:

1. Practitioners should work with vendors who will work with them—and forget the rest.
2. Practitioners should buy what sells rather than what they like.
3. Purchasers should stick to a buying plan rather than buy the plan of a sales representative.
4. Although a buying plan should be consistent, it should be periodically reviewed to determine if results (e.g., returns, cancelled orders) might require a revision.
5. If revisions are required, an alternative plan should be devised, followed, and monitored.

Supplying ophthalmic frames and lenses to patients is an important part of the optometric service. The use of quality materials and efficient laboratory service will help satisfy patients' expectations. Careful pricing of materials will keep the practice competitive.

QUALITY CONTROL

Standards for prescription dress eyewear have been established by the American National Standards Institute (ANSI); impact resistance standards for dress lenses have been adopted by the U.S. Food and Drug Administration. Accepted lens tolerances can be found in ANSI–Z80.1–1995, the current version of the dress eyewear standards (Tables 13.1 through 13.5).

To ensure the quality of lenses being dispensed, in-office lens (and frame) inspection and verification must be performed. The most important considerations are lens power and centering. Attention should also be given to surface lens defects and the edge finish. Lenses at the tolerance limit should be rejected if they could cause a problem for the patient. Lenses beyond the tolerance limit should be routinely rejected. Procedures for the return of rejected lenses should be discussed with the laboratory, which should be willing to correct defects promptly. With the state-of-the-art, high-tech equipment most laboratories use to lay out and edge lenses, quality should not be a problem. If it is, another laboratory should be considered.

LABORATORY SERVICE

Patients expect a reasonable delivery time on their eyewear. The time required for an individual order will depend on the efficiency of the laboratory fabricating the eyewear and the method of delivery to the office. Assuming the laboratory has a good lens blank inventory, all orders should be ready to deliver within 48 hours. Lenses requiring special treatment or a coating that cannot be provided by the laboratory are the exception.

Surveys of laboratories reveal that the most frequent methods of delivery are United Parcel Service, the U.S. mail, overnight express, and the

Table 13.2. Tolerances for Progressive and Aspheric Lenses*

Meridian of highest absolute power	Tolerance on each meridian (A)	Tolerance on nominal value of the cylinder (B)			
		0.00 up to 0.75	>0.75 up to 4.00	>4.00 up to 6.00	>6.00
0.00 up to 3.00	±0.12	±0.12	±0.18	±0.18	±0.25
>3.00 up to 6.00	±0.12	±0.12	±0.18	±0.18	±0.25
>6.00 up to 9.00	±0.18	±0.18	±0.25	±0.25	±0.25
>9.00 up to 12.00	±0.18	±0.18	±0.25	±0.25	±0.25
>12.00 up to 20.00	±0.25	±0.18	±0.25	±0.25	±0.25
>20.00	±0.37	±0.25	±0.25	±0.37	±0.37

*The distance refractive power imbalance between a pair of lenses in each meridian shall not exceed ⅔ of the sum of the tolerances for each lens for that meridian.
Source: Adapted from American National Standards Institute. Prescription Ophthalmic Lenses—Recommendations. ANSI Z80.1-1995. Available from the American National Standards Institute, 11 West 42nd Street, New York, NY 10036. Reprinted with permission.

Table 13.3. Tolerances on the Direction of Cylinder Axis

Nominal value of the cylinder power (D)	up to 0.37	>0.37 up to 0.75	>0.75 up to 1.50	>1.50
Tolerance of the axis (degrees)	±7	±5	±3	±2

Source: Adapted from American National Standards Institute. Prescription Ophthalmic Lenses—Recommendations. ANSI Z80.1-1995. Available from the American National Standards Institute, 11 West 42nd Street, New York, NY 10036. Reprinted with permission.

laboratory's own delivery service. The best method for any one practice will depend on where the practice is located. Delivery of orders should be discussed with the laboratory representative, and the method providing the quickest and most consistent delivery time should be used. Alternative methods for "rush jobs" should also be explored. Considerable cost can be attached to the delivery of orders, and this cost will be passed on to the patient either directly or indirectly. This factor should be considered and discussed when meeting with a laboratory representative.

Availability of frames is an important measure of service to patients. The inability of a laboratory to provide frames on a timely basis can be measured by the number of "back orders" or the length of time needed to complete orders because certain frames are unavailable. Frame lines that cannot be obtained in a timely manner and laboratories that cannot deliver frames should be discontinued. Patients should not be shown the frames of suppliers who do not have a stock of frames adequate to service the account.

COMPARING PRICES FOR FRAMES

Quality of materials and service from laboratories should be the most important factors in obtaining eyewear for patients. However, price is also a consideration. There is competition between quality laboratories, and there is often a difference in how they price their materials.

Basic lens charges among laboratories are easy to compare because laboratories publish price lists. Add-on costs for certain lens powers, special base curves, oversize blanks, specific lens centering, prism, tints, coatings, and similar considerations are harder to compare. When these additional charges are added to the order by the laboratory, they must be passed on to the patient. Thus, the practitioner must know how much these charges are and when they apply, because they must be built into the fee schedule used for patients. If two or more laboratories provide services, the practitioner should compare the invoices for similar prescriptions and determine the most reasonable fee for the services.

Table 13.4. Tolerance on Addition Power for Multifocal and Progressive Addition Lenses*

Nominal value of addition power (D)	Up to 4.00	>4.00
Nominal value of the tolerance on the addition power (D)	±0.12	±0.18

*If the manufacturer applies corrections to compensate for the as-worn position, then the tolerances apply to the corrected value and this corrected value must also be stated in the documentation.
Source: Adapted from American National Standards Institute. Prescription Ophthalmic Lenses—Recommendations. ANSI Z80.1-1995. Available from the American National Standards Institute, 11 West 42nd Street, New York, NY 10036. Reprinted with permission.

Table 13.5. Tolerances on Prism Reference Point Location and Prismatic Power

Prismatic power (Δ)	Tolerance (Δ)
0.00 up to 2.00	±0.25
over 2.00 up to 10.00	±0.37
over 10.00	±0.50

Source: Adapted from American National Standards Institute. Prescription Ophthalmic Lenses—Recommendations. ANSI Z80.1-1995. Available from the American National Standards Institute, 11 West 42nd Street, New York, NY 10036. Reprinted with permission.

It is standard practice for laboratories to award discounts to practitioners who pay their laboratory bills promptly. Many laboratories also offer different prices based on the volume of orders. These business practices encourage optometrists to use a single source for all laboratory work. These advantages should always be discussed and explored with laboratory sales representatives.

Use of discounting techniques can make a big difference in the pricing of ophthalmic materials and in the contribution of the sales of materials to practice income and profit. Ideally, an internal accounting system (e.g., pegboard, computer) should be able to identify profit and cost centers in the practice. Comparing the cost for materials in the practice to average costs for the profession is one method of evaluating fees for materials and laboratory bills. Surveys of laboratory costs usually report their findings by comparing the cost of materials to the practice gross income. Over the years, surveys of optometrists have shown that laboratory bills constitute 28–30% of gross income. If the cost of materials exceeds $35,000 for every $100,000 of gross income the practice produces, the material costs are too high or the fees for materials are too low (see Chapter 21 for a further discussion).

UNDERSTANDING LABORATORY PRACTICES

Many laboratories have policy statements regarding the management of practitioner accounts. These policies should be reviewed with the laboratory representative. Some manufacturers will guarantee patient satisfaction—often in the form of warranties—to encourage the prescribing or dispensing of new products to patients. The laboratory is given the responsibility of ensuring that these policies are properly administered. Does the policy mean the laboratory will remake an order in another lens material at no charge? Will a credit be given to the account if the new lens material is more expensive? Will a voucher or certificate be issued by the manufacturer? Practitioners should understand laboratory policies before using any products being presented.

Laboratory policies vary on remake orders and doctor errors. Any remakes that are necessary because the ophthalmic materials do not satisfy ANSI tolerances should be performed on a no-charge basis. Some laboratories will charge 50% or less on the remake if an order is transmitted incorrectly by the practitioner. The same policy is often offered if it is necessary to modify an order after the spectacles have been dispensed to the patient because of doctor error. These policies should be clarified when a practitioner first establishes a working relationship with a laboratory. They can make a difference in satisfaction with the laboratory and also in the cost of doing business.

PLACING LABORATORY ORDERS

Transmission of orders in an expedient, accurate, and complete manner is a joint responsibility of the practitioner and the laboratory. Before the advent of toll-free telephone numbers and facsimile transmission, and in the days of dependable mail service, laboratory orders were mailed at the end of the day. The use of mail was more likely if the optometrist was in a different city or state than the laboratory. Many laboratories still encourage the use of mail since written orders can be processed as they are received, when personnel are available. Mail delivery also reduces the expense of needing staff to take phone orders. The advantage of telephone orders is that they enable the laboratory to maintain personal contact with the optometrist or office staff while ensuring that all information to fabricate the eyewear will be received. In addition, laboratories with a computer inventory of frames can alert the caller to any possible delays in the order or can request that the frame be sent if it is not in stock.

Currently, the preferred method for communicating laboratory orders is by facsimile transmission. While the use of facsimile transmission saves staff time at both the office and the laboratory, it also requires that orders be complete and legible. There are times when UPS, U.S. mail, or an express service might be required for an order—for instance, when using a laboratory that does not supply frames or if using a large number of frames from other vendors. In these instances, the most expedient way to get the order completed is to send the frame, from stock, to the laboratory. Ordering the frame from another vendor and having it sent directly to the laboratory might also be necessary. If the frame received is the incorrect color or size, the error cannot be recognized by the fabricating laboratory. A practitioner must inspect and verify orders before the eyewear is dispensed to patients, however, and the in-office inspection by the staff should

detect the error before the eyewear is dispensed to the patient.

CONCLUSION

The dispensing of eyewear has been the basis of optometry's unified service to the public. Although there are many challenges in carrying out this important professional function, the selection and use of efficient laboratories and ophthalmic suppliers will contribute greatly to making this a satisfying part of practice.

BIBLIOGRAPHY

Allergan, Inc. Pathways in Optometry. Irvine, CA: Allergan, 1990.

American Optometric Association. Caring for the Eyes of America: a Profile of the Optometric Profession. St. Louis: American Optometric Association, 1992.

Anonymous. Eight ways to improve your spectacle dispensing. Rev Optom 1994;138(10):18–9.

Anonymous. Ophthalmic suppliers and sources directory: optical laboratory supplies. Rev Optom 1994;1 31(3):115–9.

Aron F, Bennett I. The 1990s, a decade for ophthalmic lenses: results of AOA surveys of laboratories and practitioners. Optom Econ 1992;2(10):17–21.

Bargman B, Yoho A. Get more out of your optical lab. Optom Manage 1993;28(5):33–6.

Bennett I. Management for the Eyecare Practitioner. Stoneham, MA: Butterworth, 1993.

Bennett I. Pricing ophthalmic frames. Optom Manage 1988;23(11):101–3.

Bierstock SR. Inventory control for the optical dispensary. Ocular Surg News 1994;12(6):23.

Brassfield A. We tamed the frame game. Optom Manage 1994;29(9):83–6.

Brogan R. After the implementation: increased patient returns and a higher level of quality dispensings. Optician 1993;205(5399):19–20.

Bruneni JL. Dispensing new frame materials. Optom Econ 1993;3(9):10–5.

Carlson AS. The importance of good dispensing in the modern optometric practice. S Afr Optom 1993;52(3):15.

Edlow R, Aron F. Labs, frames, buying groups: results of three AOA practice characteristics surveys. Optom Econ 1991;1(3):33–5.

Fanelli J. How to stock your primary care practice. Rev Optom 1989;126(2):73–6.

Gailmard NB. Consultant's corner: make your patients start seeing double. Imaging system helps patients decide on frames. Rev Optom 1994;131(9):27.

Gregg CP. The optical laboratory: state of the art today. Eyecare Tech 1993(Suppl);3(1):42–4.

Gottlieb H. Finding lost profits in ophthalmology: medical eyewear dispensing requires service-oriented mindsets. Ocular Surg News 1994;12(10):18.

Kirkner R. Frames market outlook: time to pay the piper—get ready for higher prices and standardized bar coding. Rev Optom 1992;129(9):59–65.

Lee J. How to avoid the "7 deadly sins" of dispensing. Optom Manage 1994;29(6):44–6.

Maul JR. Getting control of your frames. Optom Econ 1991;1(5):22–3.

Outcault RF, Johnson PM. Setting up to sell: is your dispensary merchandising keeping pace with the demands of today's patients? Optom Econ 1994;4(9):27–8.

Schwartz CA. Minimize inventory and maximize return: put stock where it's needed, when it's needed. Rev Optom 1992;129(9):51–4.

Chapter 14

In-House Laboratories

Donald H. Lakin

Don't be penny wise and pound foolish.

—Benjamin Franklin
Poor Richard's Almanac

At the time Benjamin Franklin wrote the often-quoted words above, the predecessors of modern optometrists were laboring in optical shops. In these shops, run by opticians, the need for vision testing became apparent, and during the nineteenth century the "refracting" optician emerged. When, at the end of the nineteenth century, these individuals sought legal recognition as an independent profession, they separated themselves from "dispensing" opticians. Through the years a guiding principle of clinical optometry has been that the practitioner who performs the examination is the best individual to determine the suitability of the eyewear prescribed. For this reason, the fabrication of eyewear has been a consistent part of optometric practice. Even though optometry has continued to evolve into a primary eye care profession, the fabrication and dispensing of ophthalmic materials has remained an important part of an optometrist's service to the public.

Surveys of practice patterns conducted during the 1980s and 1990s indicated that optometrists are increasing fabrication and dispensing services so that they can provide the quickly produced, cost-efficient, high-quality eyewear demanded by today's consumers. An essential part of the effort to provide these services is to establish an in-office finishing laboratory. Surveys in the mid-1990s of optometrists who own these in-house laboratories revealed that:

- 50% of practitioners edge their own lenses
- 65% tint lenses themselves
- 28% provide coatings (e.g., ultraviolet, scratch-resistance)

It seems likely that these numbers will only increase in succeeding years.

There are several considerations regarding patient care, equipment needs and costs, staffing, lens inventory maintenance, space requirements, and liability issues that influence the use of in-house laboratories. Perhaps the most important consideration, however, is the improved service that can be offered to patients. Optometrists who would require several days to deliver eyewear to patients can reduce the period to 1–2 days, or even a matter of hours if necessary. The "1-hour" service promoted by large chains and optical corporations is not demanded by most patients. In fact, patients are often skeptical of immediate service and worry that the quality will be inferior to eyewear that requires more time to fabricate. Optometrists in private practice can assure patients of quality service, and they also can control the timing of orders. If there is a need for a particular order to be completed rapidly, it can be given precedence. Patients are particularly grateful for timely service during emergencies. This capacity can assist greatly in the effort to maintain a patient's loyalty to the practitioner.

There is also marketing potential in having an in-house laboratory. Even without promotion, most patients perceive an in-office laboratory as being an asset. Patients assume that the practitioner has become more up-to-date and that a more efficient service will be provided. Optometrists who have in-house laboratories might find that the quality of ophthalmic materials is more consistent than when materials are obtained from outside laboratories. Certainly, the level of responsibility for eyewear increases when there is an in-house laboratory. The same strict tolerances for lens powers, lens centering, and finishing work must be provided by the in-house laboratory as would be expected if the work were done independently. That means there will be a "spoilage rate" as part of the cost of doing business. In well-run laboratories, this rate should be no more than 2–4%. To maintain a low rate, there must be a commitment, by the individuals performing the laboratory work, to the delivery of high-quality materials. If work is produced that does not meet accepted tolerances (see Chapter 13), however, it must be rejected and remade. In fact, this work is more rapidly performed and better controlled if it is performed in-house; reinspection and dispensing can more likely be provided within the time frame expected by the patient than if an outside laboratory has to remake, reinspect, and redeliver the order.

Cost is also a factor in deciding to install an in-office laboratory. The escalating fabrication costs for eyewear obtained from outside laboratories is cited by many optometrists as a key reason for establishing an in-house laboratory. When using outside laboratories for all fabrication work, the cost of ophthalmic materials averages 28–30% of gross income. This expenditure is obviously sizable, but is the effort to reduce laboratory costs "penny-wise and pound-foolish"? The costs of maintenance for machinery and of ophthalmic materials can cut—or even eliminate—profits, especially in practices with low lens volumes. The number of lenses that will be finished in-house is an important factor in determining if the laboratory will be worth the financial commitment. Recordkeeping will be necessary to determine if profit is being realized. Sound financial management demands that the optometrist determine the costs of operating a laboratory and make an effort to control these costs. There will be capital outlay for equipment, expenses related to maintenance, costs related to the purchase of materials, additional expenditures for utilities (e.g., electricity, water), and wages to be paid for labor.

Even considering all the aforementioned factors, many optometrists have found the operation of an in-house laboratory to be highly successful, although profitability is directly tied to the number of lenses finished per week. For example, in practices that finish 40–60 pairs of lenses per week, optometrists report savings of $6–8 per pair on stock single vision lenses and $10–12 per pair on bifocals. These savings can also make the optometrist more competitive in terms of the prices for ophthalmic materials.

Labor costs will affect economic projections considerably. In practices with a low volume of orders, it might be appropriate to use the "unfilled" time of office staff or to have the finishing work performed by the optometrist rather than to hire another employee. Optometrists just beginning a practice will most likely not have the patient volume to justify setting up an in-house laboratory. As the practice becomes established, however, the viability of a laboratory becomes more certain. In fact, there are cases in which optometrists in young practices have found that working in their own laboratories contributed to availability, service, and cost containment more than working for other practitioners outside the office 1 or 2 days a week.

In a multipractitioner office, an in-house laboratory can be quite successful. The per-unit cost can be competitive, not only with the costs of outside laboratories but also with those of buying cooperatives composed of groups of optometrists. A full-time employee—often an optician—will probably be necessary because of the volume of orders. Overhead costs should be computed so that the "break even" volume can be determined. For example, it can be calculated that 300 pairs of lenses must be finished per month to break even. All orders above that figure represent profit. The effect of a financially successful in-house laboratory will be to lower the cost of ophthalmic materials below the 28–30% of gross income that is typical for most practices; in fact, material costs can drop considerably below 30% when volume is high. Optometrists successfully using in-house laboratories routinely report savings of up to 25–35% of laboratory costs.

Figure 14.1. View of an in-office laboratory.

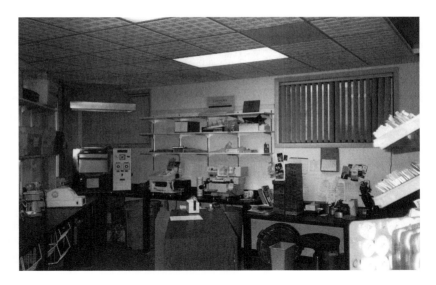

Figure 14.2. Lens-tinting device.

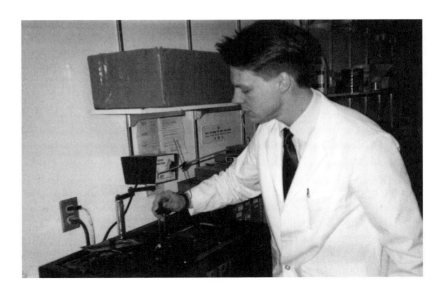

The availability of these laboratory services, when combined with a quality product, will inevitably contribute to practice growth.

The usual interest is in finishing laboratories, but, with the newer available equipment, which allows a practitioner to control the entire service, the surfacing function of lens fabrication has been added to some in-office laboratories. The use of surfacing equipment requires a higher volume to break even or generate a profit for the practice.

EQUIPMENT NEED AND COSTS

There is considerable variance in the cost of equipment needed to set up a finishing laboratory (Figure 14.1). Costs will depend on the functions to be performed—edging, tinting, coating, or all three—and whether new or used equipment is purchased (Figure 14.2). A practitioner must consider if it is wise to spend the money required to purchase mod-

Table 14.1. Basic Equipment For an
In-House Finishing Laboratory

Edger: Cuts the unfinished lens to the shape of the frame. An extra set of diamond wheels is suggested, for use when the regular wheels must be sharpened. Many edgers are available that dry edge CR-39 and polycarbonate lenses with all types of finishes— groove, facet, bevel—in about 40 seconds.

Lens groover: Used for nylon suspension frames.

Layout marker: Marks the optical center of the lens.

Layout blockers: Holds the lens in place during layout marking.

Blocker: Holds the lens in place during edging or grooving.

Frame warmer: Available with many different types of heat conductors; some also have coolers.

Lensmeter: Internal-reading models and projection-type models available.

Lensclock: Measures the base curves of the lens.

Dying tank/tinting unit: For tinting lenses.

Coating machine (open): For special lens coatings.

Drop ball testing apparatus: To verify impact resistance.

---

ern high-tech equipment. At optical shows for optometrists, at least one out of eight exhibitors will display new optical laboratory equipment. Patternless edgers can be purchased with computer memory and different types of finish; such an item can be the centerpiece of a laboratory. Much of this equipment does not require the skills of a trained laboratory optician to operate and can be a good investment. Surveys of optometrists with in-house laboratories indicate that the cost of finishing laboratory equipment ranges between $7,000 and $20,000. A list of basic equipment needed to start a finishing laboratory and a brief description of the function of each piece of equipment can be found in Table 14.1. With more than 80% of the ophthalmic lenses sold today being made of plastic (including polycarbonate), many practitioners choose not to fabricate glass lens orders and thus do not invest in chemical treating units. Table 14.1 does not include a heat treatment or chemical hardening unit. If a practitioner decides to include glass lenses, a chemical treating unit should be considered. A realistic projection of the number of glass lenses that will be fabricated should be undertaken before investing in this equipment.

The cost of a surfacing laboratory is also dependent on the range of equipment purchased.

Most optometrists put this cost at between $40,000 and $80,000. A surfacing generator, two cylinder machines, a computer, and a layout blocker make up the largest part of this investment. When put into operation, the surfacing laboratory will realize savings of up to 70%, as compared to outside laboratory costs for bifocal, progressive, polarized, and high-index lenses. To break even, approximately 25–30 pairs of lenses must be surfaced each day. There are a number of injection mold systems for plastic lenses on the market. Some questions about the ability of this method to consistently provide a quality product remain unresolved. The same thing can also be said of wafer systems. The optometrist considering these two methods should explore the equipment currently on the market, and, before making a purchase, the practitioner should visit the offices of optometrists who are already using the equipment.

As of 1992, approximately 6% of optometrists performed lens surfacing themselves (Figure 14.3). About 75% of these practitioners did the work in the office; the other 25% sent the work to a separate facility. Less than 2% of all optometrists offer lens coating services. Of these practitioners, a little more than half do the work in-office, and the remainder send the work to a separate facility that they own.

No matter what equipment is purchased, if something goes wrong with it, a service representative should be available right away. The ability to troubleshoot and operate equipment is usually acquired with experience. Optometrists who are novices at working with laboratory equipment should probably purchase it new. Often, when new equipment is delivered, it is set up by the seller, who will also provide instruction to the practitioner and the staff.

LABORATORY STAFF

The first step in human resource management is to have a plan. In Chapters 16 and 17, the economic aspects of quantifying the personnel needs of a practice are discussed. If an in-house laboratory is to be a service and profit center for the practice, economic planning is critical. A full-time employee might not be necessary for this service. The employee's status is usually dependent on the size

Figure 14.3. Hand polishing lens edges.

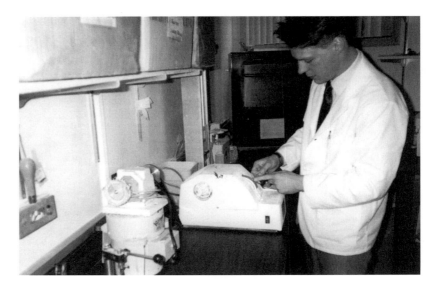

of the laboratory. When beginning a laboratory, if a technician or optician currently employed by the practice has the necessary technical background or is interested in running a laboratory, this individual can be assigned laboratory duties part-time. This person should possess good organizational skills and be able to run the laboratory as an assembly line, keeping several jobs in progress at one time. This person should also be orderly and efficient and take as much pride in the work produced as the practitioner. The time devoted to laboratory functions should be charged to optical supplies to run the laboratory as a separate profit center (Figure 14.4). The time charged to optical supplies should be equal to the time actually spent on laboratory work. It is best to have the laboratory person responsible for ordering uncut lenses and maintaining stock lenses.

In some practices, workers from other offices or optical laboratories can be chosen to "moonlight" when the laboratory is first started. If the optometrist does not have the time or background to train a staff member, an experienced optician can serve as a coach for a staff member who wants to learn laboratory work. Equipment manufacturers and distributors usually offer optometrists an in-office training program for the staff. Training can include instruction on how to use the equipment and in pertinent nomenclature.

Knowledge of parts facilitates repair—especially when that repair must be performed by telephone—since the technician can describe precisely the part or function that requires repair.

If there is enough work to keep an employee busy full-time, and the practitioner is fortunate enough to hire a trained laboratory optician, it might be necessary to orient this person to the private practice environment. Most successful optical laboratories are very production oriented. Although skilled and efficient, a laboratory optician might have a factory attitude toward work. It is hoped that a practice will be service oriented; desired work patterns and practice goals should be discussed at the time of hiring.

Finding trained laboratory technicians can be a problem, especially in smaller communities. Some larger cities will have optical laboratory technician programs that are taught in trade schools. These schools are good sources for employees. Often, individuals working in large laboratories want to move into a clinical environment. An in-house laboratory will provide an opportunity to make this move, and an offer for the individual to participate in dispensing can prove to be an additional inducement. A help wanted advertisement, or an advertisement offering to train a qualified applicant, will often bring additional individuals into the applicant pool. The ophthalmic industry is a relatively small

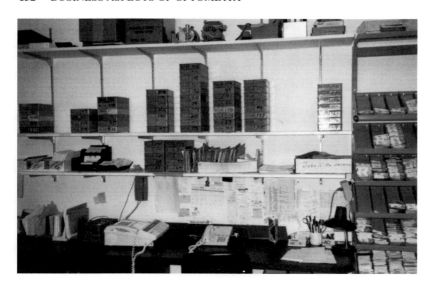

Figure 14.4. In-office ordering desk and stock area.

community, and a conversation with local optometrists, frame sales representatives, or employees of the practice can result in the recommendation of qualified individuals.

LENS INVENTORY

To intelligently develop a plan for lens inventory, it is necessary to know what materials will be prescribed and the relative frequency with which they will be used. Many in-house laboratories will limit inventory to plastic and polycarbonate lenses because glass lenses must be hardened to impart impact resistance to the lenses. Lenses purchased for stock can be bought in quantity at a lower price than on a per lens basis. Usually an optical supply house will offer the best price on quantities of 75 pairs or more. When the initial order is made, and continuous re-ordering for stock is anticipated, the practitioner can usually negotiate with the seller to obtain the same per unit price on reorders for stock or to buy lenses out of the stock range. As stock is taken from inventory, lens envelopes should be used to place re-orders, which can be daily, or at least weekly, based on volume.

Most in-office laboratories start with two pairs of lenses for each parameter stocked. In plastic, stock should be maintained up to plus or minus 3

diopters for spherical lenses and up to 2 diopters for cylindrical lenses. If scratch-resistant coatings are frequently used in the practice, coated blanks should be considered, for they are the least expensive way to offer coated lenses. Pricing should be investigated for various size lens blanks. Because the minimum thickness of minus lenses is in the center, using larger blanks than needed will not affect the quality of the work. With plus lenses, larger blanks will affect quality, because smaller lenses are needed for smaller eye sizes. Depending on the number of lenses that will be needed, and the variables chosen, the cost of a plastic lens inventory can vary somewhat from practitioner to practitioner.

If polycarbonate and high-index plastic lenses are not used frequently, they should be ordered on a per case basis. Because of safety considerations, many practitioners routinely prescribe polycarbonate lenses for all children, monocular patients, active adults, and athletic use. If polycarbonate materials are frequently prescribed, they should be stocked in the same manner as other plastic lenses. Polycarbonate and other high-index materials used for high prescriptions are usually ordered on a per case basis, since they are often beyond stock range and need to be surfaced. Because of the higher unit cost of polycarbonate lenses, a polycarbonate lens stock will require a slightly higher investment.

If a practitioner decides to fabricate glass lenses, stock should include spherical lenses up to plus and minus 2 diopters and up to 2 diopters of cylinder for each power. Today, glass is frequently prescribed as a photochromatic lens; in some practices, the percentage of photochromatic lenses is as high as 70%. For practitioners who have made the additional investment of a chemical treating unit, it can be advantageous to stock photochromatic blanks.

Compound multifocals are all surfaced lenses. Stock multifocal spherical lenses are usually available in plus powers only. Most in-house laboratories do not stock these lenses. Practitioners must know the ranges stocked by optical supply houses and use them when patients require this type of lens. Stock multifocal spherical lenses are usually less expensive than surfaced bifocal blanks. When buying uncut surfaced lens blanks in multifocals or single-vision lenses beyond stock ranges, laboratory representatives should be asked for their volume uncut price list. Many full-service laboratories have a small differential in price between uncut blanks and complete prescriptions to maintain the same profit margin on both. Laboratories with greater surfacing capabilities and an awareness of the market niche of in-house fabricating practices will be considerably more competitive in pricing uncut lens blanks.

These considerations should be explored, and the practice volume should be realistically evaluated before investing in a lens surfacing operation. If another practice has invested in a surfacing or lens molding system and has a surfacing capacity beyond their needs, this situation could also be a good source to explore.

SPACE REQUIREMENTS

The location of the laboratory and its space requirements will vary considerably, depending on volume and how fabrication is perceived as part of the optometric product. Ideally, the laboratory should occupy a separate room, at least 10 feet × 10 feet, with adequate ventilation (for chemicals). The laboratory will require several counter-top electrical outlets, and these outlets should be on two or three different circuit breakers to avoid blowing fuses. Since a finishing laboratory tends to be noisy, it should be located as far from the examination room as possible.

For a busy practice with a full-time employee performing both glass and plastic lens finishing and a second employee performing the ordering, there should be at least 400 square feet of space. If lens surfacing is included, 1,000 will be needed. In computing the cost of materials sold, the expense of this space (and maintaining it) must be considered.

When planning an office that includes a laboratory, these location and space requirements should be discussed with the designer. Some practitioners might plan the location of the laboratory adjacent to the frame room, with a window that allows patients to look into the laboratory; this emphasizes the image of a "complete" eye care facility. In such cases, the laboratory can even be located in the front of the office and enclosed with a soundproof glass window so that, on entering the facility, patients can see that eyewear fabrication is part of the service. Other practitioners might want the laboratory placed out of sight in the back of the facility to maintain a more "professional" image. This function of optometric practice often polarizes practitioners, who want optometry to be accepted as a primary eye care profession while continuing to meet the needs of patients for quality eyewear. Only a realistic assessment of the marketplace will lead to the "right" decision for any one practice.

LIABILITY ISSUES

The advantages of having an in-house laboratory are affected by the added legal responsibility of fabricating lenses that are sold directly to patients. From a liability standpoint, the most important consideration is impact resistance.

Federal regulations regarding impact resistance—which have been incorporated into ANSI standard Z80.1–1995—state that all dress lenses "shall be capable of" withstanding a drop ball test. The standard provides, however, that plastic lenses, laminated lenses, and raised edge multifocal lenses can be tested in statistically significant samples by the manufacturer. Therefore, only glass lenses have to be tested individually for impact resistance by the fabricator of the eyewear.

If prescription safety eyewear is provided, a different set of requirements must be met. The requirements for safety lenses—which are derived from ANSI standard Z87.1–1989—require a drop ball test, a minimum lens thickness (3 mm), and the use of a logo, which must be placed on the lens edge by the lens fabricator. Safety lenses must be placed in a safety frame (identified by the Z87 logo) to constitute "safety glasses."

All optometrists should have adequate professional liability insurance. Practitioners who dispense eyewear should have coverage for both negligence and professional liability claims. Because assistants or opticians are frequently involved with the fabrication and dispensing of ophthalmic materials, the policy should cover claims arising out of their actions. Coverage should also provide for instances in which these employees are injured (e.g., from accidents occurring during the fabrication or dyeing of eyewear). All optometrists who fabricate materials in the office should be sure that liability insurance covers these eventualities. The best way to check insurance coverage is to review the policy with an insurance agent and to have the agent identify the specific language that provides coverage.

Liability claims involving the fabrication of eyewear are not common, because optometrists are required to inspect eyewear to ensure that it meets legal standards for impact resistance. Optometrists who establish in-house laboratories should make certain that these obligations are met before eyewear is dispensed.

BIBLIOGRAPHY

American Optometric Association. Caring for the Eyes of America: a Profile of the Optometric Profession. St. Louis: American Optometric Association, 1992.

Anonymous. Practice management, retail and lab software. Eyecare Tech 1993;3(2):17–19, 22–5, 34.

Aron F, Bennett I. The 1990s, a decade for ophthalmic lenses: results of AOA surveys of laboratories and practitioners. Optom Econ 1992;2(10):17–21.

Barnett D. The building blocks of an in-office lens lab. Rev Optom 1992;129(10):37–40.

Bostick D. Surfacing solo: making a lab work for you. Optom Manage 1990;25(4):59–62.

Bulmlein S. Introducing in-practice prescription laboratories. Optician 1991;201(5300):18–21.

Hunter MA. Profile of Greames Optical: full comprehensive prescription laboratory. Optom Today (Britain) 1993; 33(19):22.

Kloos SA. Running your own in-office lab, ups and downs. Optom Manage 1989;24(5):57–60.

Legerton JA. In-office laboratories: control or chaos? Optom Econ 1993;3(10):24–8.

Maino JH. Moving the in-house lab into the 21st century. Computers in Eyecare 1992;2(3):51–4.

Ossip G. Should you start a finishing lab? Optom Manage 1993;28(10):32–4.

Rusynko T. Don't lose your edge with an on-site lab—they're not for everyone. Rev Optom 1993;130(9):45–8.

Underwood WB. Setting up your own in-office lab: what you should know. Eyecare Tech 1994;4(1):63–4.

Part III
Practice Administration

Chapter 15

Organizing an Office

Craig Hisaka, John Rumpakis, John G. Classé, and C. Thomas Crooks, III

Good order is the foundation of all good things.

—Edmund Burke
Reflections on the Revolution in France

In the past, it was possible for practitioners to completely ignore the business operation of a practice and concentrate on serving patients, yet still earn a comfortable income. Today, with the soaring cost of operating an optometric practice, the decrease in third-party reimbursement rates, a competitive marketplace, the expanding scope of optometric care, and the influence of managed care organizations on health care services, if the business aspect of a practice is neglected, the effect will be to create an inefficient practice. This lack of efficiency will require the practitioner to work longer hours to meet expenses and will cause an erosion of the quality of care.

There are two components of an optometric practice: a professional component and a business component. The professional component involves the practitioner's efforts at providing quality care to patients. The optometrist is trained to provide care; thus, a practitioner spends most of the day in this area. To provide quality care, the practitioner invests time and money to improve technical skills and purchases modern instrumentation to improve accuracy and efficiency of testing. The business component involves the administration of the practice. Even though the optometrist might not be trained in this area, it should be given as much time, effort, and energy as the professional component. The skills and personality needed to be an effective manager and administrator are dif-

ferent from the skills required to be an effective health care practitioner. Maximizing the efficiency of the business component of a practice will result in an environment in which the practitioner will be able to provide the best quality of care for patients. If a practice is not efficient, organized, and properly managed, the quality of care will eventually be compromised. In any community, the most successful practitioners are those who provide a high quality of care due to the acceptance and integration of successful business concepts into the practice.

The purpose of this chapter is to provide basic guidelines for organizing a private practice. Ideally, if a practitioner spends 40 hours seeing patients, the practitioner should spend the same amount of time—40 hours—in office administration. However, the reality is that most practice time will be allocated to patient care. Despite the burdens of these professional duties, there are some essential administrative tasks that must be performed. If the practice is new, there are a number of responsibilities that the practitioner faces in just preparing the practice to open for business.

GETTING STARTED

When beginning a private practice it is essential that the practitioner obtain a support network of advisors.

137

Professional consultants can provide valuable advice, and good business strategies are as important to the stability of a practice as satisfied patients. The practitioner should establish relationships with a banker, attorney, accountant, and insurance agent. These relationships are essential to the organization of a practice. A banker is needed because loans and business and personal checking accounts need to be obtained at a full-service bank. An attorney can be consulted for advice and assistance related to the type of business organization being formed (i.e., sole proprietorship, partnership, professional association or corporation) and the legal steps required to begin the business. An accountant will be needed to provide advice and assistance about the withholding and paying of taxes. An insurance agent should be consulted to obtain office contents insurance, disability insurance, office overhead insurance, life insurance, premises liability insurance, malpractice coverage, or any other insurance coverage needed for the protection of health, home, and personal property.

One of the most valuable means of evaluating a potential advisor is simply asking other professionals about the advisor's reputation. If other health care providers have found the advisor's services to be helpful and reasonable, it is a good sign. A meeting should be scheduled to discuss how the advisor can be helpful and the cost of the advisor's assistance. At this meeting it is appropriate to inquire about the advisor's years of experience and how the advisor keeps up-to-date with current trends, legislation, and clients' needs.

A key task for the beginning practitioner is the formation of an office staff. To identify potential staff members, advertisements or other means of contacting qualified applicants should be used. The standard process of interview and evaluation of candidates should be followed (see Chapter 16).

Another important task is to contact representatives of optical laboratory and frame and contact lens manufacturers. A frame and contact lens inventory must be assembled, and accounts must be opened at the optical laboratories with which the practice will be doing business. In addition, inventories of supplies—such as ophthalmic drugs and solutions, stationery, business cards, appointment reminder cards, recall notices, magazine subscriptions, prescription pads, examination forms, and record folders—should be ordered. Fee schedules also need to be set.

The practitioner must enroll as a provider in third-party health care plans such as Medicare, Medicaid, Vision Service Plan, and medical insurance (e.g., Blue Cross/Blue Shield). If there are health maintenance organizations or other types of managed care panels in which the practitioner wishes to participate, enrollment should be solicited. If the practitioner is not already a member of the state optometric association, an application should be obtained and submitted.

Telephone service should be initiated (deadlines for inclusion in the annual directory need to be ascertained), and accounts with utility companies (electricity, gas, water) should be opened. Answering and paging services should be contacted, and janitorial services need to be obtained.

The visibility of the practice is important in attracting patients. Signs for the office, announcements of the opening in the newspaper, Yellow Pages listings, and other means of putting the public on notice should be secured.

These are but a few of the many tasks that await the new practitioner. A checklist should be devised so that omissions are kept to a minimum (Table 15.1).

PATIENT MANAGEMENT

Efficient patient management requires a coordinated effort from both practitioner and staff—combined with a well-rehearsed patient flow, effective communication, scrupulous bookkeeping, and conscientious attention to detail. To provide orderly management, the practitioner must organize the facility, the staff, and the paperwork. Staff members must be instructed about how the system is to be run. Ongoing evaluation is an integral part of an efficient office; regular meetings between practitioner and staff to identify and eliminate deficiencies are necessary. Coordination of effort can be achieved with adequate planning and experience, but cohesion between practitioner and staff requires a different form of interaction: trust. The staff must trust the practitioner to establish a workable plan, and the practitioner must trust the staff to carry it out. The trust between practitioner and staff must be mutual; if it is not, it will be apparent to patients that such is the case. Patients seek a satisfying relationship with both practitioner and

Table 15.1. Timetable of Things to Do When Starting a Private Practice

1 year before starting a practice

__ Obtain demographic and health resource data on the chosen practice location from books, guides, and the local chamber of commerce.

__ Visit the community to discuss the need for optometric services (optometrists, dentists, physicians, pharmacists, bankers, teachers, school nurses, real estate agents).

__ Talk with representatives from ophthalmic laboratories about opening a practice in the community.

__ Make site visits to determine the practice location. If possible, make a final decision on the practice location.

__ Contact the state Board of Optometry about the requirements for licensure. Obtain a copy of the state optometry laws.

__ Check on membership in local, state, and national professional societies.

__ Determine the date that information must be submitted to be included in the white and yellow page telephone directories. If possible, reserve an office telephone number.

__ Visit banks to meet bank officers. Obtain a loan application from the loan officer and determine the information and format needed to submit a proposal to obtain practice financing.

__ At the bank selected, open personal and business checking accounts.

__ Prepare a loan proposal to obtain the necessary capital for equipment and operation of the practice. Submit the application within the appropriate deadline.

9 months before starting a practice

__ Check the office site and determine if leasehold improvements will be needed. Obtain necessary estimates for the improvements.

__ Check with the local city hall or zoning board to determine the requirements of zoning ordinances that apply to the site chosen.

__ Determine office layout and design.

__ Determine office and professional equipment that will be needed.

__ Select professional advisors (accountant, attorney, banker, insurance agent, real estate agent).

__ Obtain bids on the purchase of office and professional equipment. Compare leasing vs. purchasing.

6 months before starting a practice

__ Obtain the services of an answering service (physician's exchange, beeper service, call forwarding).

__ Meet or talk with representatives of Medicare, Medicaid, and other third-party insurance carriers. Obtain provider numbers, prevailing fee schedule (Medicare), insurance claim forms, and copies of procedure codes (CPD-4) and diagnostic codes (ICD-9).

__ Obtain application for hospital privileges.

__ Order office record system.

__ Plan and order an accounts receivable or payable system.

__ Plan and order payroll accounting system.

__ Order sign for office.

__ Notify frame, contact lens, and pharmaceutical representatives of the practice.

__ Obtain county and city occupational licenses (from the county or city clerk or city hall).

3 months before starting a practice

__ Obtain professional liability insurance coverage.

__ Obtain office insurance (office overhead coverage, office liability, business interruption, employee fidelity bond, office contents). Umbrella coverage provides comprehensive catastrophic coverage for liability claims that are beyond the limits of regular insurance.

__ Determine if worker's compensation is required by state law by consulting with the state worker's compensation board or industrial commission.

__ Obtain health and accident insurance coverage for yourself and employees.

__ Obtain disability insurance coverage.

__ Obtain life insurance coverage.

__ Obtain automobile insurance coverage.

__ Arrange for telephone service and installation. Determine the telephone equipment and system to be purchased.

__ Consider credit arrangements for the office (American Express, Mastercard, Visa) and arrange for accounts to be established.

__ Order office opening announcements. Discuss the placement of advertisements in local newspapers.

__ Meet with local physicians who are potential referral sources. Send follow-up letters.

__ If there is a local referral service through the optometric society, provide the information needed to be listed.

__ Check on membership in local civic and religious organizations and join as appropriate.

__ Write to the state Department of Labor to obtain state employment regulations and wage and hour information.

__ Arrange for movers, if necessary.

__ Write preliminary job descriptions for employees. Obtain a specimen office procedures manual.

__ Begin the effort to locate employees for the office (advertising, interviewing).

__ Apply for your Federal Employer Identification Number from the Internal Revenue Service (form SS-4).

__ Apply for your state employer identification number through the state employment office or Department of Labor.

__ Obtain the Small Business Tax Guide (publication 334) and Your Federal Income Tax Guide (publication 17) from the Internal Revenue Service. Obtain the appropriate tax forms from the IRS and the state employment office or Department of Labor.

__ Obtain payroll withholding booklets for federal, state, and local taxes from the IRS.

__ Review tax withholding and reporting requirements with an accountant or tax attorney.

__ Choose and order an appointment scheduling book or system.

__ Arrange for appropriate office support services as needed (janitorial, snow removal, laundry service, lawn care).

__ Order clinical supplies and set up an inventory control system.

__ Order necessary business supplies (appointment cards, business cards, letterhead stationery and envelopes, patient recall notices, petty cash vouchers, deposit stamps for checks, prescription pads, purchase orders, preprinted telephone message pads).

__ If desired, meet with collections attorneys or agencies about the collection of unpaid accounts.

__ Determine fee schedule.

__ Select and order magazines for the reception area. Also select and order professional journals.

__ Purchase office equipment and furniture and arrange for their delivery to the office.

__ Arrange for laboratory services at optical laboratories.

__ Notify area pharmacies that you are starting a practice.

__ Select any patient information materials and have them printed or delivered.

__ Obtain a postage meter and a bulk mail permit, if necessary.

1 Month Before Starting a Practice

__ Start setting up the office.

__ If necessary, have the utilities turned on.

__ If not previously arranged, have signage displayed.

__ Hire and begin training office personnel, with emphasis on telephone techniques, appointments, collections procedures, office policies.

__ Begin making appointments.

__ Establish a petty cash fund.

__ Have announcements of the office opening published in the local news media.

__ Mail out announcements of the opening to local physicians, pharmacists, health groups, school nurses, and others as appropriate.

__ Hold an "open house."

__ Begin seeing patients.

Source: Adapted from DL Park. Optimum Timetable for Starting Your Practice. Uriah, CA: 1990.

staff. This requires that they be treated with respect, be rendered competent service, and be given individual attention. When these objectives are achieved, trust is the result. Trust is the cornerstone of patient loyalty, and it is an inevitable ally of efficient management.

The four cornerstones of effective patient management are availability, efficient patient flow, communication, and troubleshooting.

AVAILABILITY

Inefficient appointment schedules have long been a problem for optometrists. The availability of the practitioner is based on the policy decisions adopted by the practice:

- What days will the office be open?
- What will be the office hours?

- How much time will be allocated for each appointment?
- How will the practitioner's absences be managed?
- How will emergencies or "walk-ins" be served?

These are decisions that must be made at the outset of a new practice. Modifications can be incorporated into the schedule as the dictates of time permit.

Office Hours

Determining the days and hours available for patient examination depends on several factors: the cost of staff and office overhead, the needs of the patient population being served, the quality of life the practitioner wishes to enjoy, and similar considerations. When debating the scheduling of weekend or evening office hours, the practitioner should consider the long-term ramifications. Once these times are offered, it can be difficult to eliminate them. In competitive areas, where it is common to have two working spouses, it might be necessary to offer expanded hours of operation.

In many practices, the newest associates see patients in the evenings and on Saturdays. Since about 70% of U.S. family households have both the husband and wife working outside the home during the daytime hours, evening and weekend appointments are highly desirable in many communities. In fact, seeing patients in the evenings and on weekends allows new associates to develop their skills sooner and become partners. More important, patients deeply appreciate the extended office hours, and being open during unconventional business hours shows that the practitioner cares about the patients' needs.

Patient Scheduling

The allocation of time for appointments will differ according to service. Contact lens fits, eye health assessments, glaucoma follow-ups, and low vision examinations all require different amounts of time. The practitioner must determine the time to be allocated for each service, and the receptionist who schedules appointments must be told how to provide the proper amount of time for each patient. Of particular importance is the use of pupillary dilation, which adds time to the examination and changes the flow of patients.

Patient scheduling is a reflection of the philosophy of care. In many practices, each patient is scheduled for 45 minutes to an hour. The visual analysis not only consists of the traditional optometric procedures but also includes routine pupillary dilation and examination using the binocular indirect ophthalmoscope, assessment with a 60 D, 78 D, or 90 D fundus lens, Goldmann tonometry, blood pressure measurements, automated perimetry, and other tests. It is common to recall patients every 2 years for a routine visual analysis.

Checkup visits for contact lenses are typically scheduled for 30 minutes. A patient who is interested in being fitted for contact lenses is scheduled for a 1½-hour examination. Office visits are usually 30 minutes. There are two basic scheduling methods: The "stream" method of patient scheduling requires appointments to be equally spaced throughout the day in 1-hour or ½-hour intervals. The "wave" method entails scheduling patients in groups—for example, two patients are scheduled at 8:00 AM; one, at 8:45; and two, at 9:30. If one patient is late or if the optometrist needs more time with a patient, the wave will help average the time spent with each patient.

The use of pupillary dilation extends the amount of time needed for examination and disrupts the examination sequence. During the 15–30 minutes needed to achieve adequate dilation, the patient should be removed from the examination room so that it can be used for the evaluation of another patient. A special room can be set aside for patients who are waiting for dilation. They can be taken to the dispensary, they can be given a visual field test, or they can be returned to the waiting room. Management must be coordinated between practitioner and staff to ensure that efficient use is made of this time and that unnecessary delays are avoided.

It might be necessary to rehearse the movement of patients on a drawing of the office layout and to have "walk throughs" to ensure that patient flow is properly controlled. Meetings between the practitioner and staff members can also be used to identify problems and arrive at solutions.

Absence of the Practitioner

Practitioner absence not only affects availability but also disrupts continuity of care. If a practitioner is not available because of vacation, illness, or continuing education, a patient in need of care must seek another eye care provider. Coverage by other practitioners during these periods must be planned, and patients calling for care must be appropriately notified or directed to substitute clinicians by the practitioner's staff.

Patients seeking emergency or urgent care do not often call for appointments. An efficient office must be able to offer services to "walk-in" patients who require timely diagnosis and treatment. To manage these patients, many offices leave appointment slots open just before lunch and in the late afternoon, to ensure that time is available for examination.

When a patient calls for an appointment, the preferred method of scheduling is to offer the patient two specific dates and times and to permit the patient to choose the one that is most convenient. If neither time is acceptable, a third, compromise choice can be offered. The patient's name, status (new or former patient), and telephone number should be noted in the appointment log. Because changes in scheduling of appointments are inevitable, this information is written in pencil. Erasures can be used when necessary to change and refill appointment slots. Computerized appointment systems should also be flexible.

The patient should be reminded of the appointment prior to the scheduled time, and the receptionist should note in the log that this reminder has been given. A list of each day's appointments should be prepared for the practitioner and posted in the examination room or on the door to the room. A master list of patients can be maintained on computer, which can also keep track of "no shows," recalls, and referrals.

PATIENT FLOW

Patient flow for a new practice can be divided into three phases: the initial buildup of a patient base, which generally requires 5–7 years; the plateau, a period of two or three decades during which the practitioner enjoys a fairly stable patient base and income; and the preretirement phase, a period of declining practitioner involvement and patient flow, which can last 5–10 years.

For each of these phases, the demands of patient flow are different. This discussion describes general principles that can be applicable to any phase of practice.

Efficient movement of patients through the office is necessary to reduce patient waiting time, eliminate unnecessary delays, and keep "chair time" to a reasonable level. Efficiency is especially desirable when a practitioner has only one examination room. Of particular importance is the scheduling of patients. This has to be carefully planned but can be disrupted by the cancellation of appointments, appearance of unexpected "walk-ins," late arrival of patients, or misallocation of time for examination.

As soon as a patient enters the office, management is necessary. Time spent waiting to be examined should be kept to a reasonable minimum. This time can be used for the filling of forms and providing pertinent information. If a technician is available to assist the practitioner, the patient can be moved to a room for preliminary testing. This room can be an examination room or another room used for the purpose of initial evaluation. Then the patient can be moved to the examination room so that the practitioner can perform the necessary testing. After the practitioner has finished, the patient must usually be taken to the dispensary and, after that, to the waiting room or administrative office where financial details can be settled.

PATIENT COMMUNICATION

Nonverbal communication is of well-established importance: dress, conduct, and physical environment all assist in creating an impression—favorable or unfavorable—of the practitioner. Various written and verbal communications are also influential in forming a favorable impression of practitioner and practice. The most important forms of communication include:

• Reception of patients in the office
• Telephone conversations with patients
• Oral and written communications in the office
• Mailings to the patient

Each of these communication problems requires a brief commentary.

Reception of Patients

The reception room should be comfortable, clean, and capable of putting the patient at ease. Numerous decisions must be made to create an environment that achieves these goals. Is smoking permitted? Is there a play area for children? Is there adequate room for all patients? Are toilet facilities conveniently available? Is there a wide range of current reading material? Similar questions also need to be asked with regard to the decor of the reception room and the conduct of the receptionist. Unless all these considerations are planned (and evaluated periodically), an undesirable impression can be conveyed.

Telephone Conversations

The manner in which telephone queries are handled by a receptionist is of great significance; patients are frequently won or lost on the basis of these brief conversations. Practitioners must ensure that receptionists receive proper training in this vital area of patient communication. Many sources can be consulted to obtain this training, including telephone companies, practice management consultants, and various publications. Some basic considerations include:

- The telephone voice and personality of the receptionist should be an asset at all times.
- Telephone "busy signals" should be avoided with the use of the proper telephone technology.
- The receptionist should be capable of succinctly answering patient questions about examination fees and charges for materials.
- Telephones should be available in key areas of the office, such as the reception desk, the dispensary, and the practitioner's office.
- Receptionists should be able to triage patient complaints and schedule patients who require emergency or urgent care for same day examinations.

Receptionists are often questioned by patients about matters of clinical care that are outside their area of expertise. Receptionists should understand how to manage these situations so that patients are not offended and so that erroneous information is not conveyed.

Paper Flow

The average office has three typical avenues of distribution and dissemination of paper: information given directly to patients, prescriptions and other records of care, and follow-up mailings such as bills, recall notices, and newsletters.

Patient information includes brochures, instructional booklets, fitting agreements for contact lenses, and similar documents. These items can be especially useful with contact lens patients, when medicines are prescribed, or if patient education is needed for a complex condition such as glaucoma.

Records should be carefully controlled. Although the practitioner is the owner of the record, the patient generally has a right to review the information in the record, and that right should be respected. Policies for the release of contact lens prescriptions should be adopted in all offices and should conform with the requirements of state law. When patients move or change practitioners and request the transfer of records, it is preferable to provide a summary rather than a verbatim copy. The practitioner should always retain the original record for the period of time required by law.

Follow-up mailings such as newsletters can be used to provide information on new services or instruments, while cards thanking a source of referrals can be used as a practice builder, and computer-generated reminder notices can personalize the effort to provide recall. The ways in which follow-up mailings can be used to communicate more effectively with patients is limited only by the ingenuity of the practitioner.

Management does not end after a patient leaves the office. It might be necessary to schedule the patient to return for the dispensing of ophthalmic materials, to recall the patient for further examination, or to refer the patient to another health care provider. The appropriate steps must be taken to ensure that the patient understands when and where to go. Patient communication is an integral part of efficient management.

TROUBLESHOOTING

It is inevitable that, occasionally, difficulties will arise in the management of patients and that troubleshooting will be required. These problems are often of acute onset, trying to both the practitioner and the staff, and difficult to resolve. If managed improperly, the effect can involve not just one patient, but several. Patient control is more easily achieved if procedures have been developed for management. Also, patient satisfaction is more likely.

Although there are numerous potential sources of conflict with patients, the most common situations involve fees, ophthalmic materials, and prescriptions. Some pointers for troubleshooting in these situations:

- With the complexities of third-party care, mistakes do occur. Make sure a knowledgeable staff member (or the practitioner) reviews the billing before telling the patient no mistake was made.
- Complaints about fees should be answered honestly and openly; candor is never inappropriate in such a situation.
- Be certain that spectacles are correct before debating the fact with a patient.
- Do not be reluctant to recheck refractions or other sources of patient dissatisfaction.
- If ophthalmic materials are incorrect, make them right.
- Try to resolve patient disputes in an amicable fashion. Arguments do not contribute to the benefit of the practice.
- Establish a written office policy for the release of contact lens prescriptions.
- To reduce conflicts over contact lens prescriptions, de-emphasize charges for materials such as contact lenses and place more emphasis on fees for services.
- Use prepaid service agreements for contact lens patients.
- Offer patients a spectacle prescription (if needed) after the examination is concluded.

One of the keys to effective troubleshooting is to project confidence when dealing with the patient. Although confidence is an attribute that is easily communicated to a patient, it is also one that is just as evident in its absence. To feel confident, technical expertise is required. Education does not end after graduation from school; it persists throughout the professional lifetime of the practitioner. Knowledge is often the difference between settling a problem and leaving the patient dissatisfied. Optometrists should work diligently to keep up with technical developments and to use them for the benefit of those they serve.

Another key to projecting confidence is to have an established method for management of the problem. Such methodology is usually the result of experience or of trial and error, but common sense will often go a long way in attempting to resolve patient disputes. Both practitioner and staff must discuss and develop ways of efficiently dealing with patient management problems. Efficiency is a learned skill that repays many times the time spent in its acquisition. It is of unquestionable assistance in developing effective patient control.

PERSONNEL MANAGEMENT

Undisputedly, among the most challenging tasks faced by a practitioner are the hiring, training, supervision, and dismissal of personnel. These tasks are described in detail in Chapters 16 and 17. The organization of personnel and the description of their duties is best achieved through the use of an office procedures manual. This manual should outline the standard operating procedures that have been agreed on for the orderly, day-to-day management of the practice. The specific duties assigned to each employee, employee compensation, procedures for personnel evaluation and dismissal, and many other items are described in the manual. It is a necessary first step in the management of a practice's greatest resource, the people who work in it. Exemplar manuals can be obtained from various sources and can be used as the "template" for a manual specifically written for the practice.

Table 15.2. Typical Monthly Expenses

Rent
Health and dental insurance
Loans and interest for loans
Life insurance
Salaries
Payroll taxes
Answering services
Janitorial services
Pension and profit-sharing plans
Utilities
Telephone service
Postage
Office supplies
Printing
Computer supplies
Legal and professional fees
Lease payment
Convention and seminar fees
Promotional and advertising fees
Donations
Subscriptions to magazines and professional materials
Dues for professional organizations
Business and property tax
Automobile expenses
Unemployment insurance
Miscellaneous expenses

FINANCIAL MANAGEMENT

In an efficiently run office, procedures are established to manage the finances of the practice. In general, the practitioner must set reasonable fees, ensure that they are properly billed and collected, monitor practice expenses and adjust them as necessary, exercise control over inventories of ophthalmic materials and supplies, and guard against loss from waste and theft.

Fees

After fees have been initially established, the practitioner must monitor costs and expenses to determine when fees should be increased. The decision to change fees must be adequately explained to staff members so that they can answer patient queries properly. Because fees are among the most common causes of conflict with patients, staff members must be able to explain clearly what charges are for and how they can be paid.

It is not unusual for the fee schedule to include "professional courtesy," which is a means of reducing or eliminating the fees charged to certain individuals—usually other health care providers—who, in return, provide a similar courtesy to the optometrist. Immediate family members are usually included in the arrangement.

Fee schedules set by third-party health care programs such as Medicare and Medicaid and by vision and medical service plans are invariably different from those charged by the practitioner on a fee-for-service basis.

Billing and Collections

Office policies must be set for the awarding of credit and for the billing of accounts (see Chapter 24). Staff members responsible for the collection of payment must understand these policies and apply them fairly and uniformly. Because of the complexity of third-party reimbursement plans, in a busy office it will be necessary to have a staff member assigned to the billing and collection of these accounts. Changes in billing methods are frequent, and reimbursement problems can arise quickly if appropriate attention is not devoted to program details.

An office policy for the collection of unpaid accounts must be set by the practitioner. Accounts receivable should be monitored monthly to ensure that these procedures are effective and that a disproportionate number of accounts do not go uncollected.

Periodic Economic Evaluation

It is essential to list monthly expenses so that they can be properly monitored for any significant changes. Typical monthly expenses involve quite a number of items (Table 15.2).

Ideally, the expenses on the monthly expense sheet should be monitored each week. If an expense is unusually high, it will be necessary to review the records for the past 12 months and compare the amounts. For example, if health insurance costs for employees increase substantially from the previous year, the person in charge of the office's insurance plans should call insurance agents and try to get a more cost-effective health plan. Observing present trends can provide valuable information in planning for the future. For instance, by refinancing loans at lower rates, the practitioner can reduce monthly expenses. Variable expenses should be monitored to minimize the likelihood of being forced to make large increases in fees or to see more patients to offset the increase in expenses.

An economic analysis should be performed periodically to determine the progress of the practice toward reaching its financial goals (see Chapter 28). Fees must be periodically evaluated and adjusted to compensate for added costs and expenses.

Inventory Control

Because optometrists sell spectacles and contact lenses, inventories must be maintained for these ophthalmic materials. An inventory control system—utilizing a ledger or a computer—must be established (see Chapters 12 and 21).

Protection Against Embezzlement

A surprising number of optometry practices are plagued by employee theft. Few optometrists think about this possibility before it occurs and therefore do not have office procedures to prevent employee theft. Preventive policies should be effective, but not offensive to employees.

The simplest and least intrusive method of protecting against loss by embezzlement is to obtain appropriate insurance coverage. If economic loss is incurred, the policy will provide reimbursement.

CONCLUSION

When an optometry school graduate enters private practice, there will inevitably be a "learning curve," as the graduate acquires needed experience with office administration and patient management. The young practitioner might have to spend just as much time attending to the business tasks of a practice as is spent actually seeing patients. Being involved with office administration might seem to be an un-

desirable task for many practitioners; however, for those who become owners of practices, knowledgeable administrative techniques and prudent business strategies are necessary for a practice to operate smoothly and efficiently. Such practices enjoy a high level of morale—on the part of the practitioner as well as the staff. Just as important, these practices are perceived as "patient friendly" by patients and are inevitably popular and successful.

BIBLIOGRAPHY

Allergan. Pathways in Optometry. Irvine, CA: Allergan, 1992.

Andrews FJ. Choosing your "experts" wisely. Optom Manage 1988;24(7):64–8.

Baldwin BL, Christensen B, Melton T. Rx for Success. Midwest City, OK: Vision Publications, 1982.

Bennett I. Dealing with patient complaints, remakes. Optom Manage 1988;24(2):94.

Bennett I. Keeping your office expenses in line. Optom Manage 1988;24(5):29–39.

Bennett I. Management for the Eyecare Practitioner. Boston: Butterworth-Heinemann, 1993.

Christensen B. Personalities: can you mix and match? Optom Manage 1989;25(12):29–33.

Coleman DL. Protect yourself from employment lawsuits. Optom Econ 1991;1(11):47–8.

Coleman DL. Your new ophthalmic equipment (first decide which is better for you. Then make sure you know the rules). Optom Econ 1992;2(4):30–3.

Day J. Turning the heat on employee pilfering. Optom Manage 1989;25(9):84–91.

Fischer BA. Fine tuning the message. Optom Econ 1992; 2(1):12–21.

Gailmard NB. Guide to diagnostic instruments and equipment. Rev Optom 1993;130(3):111–28.

Goldberg F. Foolproof records that stand up in court. Optom Manage 1990;25(11):59–70.

Goldsborough R. Five ways to ease the strain of opening cold. Rev Optom 1987;124(5):97–103.

Handler G. Remember the person behind the eyes. Optom Manage 1989;25(2):88–92.

Hayes J. How much to spend on new instruments. Optom Manage 1993;28(4):15.

Legerton JA. Sound purchasing decisions (analyzing the what, when, why and how of purchasing ophthalmic equipment). Optom Econ 1992;2(10):34–8.

Melton JW, Phillips JH, Plank KE. Answers for success. Optom Econ 1992;2(4):34–6.

Miller PJ. How to prevent employee theft. Optom Manage 1988;24(9):62–6.

Morrison RJ. Quality, caring, and marketing. Optom Econ 1991;1(6):28–31.

Palmer DM. Telephone techniques. Optom Econ 1991; 1(3):18–21.

Practice Enhancement Program. Optimize Your Professional Opportunities through Patient Communication in Your Practice. Professional Enhancement Monograph, MN 17. St. Louis: American Optometric Association, 1986.

Practice Enhancement Program. Optimize Your Professional Opportunities through Patient Communication in Your Community. Professional Enhancement Monograph, MN 18. St. Louis: American Optometric Association, 1986.

Practice Enhancement Program II. Professional Enhancement Module, Managing Your Practice Plan, Precourse Workbook. St. Louis: American Optometric Association, 1986.

Schulman E. What patients need to know. Optom Econ 1991;1(9):12–15.

Sherburne SO. Handling the problem patient. Optom Econ 1991;1(11):25–7.

Stein H. Communication skills: do you rate a ten? Optom Manage 1991; 26(1):65.

Stein H. Communication skills, part 2: opportunities for success. Optom Manage 1991; 26(2):59.

Chapter 16

Selecting an Office Staff

Donald H. Lakin, Ronald S. Rounds, Peter Shaw-McMinn, and Craig Hisaka

People who produce good results feel good about themselves.

—Kenneth Blanchard
One Minute Manager

In successful human resource management, all basic functions of management must be considered. These functions are: planning, organizing, directing, and controlling. Many classic business texts add a fifth consideration—staffing—to this list. These five basic functions are considered in this discussion of human resource management for an optometric practice.

Management is defined as the process of accomplishing objectives through these five functions. The objective that will be addressed in this chapter is development and maintenance of an efficient, enthusiastic staff. There is no office in which the instruments used, procedures performed, or materials dispensed contribute to the success of the practice and the goodwill of patients more than the staff. When in place and functioning properly, the staff of an optometric office adds services to patients, assists with marketing efforts inside and outside the office, increases efficiency and productivity of the practice, and elevates the personal aspects of eye care.

When the five functions of management are described, there is inevitably some overlapping and considerable interdependence. All these functions must be addressed, however, to achieve the goal of implementing a management plan that will result in developing and maintaining an efficient, enthusiastic staff. In considering the goal of developing and maintaining such a staff, it might be asked, "Are the two related?" The answer is clearly "yes." By producing good results (being efficient), people acquire a feeling of achievement (enthusiasm). This enthusiasm permeates the person, the practice, and the care being rendered to patients.

There are six things that all employees need to know and feel if they are to be enthusiastic. They are to:

- Know they are needed
- Know what is expected of them and how to meet these expectations (proper training)
- Know there is a possibility for growth
- Know they are compensated fairly
- Know they are appreciated (recognition)
- Feel they are involved in the delivery of care and the growth of the practice (ownership)

These six things should be kept in mind as a management plan is developed.

PLANNING

To acquire an office staff, planning is a necessary first step. The planning process is used to determine the need for and qualifications of new staff members.

Need for Staff

Before hiring an employee, it is essential to determine the needs of the practice that the employee will fulfill. What responsibilities will this staff person have? In traditional personnel terms, what will be the work load of this employee? In this planning phase, it is necessary to determine how and why specific work functions are performed and to quantitate their significance in terms of time and value to the practice. For an optometrist starting a practice with one employee, the primary responsibilities will probably be those of a receptionist. Even at this early stage of practice, however, a list of responsibilities should be developed. One optometric text on practice management has listed 27 responsibilities for this job classification. The determination and listing of these responsibilities become part of the organizational aspect of the management plan.

When a new position is to be added to the staff, input should be obtained from current staff members (beyond the familiar cry of "we need more help"). Asking the staff to assess the responsibilities currently being performed by individual members—through the use of daily logs or time management sheets—permits quantitation of the allocation of time and duties and helps to identify needs. This process also provides a role for employees in the planning process and serves as an occasion for employees to do a self-evaluation of their contribution to the delivery of care.

When a new position is created, the use of an appropriate title often helps the person fit into the staff. For example, if a second optometric technician were hired, with primary responsibilities in styling and dispensing, the appropriate title might be ophthalmic technician. For the first technician, if he or she has demonstrated leadership qualities, the title might be changed to senior technician.

In planning for the addition of a staff member, the economics of delivering care must be considered. As stated in the introduction to this chapter, there is no aspect of a practice that is more important to its success than the staff. It can also be the most expensive aspect of a practice if not planned wisely. From an economic standpoint, both original or additional staff members should increase the productivity of the practice. Increased productivity can be achieved by the delegation of responsibilities to staff members so that the practitioner's time is better utilized for the delivery of income-producing professional services. (This assumes that there is potential for the practitioner's time to be used more productively.)

Optometry students and new graduates often think they must work with a full range of paraoptometric personnel, but during the developmental phase of a practice the use of a large staff is not economically sound.

Findings obtained by recent American Optometric Association (AOA) Economic Surveys reveal that staff costs should average about 15% of the total gross income of a practice, with a range of 12–18%. Another guideline for staff costs is also based on practice income; it holds that a practice should have one full-time staff person for every $150,000 of gross income. A model for staff productivity has been proposed, using dollar productivity per hour per employee. Of course, actual figures will vary considerably with the type of practice and the optometric product being delivered. A practice performing a significant amount of in-office visual training that uses technicians would be labor-intensive and would have a higher percentage of gross income devoted to staff than a primary care practice.

QUALIFICATIONS OF APPLICANTS

During the planning phase, the qualifications of applicants should be carefully considered. These qualifications need to be commensurate with the specific staff responsibilities to be assumed. Although screening for these qualifications is clearly a part of staffing, the better the planning, the better the chance of finding someone who has these qualifications in the applicant pool. Each position will require a different prioritization of general abilities, in addition to specific knowledge or skills. General abilities needed might include dexterity, memory, verbal and nonverbal communication skills, ability to handle people, and telephone voice. Telephone voice would probably be the top priority if the position was for a receptionist with appointing responsibilities. If preparing reports was part of this same job, specific skills in typing or using a word processor would be critical. Minimum hiring standards should be part of planning. In busy offices that need a person to assume specific duties with minimum training, experience might be essential. A person with the right education and training will usually be an efficient and enthusiastic employee much sooner than someone trained on the job. The meeting of these standards will depend on the applicant pool, wage level, and competition for people with similar skills from other industries. People who are working as optometric technicians and who have formal academic training only account for 18% of the individuals filling these positions.

ORGANIZATION

Organization is the management function of relating people, tasks (or activities), and resources to each other so that the practice can accomplish its objectives. Plans are carried out through the organizing process. Table 16.1 is an example of one organization model for optometric personnel.

In most optometric offices, a staff person will be needed to perform the functions of a receptionist, ophthalmic technician, frame stylist, typist, and office manager (see top, Table 16.1). There are optometric practices in which all of these functions are performed by one or two staff members and also by the optometrist. In larger group optometric practices, one or more staff people can be found performing each function, and there might be added areas of responsibility. For instance, ophthalmic assistants or optometric technicians could perform pretesting procedures, another staff member might perform all the insurance billings, and so forth. The organizational chart needs to describe the specific areas of responsibility for each position. For example, in Table 16.1 the "primary patient needs" of the receptionist will be to answer the phone, make and confirm appointments, prepare patient files, and manage related duties.

Personality traits should also be considered. In Table 16.1, the "qualities" that are required to perform the "primary patient needs" are listed. For example, for a receptionist to perform "primary patient needs," he or she would need "qualities" associated with performing those tasks—such as being friendly, pleasant, polite, consistent, and patient with people.

Another consideration is the secondary skills required for a position. In Table 16.1 "secondary patient needs" and "management skills" required by the receptionist, ophthalmic technician, and office manager are described. Under "qualities," some of the personality traits required to perform those specific tasks are listed.

Whether it is a first or a subsequent employee that is being selected, a careful assessment should be made of the prospective employee's strengths and personality traits to determine the person's suitability for the position. It has often been said, "One can teach skills, but it is difficult to change a personality." Inappropriate matching of personality traits and staff positions will lead to stress, conflicts, high turnover rate, and a detrimental influence on the overall growth of the practice. Patients will be quick to notice changes and conflicts within the practice, and, although they will return to the office for optometric care, their enthusiasm to refer other patients to the practice will diminish.

Through the years three basic types of staff organizations have developed in the practice of optometry. They are referred to as type I, type II, and type III.

Type I Staff Organization

Type I is referred to as the "family" staff organization. It is composed of a solo practitioner and one full-time staff person, who performs most of the staff functions. The optometrist also helps in the dispensing and adjusting of glasses. In addition, there can be a part-time staff person, and the spouse of the optometrist is usually part of the office staff. The full-time staff person has been in the practice for many years and is an excellent employee but is not necessarily a "team player." The outstanding characteristic of this practice for the staff member is the closeness, friendship, and loyalties between the employer and the employee. If there are personal problems or tragedies, the support systems function just like those of a family. The staff wages and benefits might be less than other offices. The overall office efficiency and organization is not the strength of this type of practice. The gross income of this type of practice does not change significantly over the years. In the type I practice there is a strong resistance to changes in staff organization and to the incorporation of changes in examination procedures. Because of the inflexibility of the type I practice, there is little acquisition and use of modern instrumentation or equipment.

Table 16.1. Organizational Model for Optometric Personnel

	Receptionist	Ophthalmic Technician	Frame Stylist	Typist	Office Manager
Primary patient needs	Answer phone Make/confirm appointments Prepare patient files Greet patients Record charges Deposit money and handle banking Bill patients	Order prescription contact lenses Verify prescription contact lenses Deliver prescription contact lenses	Select frames	Type	
Qualities	Friendly Pleasant Polite Consistent Patient Courteous	Able to verbally instruct Mechanically aptitudinal Patient Skilled in time management	Fashion and color sensible Patient Perceptive Detail oriented Sensitive	Organized Efficient	
Secondary patient needs	Bill insurance Record insurance payment Recall patient File charts Restock office supplies	Repair and adjust prescriptions Train patients in contact lens wear			
Qualities	Organized Efficient	Methodical			
Management skills	Manage and control accounts receivable	Log and monitor prescriptions Restock contact lenses Restock contact lens solutions			Supervise Purchase frames Pay taxes and bills Reconcile bank accounts Resolve aging accounts receivable Maintain bookkeeping and accounting
Qualities	Decisive Direct Relentless "Respectable vs. likable"	Resourceful Creative Organized Judicious			Organized Respected Supportive of sharing goals Administrant Managemental Stable; Consistent

◄──────────────── CROSS TRAINING ────────────────►

Type II Staff Organization

The type II practice is referred to as the "saturated" practice. There is usually a solo practitioner and an associate optometrist, who works several days at the practice. The staff organization, staff salaries, and benefits are at higher levels than the type I practice.

There are often three full-time and permanent staff members (or the part-time equivalent of three full-time staff members), and staff functions are divided among the three staff members, each having a primary area of responsibility. The staff members are excellent "team players," with one staff person extremely strong and perceived as the "leader."

The outstanding characteristic of the type II office is the efficiency of the office and the harmony. The office continues to grow and develop, and the instrumentation and equipment are usually updated. However, in general, the support systems, friendship, and closeness do not compare to the type I practice.

Type III Staff Organization

The type III practice, referred to as "the group," represents only a minority of optometric practices. There are at least three or more partners. The staff organization, salaries, and benefits are at the highest level of optometric practices. However, due to the large volume of patients and the use of many staff members, there is a limited time in which to cultivate the friendship, loyalties, and closeness found in the type I (and, to a lesser degree, in type II) practice.

DEVELOPING AN OFFICE MANUAL FOR EMPLOYEES

After a thorough evaluation of the staff needs has been performed and the appropriate organization has been determined, it is mandatory that an office policy manual be written. If the office does not have a manual, the time should be taken to develop one. Even if a solo practice is started "cold," it should have a manual. The employment policy manual should include several basic topics (Table 16.2).

The AOA (and individual authors) have published guidebooks that go through each step of manual development. These sources should be consulted before attempting to draft a manual for a specific office.

DESIGNATION OF THE PERSONNEL ADMINISTRATOR

One of the significant advantages of a group practice is that one of the partners can be responsible for the management of the staff. Often this position merits special compensation because of the time commitment, stress, and pressure. In some practices, this administrator might give a performance

Table 16.2. Topics to be Included in an Office Manual

Philosophy of care and of the office
Employee classification
    Full-time, part-time, probationary
Equal opportunity statement
    Policy of nondiscrimination
Duties and responsibilities of employees: staff functions
Employee conduct
    May include personal conduct, dress code, personal calls, personal visitors, punctuality, smoking, eating, drinking, chewing gum, grooming and attire, and so forth
Working hours
Vacations, holidays, and leaves of absence
    May include paid vacations, holidays, sick or absence, emergency leave, leaves without pay, and similar issues
Payroll and employee benefits
Safety
Confidentiality
    May include provision that "violation of patient confidentiality" will be grounds for immediate dismissal
Performance and salary review
Patient complaints
Termination
    Voluntary, mutual, and involuntary
Jury duty
Bereavement leave

review and evaluation for each staff member every 6 months, or at least once a year. During this review the administrator discusses the job description with the employee and measures performance against expectation, develops with the employee a plan for improvement, and provides feedback on employee strengths and weaknesses.

The personnel administrator also listens to staff complaints about the practitioners and the office. These complaints are then transmitted to the practitioners, who meet weekly to discuss issues as they occur. There should also be a staff meeting at least once a month. If it is at noon, a catered lunch could be served since the staff members are giving up their lunch time for an office meeting. The chair of each meeting is rotated among the staff. The administrator also determines staff vacation time for the calendar year and monitors sick leaves, bereavement leaves, and similar periods of absence.

Other models of an office hierarchy might have an office manager or personnel administrator who is not an optometrist. These administrators operate in a manner that is very similar to the process described above, reporting frequently to the optometrist responsible for this part of the practice.

Many offices use front office coordinators or senior technicians as administrators to establish some vertical management. Whenever there is more than one employee, it is necessary to establish who is responsible to whom. Job classifications identify individual responsibilities, but there must be someone within the practice to see that these responsibilities are fulfilled on a day-to-day basis. The structure of any vertical management should be included in the practice manual or employee handbook.

LEGAL CONSIDERATIONS OF THE SELECTION OF STAFF MEMBERS

Employer-employee relationships, even in small optometric practices, are affected by a variety of both federal and state laws. Although some laws limit their application to employers having a minimum of 15–20 employees, others are more broadly applicable. The legislation therefore is applicable to most optometric practices. Because of its complexity, it is important to have competent legal counsel in dealing with these laws.

The Fair Labor Standards Act (FLSA) establishes minimum wage, overtime pay, recordkeeping, and child labor standards affecting more than 80 million full-time and part-time workers in the private sector and in federal, state, and local governments.

The Wage and Hour Division (Wage-Hour) administers and enforces FLSA with respect to private employment, state and local government employment, and federal employees of the Library of Congress, U.S. Postal Service, Postal Rate Commission, and the Tennessee Valley Authority. For example, the Office of Personnel Management is responsible for enforcement with regard to all other federal employees.

Special rules apply to state and local government employment involving fire protection and law enforcement activities, volunteer services, and compensatory time off in lieu of cash overtime pay.

Beginning in 1997, covered nonexempt workers have been entitled to a minimum wage of not less than $5.15 an hour. Overtime pay at a rate of not less than one and one-half times the regular rate of pay is required for each hour worked over 40 hours per week. Wages required by FLSA are due on the regular payday for the pay period covered. Deductions made from wages for such items as cash or merchandise shortages, employer-required uniforms, and tools of the trade are not legal to the extent that they reduce the wages of employees below the minimum rate required by FLSA or reduce the amount of overtime pay due under FLSA.

While FLSA does set basic minimum wage and overtime pay standards and regulates the employment of minors, there are a number of employment practices that FLSA does not regulate. For example, FLSA does not require:

- Vacation, holiday, severance, or sick pay
- Meal or rest periods, holidays off, or vacations
- Premium pay for weekend or holiday work
- Pay raises or fringe benefits
- A discharge notice, reason for discharge, or immediate payment of final wages to terminated employees

Also, FLSA does not limit the number of hours in a day or days in a week an employee can be required or scheduled to work, if the employee is at least 16 years old. These matters are for agreement between the employer and the employees, or their authorized representatives. Under certain conditions, employers can pay a training wage of at least 85% of the minimum wage for up to 90 days, to employees under age 20. In addition to these issues, there are other conditions and exemptions in FLSA that should be considered.

The FLSA child labor provisions are designed to protect the educational opportunities of minors and prohibit their employment under conditions or in jobs that are detrimental to their health or well being. These provisions include restrictions on hours of work for minors under age 16.

The FLSA requires employers to keep records on wages, hours, and other items, as specified in Department of Labor recordkeeping regulations. Most of the information is of the kind generally maintained by employers in ordinary business practice and in compliance with other laws and regulations. The records do not have to be kept in any particular form, and time clocks need not be used.

The Civil Rights Act of 1964 and related amendments and executive orders prohibit discrimination on the basis of race, color, religion, sex, or national origin. This legislation applies—and many state laws apply—to all employment practices, including hiring, firing, promotion, compensation, and other conditions of employment. A separate act, the Age Discrimination in Employment Act of 1967 and related amendments, requires employers to treat applicants and employees equally, regardless of age. Sexual harassment in the workplace has also become a highly sensitive issue in recent years, requiring employers to maintain a proper work environment.

SELECTION PROCESS

Five Steps for Interviewing and Hiring

One of the most frustrating aspects of private practice is personnel turnover. The finding, keeping, and training of personnel is an ongoing project and problem for most offices. Outstanding employees might move out of state to get married, have a child, or take other employment. Whatever the reason, the replacement of an employee should be regarded as an opportunity. A new face can bring a fresh attitude and ideas. Too often practitioners keep employees who are chronically late, sloppy in their work, and snippy with patients, out of fear that they will not be able to find an adequate replacement.

Step 1. Sources For Applicants

There are several resources that can be used to search for employees—including employment agencies, technicians' schools, friends, patients, newspaper advertisements, optical companies, retail sales representatives, and employee leasing agencies.

Employment Agencies. Employees obtained from an agency come with a price. It is customary to pay the agency a fee of 1% for every $1,000 of the employee's first-year salary. (This offsets the agency's costs for the advertising and screening of applicants.) If the practice is a small office, an agency can offer a discount. There is usually a 30-day trial period during which money is refunded if the employer or the employee is dissatisfied. If there is a problem within the first 90 days, the employment agency will usually guarantee to provide a replacement.

Optometric Technicians' Schools. Technicians who graduate from these schools have good background knowledge and some clinical training but are limited in number. A recent AOA survey reported that only 18% of employed optometric technicians had received formal training.

Friends. This source of employees has to be managed wisely. Hiring friends to work in an office can be a delicate situation. It can be difficult to introduce a business attitude into a relationship that has been built on an equal basis.

Patients. Satisfied patients make wonderful, enthusiastic staffers. They talk from personal experience about an office's good service and can be a great asset in promoting the office. Before a patient is hired, however, it should be determined that the patient possesses the required skills or is trainable.

Newspaper Classified Advertisements. There are several ways in which a newspaper advertisement can be used to attract applicants. One technique is to list a post office box number and request that applicants submit résumés; another is to list a private telephone number and request that applicants submit résumés. This technique can decrease the number of applicants, because many employees applying for general office work or optical work do not have résumés. An alternative technique would be to ask for a letter of application rather than a résumé. The key to attracting applicants is writing an advertisement that makes the position or office sound exciting. People read into advertisements what they want, and generally what they want is excitement, fun, and a challenge.

Optical Companies. Super-opticals and chain locations are usually open 6–7 days a week, 12 hours a day. Many talented and experienced employees are not interested in working such an extensive work week. These individuals might even be willing to accept a decrease in salary for the more convenient hours of a private practice.

Sales Representatives in Optical Industry. Ophthalmic sales representatives are in a different office every day. They hear firsthand from employees if they are unhappy or are interested in moving for one reason or another. They can be very helpful in spreading the news that the practice is in the market for a new assistant.

Cosmetic or Jewelry Sales Representatives. Retail sales people in clothing, cosmetics, and jewelry have the personality and sales ability that adapts easily to the optical area. Many times, when hiring an experienced frame stylist, one also hires the stylist's old habits, such as prejudging a patient's spending ability. Someone who knows how to provide a fresh attitude can bring a fresh approach as well.

Employee Leasing Agencies. These companies interview, hire, and pay employees, saving the hassle that comes with frequent personnel turnover, the cost of benefits, and inconvenience of paying employment taxes. A fee must be paid to the agency, however, for the services and personnel obtained from the agency.

Step 2. Screening Applicants

Screening applicants over the telephone is a crucial step in the hiring process. The interviewer should have a legal-size pad of paper by the phone, to note the applicant's name and the interviewer's first impressions. The sound and tone of the applicant's voice is one important impression. Is the voice harsh, the rate of speech too quick, or the tone of conversation false?

The "telephone personality" of the applicant should also be assessed. Close attention should be paid to the ease of conversation, the use of grammar, and any accent or dialect that is difficult to understand. During the telephone screening process, it is essential to stay in control of the conversation. The applicant's name and phone number should be obtained for future reference. (If the caller is not willing to provide this information, the conversation should be politely concluded.)

The caller will usually ask for a job description and the salary being offered. To stay in control, the interviewer should immediately ask the caller, "What are you doing presently?" This question will provide information about the caller's employment situation, such as whether the caller is unemployed and for how long that has been the situation. If the caller is working, the interviewer can find out where the caller is employed, what the caller's skills are, and the salary range expected.

Step 3. First Interview

The first interview should be handled by a senior employee. The office administrator should have applicants fill out an employment application. After all applications have been collected, the administrator can narrow the applicant field so that the practitioner only has to interview the best two or three prospects. Filling out an employment application provides not only pertinent facts about the applicants but also allows the applicant's handwriting and spelling skills to be analyzed.

One of the goals of a first interview is to size up the personal appearance of the interviewee. Note should be made of the cleanliness and neatness of clothes and hair. A professional image is desired, and the person should be evaluated on that basis. The demeanor of the person should also be considered. The handshake can provide an indication of the person's personality; so can eye contact and the person's posture. Although the professional image of a person is composed of many factors, from a legal and an ethical standpoint the person's race, religion, sex, and age should not be considered.

The interviewer should have prepared questions to ask. At the conclusion of questioning, the interviewer should ask if the interviewee has any questions.

Step 4. Questioning the Applicant

There are a number of questions that are regularly asked during job interviews (Table 16.3). Often the most important question to ask a prospective employee is, "What do you like to do best?" This question is asked to establish if the interviewee's expectations and needs match the job description.

No matter what position a person is hired for, an employee will always gravitate toward the skills he or she enjoys most. A person can be hired as a receptionist, with duties of appointment making, collections, and recall, but if the person enjoys performing computer work, he or she will find ways

Table 16.3. Fifteen of the Most Frequently Asked Interview Questions

• Tell me about yourself.
• Why are you interested in working for this company?
• Why do you want to leave your job?
• Why have you chosen this particular field?
• Why should we hire you?
• What are your long-range goals?
• What is your greatest strength?
• What is your greatest weakness?
• What is your current salary?
• What is important to you in a job?
• What do you do in your spare time?
• Which feature of the job interests you least?
• How do others describe you?
• What are your plans for continued study?
• Tell me about your schooling.

Suggested reference checklist

1. Applicant's name _____
   Date of reference check _____
2. Reference contacted _____
3. Employment dates _____to _____
4. Salary history _____
5. Type of responsibilities _____
6. Attendance/punctuality _____
7. Special skills _____
8. Reason for leaving _____
9. Notice given _____
10. Severance pay given _____
11. Unemployment compensation _____
12. Is the applicant qualified for rehire? _____
13. Other comments _____
    _____
    _____

Figure 16.1. Example reference checklist for job applicants. (Courtesy of the American Optometric Association. Reprinted with permission.)

to work at the computer, avoiding important job responsibilities. Thus it is best to determine beforehand if the prospective employee's interests and the responsibilities of the position are well matched.

Step 5. Checking References by Phone

After reviewing the applications and the results of the interviews and selecting the two best candidates, the references of these candidates should be questioned over the telephone. If the applicant works (or worked) for a large employer, someone in authority should be questioned to verify the applicant's work history and establish that the person is right for the job (Figure 16.1).

There are a number of questions that can be asked. The first question, however, should be, "Is the employee punctual?" This question provides an indication of the responsibility and dependability of the person. The last question should be, "Would you rehire this employee?" This question allows for a "no" response, while protecting the employer from possible legal entanglements.

OFFERING EMPLOYMENT

Once it has been decided that an applicant appears to suit the practice's needs, no time should be wasted in offering the position. Good employees are hard to find and can have other job offers to con-

sider. During the interview, some of the benefits of working for the practice might have been discussed. During the job offer, it is necessary to negotiate the actual terms of the agreement, and—in so doing—to reach an agreement that fits the needs of both the practice and the new employee. The areas of concern in achieving this goal are preparing for the negotiation, items open to negotiation, a written agreement stating expectations, and what was agreed to by the parties.

Preparing for the Negotiation

Most job offers today are made over the telephone. The applicant is called, the job is offered, and a starting salary is specified. This approach can be adequate if no further negotiation of the employment terms is required. In most situations, however, there are many points open to negotiation, and this can necessitate a face-to-face meeting.

As in any negotiation situation, it is best to negotiate from a position of power, and that is most readily achieved if the applicant comes to the office for the employment offer. In some situations, sitting behind a large desk might be preferred—to demonstrate a position of control. At other times, it can be better to be seated without anything between the two parties or to be seated next to one another. One of the considerations for choosing the setting is the employer's personal management style.

The terms of negotiation are based on how badly the practice wants or needs the potential employee. Employers should keep in mind that employees can be responsible for as much as two-thirds of the gross income of a practice, and that they can make or break a practice. Thus, it might be necessary to make numerous concessions for the right applicant. On the other hand, there are reasonable limits to any negotiation. The employer should determine and write down, before the negotiation, these bargaining limits. In so doing, specific limits should be decided for each of the following negotiable points:

- Responsibilities
- Hours
- Days
- Salary
- Education benefits
- Medical insurance
- Sick pay
- Vacation pay
- Personal time off
- Purchase of optical supplies
- Purchase of the practitioner's services
- Paid holidays
- Retirement plan
- Bonuses

Usually salary is the key item of interest to the new employee, particularly if the employee is young. If the employee has a family, medical insurance coverage might be more important. An older, single employee might be interested in retirement benefits. Employees over age 65 could be concerned with keeping their income lower because of Social Security benefits; they might prefer other forms of compensation, such as fringe benefits or personal time off. The employer should attempt to find out what compensation the prospective employee has decided is most important.

When making the employment offer, it is often advantageous to have a written document that can be used to record the negotiations.

Responsibilities

A responsibilities survey can be used to discuss the expectations of both sides (Figure 16.2). This survey is intended to allow the prospective employee to evaluate—on a 1–5 scale (1 being the most desirable and 5 the least)—potential or prospective work assignments. Use of such a survey can give the employer additional insight into the type of person who is being hired. Later on, if conflicts arise over work responsibilities, the survey can be used to document proof of what was discussed.

There will be a wide range of responses from the survey. Some potential employees will mark nothing below a 2; they might want to give the impression that they are willing to work in all areas. Other applicants might mark several areas with a 5. This response can indicate that the potential employee is inflexible and might not wish to change, or, perhaps he or she had some poor prior experiences. On the other hand, the response can indicate that the potential employee is straightforward and willing to communicate honestly.

The survey must be carefully reviewed by the employer. Does the completed survey of responsibilities fit the practice's needs? Do the likes and dislikes complement other employees? If not, can the practice settle for less than perfect? At what cost? The completed survey can affect the salary amount to be offered the prospective employee.

Probation Period

Since benefits do not begin until the probation period has passed, some potential employees might wish to have a shorter probation period. An offer of a lower initial salary in return for a shorter probation period might be acceptable to the potential employee.

Hours

The potential employee might prefer not to work past 5:00 P.M. If that is the case, a lower salary could be acceptable. On the other hand, if the practice requires late hours, the potential employee might feel that additional compensation is deserved. Is the practice willing to pay more? How much? How will this affect other benefits?

Areas of Responsibility

Place a 1 next to what you definitely wish to do and have done before.
Place a 2 next to what you would like to try but have never done before.
Place a 3 next to what you would do if asked.
Place a 4 next to what you don't think you'd like to do but never tried.
Place a 5 next to what you definitely don't want to do at this time.

Areas of responsibility:

- Answering the telephone
- Making appointments
- Greeting patients
- Distributing office information
- Performing hostess duties
- Seating patients in pretesting room
- Answering patient inquiries into services
- Obtaining patient case histories
- Administering preliminary testing
- Informing about office services and doctor's qualifications
- Showing videotapes
- Seating patients in exam room
- Instructing about contact lens handling
- Selecting frames
- Discussing options on lenses and additional pairs
- Writing up orders
- Checking orders
- Dispensing

- Instructing about proper maintenance and adaptation
- Explaining fee breakdown
- Designing payment schedules
- Writing up receipts and day sheet entries
- Maintaining accounts receivable
- Handling bank deposits
- Maintaining inventory
- Restocking supplies
- Maintaining instruments
- Maintaining facilities
- Typing
- Ordering office supplies
- Assembling patient information packets
- Maintaining public relations
- Performing lab technician duties
- Performing visual therapist duties
- Performing low vision therapist duties

Figure 16.2. Example employee responsibilities survey.

Days

The days of employment require a negotiation strategy similar to the one used for hours. Is the applicant willing to work on Saturdays? How will the potential employee's attitude affect the salary offer?

Salary

Salary is the one item that was most likely discussed when the potential employee first applied for the job. At that time a specific figure, or perhaps a salary range, was described. The employer must consider whether negotiations on other matters have altered the assessment of salary. Can a higher salary be traded for fewer fringe benefits? For example, the employer might be willing to pay a higher salary if the prospective employee agrees to work at particular hours or on particular days, or is willing to accept a limited number of personal leave or vacation days. The presentation of the offer is important. The employer should make the potential employee feel that the practice is willing to bend to suit the employee's needs. The employer should also stress the positive. The negotiation must stay, however, within the reasonable limits set.

The employer must constantly ask, "How far am I willing to go to hire this person?" It should be remembered that, if too much is paid, others in the office might be resentful, and that there is an important need to keep everything in equilibrium.

One way of offsetting a prospective employee's disappointment at the salary offered is to provide a bonus program. Such a program will give the confident employee a boost. The bonus system allows the employee to be paid more after the employee has demonstrated improvement in skills and thereby improvement in worth to the practice. A bonus system is often tied to the probation period. For example, an employee hired to work in the dispensary might be given the following offer: "I can pay you $6 per hour for the first month while we are training you how to do frame selection and adjustments. When you have demonstrated your proficiency at this skill, we will raise your salary to $7 per hour and begin training you in pretesting and lab work. Once you've mastered the pretesting skills, your salary will be $7.50 an hour, and then $8 an hour at the time you can complete the lab work independently."

The employee might be willing to settle for dispensing at $7 an hour and have no interest in lab work or pretesting. At other times, the new employee will spend extra time and effort learning the added skills to obtain a higher salary. In either case, the pay will be what was expected for the responsibilities performed.

Employee development probably should not be open to negotiation. No matter who is hired, some time needs to be spent in integrating new employees into the office. An initial training period, continuing education, office meetings, and office retreats offer opportunities to increase the efficiency of the employee.

After all the negotiable points have been agreed on, they should be written down, and the new employee should be given a copy of the agreement. If everything has been presented properly, the practice now has someone who knows what responsibilities are expected, knows what can be expected as payment in return, and is eager to become a part of the team.

DETERMINING COMPENSATION

To develop and maintain an efficient, enthusiastic staff the practice must offer salaries equal to or slightly above the current pay scale in the area for persons with similar skills and responsibilities. The pay scale in the area can be determined by checking with other optometrists, other health care providers, and businesses nearby. Positions with more responsibility or those that need special training will require a higher pay scale.

Salaries should be evaluated at least once each year. If an employee is exceeding the responsibilities assigned and is an asset to practice growth, that initiative should be rewarded.

Often state or local optometric associations will survey members to determine prevailing salaries and benefits. An example of this is a survey performed in West Michigan in 1992. The range for receptionists was $5.50–$10.00 per hour, with a mean rate of $7.36. The range was $6.00–$12.50 per hour for technicians, with a mean rate of $9.27. Considering inflation, these figures are close to a 1989 AOA report of pay scales for optometric assistants.

Most optometrists pay on an hourly basis rather than providing a weekly salary. There will be occasions when staff members have to remain after normal hours to fulfill responsibilities to patients. Staff members should be compensated for this time, and an hourly rate is more equitable than providing equivalent time off or adjusting the weekly or monthly pay of a salaried person. Many offices schedule full-time employees less than 40 hours a week to allow for this fluctuation in daily hours, thereby avoiding the payment of time and a half for work weeks over 40 hours.

Fringe benefits are usually based on the practice location and the size of the practice. Some offices pay bonuses, health insurance premiums, contributions to pension plans, and similar benefits. Other employers might not find it necessary to offer these types of benefits to keep satisfactory employees. An employer can offer many forms of benefits, although federal laws do not require them to be provided. If an employer decides to offer benefits, the same benefits must be offered to other employees that fall into the same employment category.

Fringe benefits are often as important to employees as salary. The West Michigan survey included various pension plans; medical, dental, and optical insurance; vacation, sick, and holiday pay; educational and travel allowances; uniforms; paid parking; child care; and various periodic incentive bonuses. These benefits should be planned and budgeted and included in the employee handbook.

CONCLUSION

Mistakes are made by everyone in hiring. Many optometrists would list employee management as the single largest headache faced by the private independent practitioner. Determining reasonable terms, negotiating terms with the employee, and putting them in writing will facilitate the integration of the new employee into the team. Time and attention to such a process can save many hours in the future, avoid disagreement, and result in a smooth running office.

BIBLIOGRAPHY

American Optometric Association. Practice Enhancement Program II, Professional Enhancement Module, Managing Your Practice Plan, Precourse Workbook. St. Louis: American Optometric Association, 1986.

American Optometric Association. Practice Enhancement Program II, Professional Enhancement Module, Your Marketing Plan Module Two, Precourse Workbook. St. Louis: American Optometric Association, 1986.

American Optometric Association. Practice Enhancement Program, MN 1, Optimize Your Professional Opportunities Through Personal and Professional Goal Setting. St. Louis: American Optometric Association, 1986.

American Optometric Association. Practice Enhancement Program, MN 5, Optimize Your Professional Opportunities Through Effective Office Staff Policies and Procedures. St. Louis: American Optometric Association, 1984.

Baldwin BL, Christensen B, Melton T. Rx for Success. Midwest City, OK: Vision Publications, 1982.

Blanchard K, Johnson S. The One Minute Manager. New York: Berkeley Publishing Group, 1982.

Blanchard K, Lorber R. Putting the One Minute Manager to Work. New York: Berkeley Publishing Group, 1985.

Carter v. Gallagher, 452 F2d 315 (8th Cir 1971).

Davis v. County of Los Angeles, 566 F2d 1334 (9th Cir 1977); vacated and remanded 440 US 625 (1979).

Dothard v. Rawlinson, 433 US 321 (1977).

Equal Employment Opportunity Commission. Age Discrimination in Employment Act Regulations, 29 CFR 1625.5.

Equal Employment Opportunity Commission. Guidelines on Discrimination Because of National Origin, 29 CFR 1601.6(a)(2).

Equal Employment Opportunity Commission. Guidelines on Discrimination Because of Religion, 29 CFR 1605.3.

Equal Employment Opportunity Commission. Guidelines on Employee Selection Procedures, 29 CFR 1607.4c(2).

Green v. Missouri Pacific RR Co., 423 F2d 1290 (8th Cir 1979).

Gregory v. Litton Systems, Inc., 316 F Supp 401 (DC Cal 1970); affirmed 472 F2d 631 (9th Cir 1972).

Griggs v. Duke Power Co., 401 US 424 (1971).

Johnson v. Pike Co., 332 F Supp 490 (CD Cal 1971).

Lewis v. Western Airlines, 9 EPD 10, 151 (ND Cal 1975).

Lea v. Cone Mills Corp., 438 F2d 86 (4th Cir 1971); affirmed in part 310 F Supp 97 (NC 1969).

Local 53, International Association of Heat and Frost Insulators and Asbestos Workers v. Vogler, 407 F2d 1047 (5th Cir 1969).

Maslow AH. Motivation and Personality. New York: Harper & Row, 1970;51.

McGregor D. The Human Side of Enterprise. New York: McGraw-Hill, 1960.

Peters TJ, Waterman RH Jr. In Search of Excellence. New York: Harper & Row, 1982;50,53–4.

Philips v. Martin Marietta Corp., 339 F Supp 906 (SD NY 1971); affirmed 413 US 634 (1973).

Stein H. Seven steps for interviewing and hiring employees. Optom Manage 1989;24(5):112–13.

Sugarman v. Dougall, 339 F Supp 906 (SD NY 1971); affirmed 413 US 634 (1973).

Tecker IJ, Tecker GH. "Big boom theory." Assoc Manage 1991;43(1):46–7.

Chapter 17

Managing an Office Staff

Donald H. Lakin, Ronald S. Rounds, Peter Shaw-McMinn, and Craig Hisaka

Nothing great was ever achieved without enthusiasm.

—Ralph Waldo Emerson
Circles

Successful human resource management requires that attention be given to the basic functions of management: planning, organizing, and directing and controlling personnel. This chapter describes the direction and control of office staff. Directing staff members begins with training.

TRAINING OF STAFF

Training of staff is an ongoing process. Technology improves, economic conditions change, and commitments need to be redefined. An efficient practice continues to evolve policies that are appropriate for the times and to reconfirm policies that work well. To remain efficient, time must be set aside for continued employee development. An American Optometric Association (AOA) survey of practicing optometrists showed that the average amount of time devoted to training per month was 2.8 hours. The same survey revealed that the minimal amount of training these optometrists thought should be provided was 6.1 hours per month. This result indicates that optometrists believe staff members do not receive as much training as is desirable. The amount of time needed by the employees of a particular practice, however, will depend on the goals set for the practice and the

abilities of both employer and employees to achieve these goals.

Goals and Objectives of Training

The AOA survey referred to above also showed that surveyed practitioners believed the objectives of training should be:

- 71% communication with patients
- 61% technical skills
- 54% ophthalmic dispensing
- 53% general knowledge
- 43% office policies

In a partnership or group practice, one way of identifying the areas to include in training is to survey the optometrists involved (and, if available, the office manager). Using a checklist can be helpful (Figure 17.1). If patient surveys or suggestions have been used, they should be checked for the areas that patients rated as below excellent. These areas should be considered for training. Another source of topics can be gleaned from looking over the evaluations of each employee. Areas of weakness within the practice can be identified and prioritized, and design objectives for training can be created to remedy

VI   YOUR STAFF

    Staff assessment checklist

Exercise 2.18

Although your primary responsibility is providing vision care for your patients, you are also an employer. Here is a checklist of staff activities. Go through it quickly, indicating your actual assessment of your staff members. Put an X in the third column if you'd like to see improvement in certain areas.

	Yes	No	Wish would improve
1. I like being in charge of my office.			
2. I like my staff members to wear uniforms.			
3. I like my staff members to make all my appointments.			
4. My receptionist has a pleasant telephone voice.			
5. My receptionist is courteous.			
6. My receptionist is patient.			
7. My receptionist knows when an emergency occurs and knows when to interrupt me.			
8. My staff members keep my files in order.			
9. My staff members keep my billings up-to-date.			
10. My staff members are well groomed and project a neat, clean appearance.			
11. My staff members know my office policies and follow them.			
12. My staff members are on time for work.			
13. My staff members respect and keep patient information confidential.			
14. My staff members get along well with patients.			
15. My staff members get along well with each other with a minimum of friction.			
16. My staff members get along well with me.			
17. My staff members know how to generate appointments for me.			
18. My staff members, on their own, know how to generate income in my office.			
19. My staff members are competent in all areas of my practice.			

Figure 17.1. Staff assessment checklist. (From American Optometric Association. Practice Enhancement Program II, Professional Enhancement Module, Managing Your Practice Plan, Precourse Workbook. St. Louis: American Optometric Association, 1986. Reprinted with permission.)

problems. An example of such a training program can be found in Table 17.1.

Training Techniques

There are several options available to the practitioner when choosing a way to train the staff in appropriate behavior. Opportune moments, performance reviews, lunch meetings, staff meetings, retreats, and continuing education seminars all provide opportunities for training employees. The choice of technique depends on the objectives and goals of training.

Opportune Moments

During the course of working with an employee, positive or negative behavior can be observed. Practitioners should look for positive behavior and reinforce it whenever possible. The reinforcement and accompanying dialogue can be used to train the correct behavior.

For example: A practitioner notices that the receptionist has appeared indifferent to telephone callers who ask for the price of contact lenses. In response to one of these calls, the receptionist gives an excellent explanation of the choices and services the office provides; this is followed by the scheduling of an appointment. The practitioner should reinforce this behavior by telling the receptionist that his or her management of the caller was exceptional. The reason for approval should be explained. In this case, the receptionist initially avoided the issue of cost by describing the advantages of using the office, educated the patient about the complexities involved in fitting contact lenses, and explained the range of fees in such a way that the patient was confident enough to set an appointment. This moment results in making the employee feel good, reinforces positive behavior, and improves patient satisfaction.

At other times it can be difficult to catch the employee doing the right thing. When the practitioner is feeling patient, and the employee is in the right mood, a poor performance should be discussed in a nonthreatening way. The practitioner should do this privately and as soon as possible after the poor performance.

Table 17.1. Design Objectives for a Sample Training Program

The staff will demonstrate patient-centered care by:
• Calling patients by name when greeting them
• Smiling when talking on the phone
• Offering choices of activities to patients waiting in the reception area
• Pinpointing patient needs when taking a history
• Educating patients about treatment options the practitioner may recommend
• Reinforcing the practitioner's recommendations with demonstrations that focus on a particular benefit to the patient's welfare
• Conducting reminder of appointment phone calls on Sunday from the employee's home for Monday patients
• Stopping by a patient's home to provide a service

These objectives are directed toward the overall goal of assisting the staff in becoming patient-centered in the offering of their services.

For example: A practitioner hears the receptionist answer a patient's inquiry about the price of contact lenses by saying, "Contacts are $400 a pair. Goodbye." This moment can be used by the practitioner to review office procedures and policies about answering such questions. It is hoped that within the near future, the receptionist will be overheard answering such inquiries more appropriately.

Lunch Meetings

Some offices have a difficult time finding a few hours to set aside for training. Since most people eat lunch at some time, lunch meetings can be held to satisfy a limited objective. There are many distractions that can occur during a lunch meeting, however, and the stress of a lunch meeting can cause fatigue in the afternoon and affect employee performance or morale. For these reasons, it is best to choose lighthearted, less important activities and objectives during a lunch meeting. An example of an appropriate topic would be a brief presentation on what it means to be "patient centered." This could be followed by a brainstorming session and the identification of staff behaviors that indicate services are patient centered.

Table 17.2. A Typical Agenda for a Staff Meeting

I. Report of results from interventions recommended at last meeting (each individual staff member)
II. What is meant by patient-centered care (senior staff member)
III. Pretest activity
IV. Discussion of pretest questions (practitioner, facilitator)
V. Recommendations for change
VI. Assignment of responsibilities
VII. Topics for next meeting

Staff Meetings

Regular staff meetings can provide the time necessary to mold a cohesive team that is consistent in providing services. Enough time must be set aside for planned objectives. Whatever time is allocated, there must be a plan with objectives and outcomes in mind. The meeting should not be left open without defined goals, for the effort to reach objectives can pay large dividends in the long run.

Examples of activities for staff meetings include:

- Role-playing sessions
- Question and answer sessions
- Surveys
- Pretesting procedures
- Discussion workshops
- Problem-solving panels
- Demonstrations
- Lectures

The activities chosen can depend on the management style in use. Too often, when using a lecture format, it is assumed that everything said will "sink in." Although lectures can be effective on some occasions, there are times when the information will not result in any behavior changes. Generally, employees will learn best by getting involved and participating in an activity.

There are two adages to keep in mind when training staff members. One is, "No one ever fell asleep while talking." The other is, "The best way to learn is to teach." These sayings reinforce an important point—the most successful sessions can be those in which the optometrist says the least.

The usual staff session will begin with a review of the previous meeting and a summary of the success of previous changes (Table 17.2). Then a staff member will be asked to provide a brief presentation. The member might be chosen because he or she understands the topic best, or because of an ability to demonstrate it most skillfully. The practitioner assists or provides resources to the staff member so that an adequate presentation can be given.

Before the presentation, a pretest can be given to staff members to determine their level of knowledge and to focus their thoughts. The order of questions can be designed to lead the group through levels of increasing awareness. Questions are designed to incite discussion and not necessarily to elicit right or wrong answers.

The practitioner then serves as the facilitator to lead the group through each question. The employees save their pretests and are allowed to jot additional notes as they go along. It is stressed that the pretest is to be used by the individual staff member and will not be seen by anyone else. If done properly, the practitioner will have very little to say other than to focus staff involvement on the questions and the ultimate goal and objectives of the meeting.

Awareness is of little value without action. Goal sheets for the meeting are prepared by the practitioner. Typical goals include behavioral changes and measurements (Figure 17.2). These changes are then discussed at the beginning of the next meeting.

Retreats

When great change is desired—and more time might be needed to reach objectives than the time afforded in a staff meeting—it can be of value to close the office for a day and hold meetings away from the office. This type of intervention is especially effective when dealing with sensitive issues or defensive staff. Part of the day can be designed as a reward to lighten the concerns of attendees. Retreats can vary from an all-expenses-paid trip to a vacation spot to a day at a local meeting facility. A sample retreat agenda is provided (Table 17.3). An information packet, typically including articles and background information on the chosen topic, is distributed to staff members a week or so before the retreat.

One of the advantages of setting aside an entire day is that the progress toward the objectives can be

```
┌─────────────────────────────────────────────────────────────┐
│                    SAMPLE GOAL SHEET                          │
│                           Today's Date_____           │
│   Specific goal:                                              │
│                                                               │
│                                                               │
│      - Specific benefits of reaching goal:                    │
│                                                               │
│                                                               │
│                                                               │
│   Target date:                                                │
│   Where am I today with regard to the goal?                   │
│                                                               │
│                                                               │
│   Obstacles to achievement:                                   │
│                                                               │
│                                                               │
│   Checkpoint dates:                                           │
│      - Intermediate Goal #1                                   │
│                                                               │
│      - Intermediate Goal #2                                   │
│                                                               │
│      - Intermediate Goal #3                                   │
│                                                               │
│      - Intermediate Goal #4                                   │
│                                                               │
│   Plans for surmounting obstacles:                            │
│                                                               │
│                                                               │
│                                                               │
│   Specific actions to take to form new habits:               │
│                                                               │
│                                                               │
│                                                               │
│                     Date Goal Was Met:_____        │
│                                                               │
│                                                               │
└─────────────────────────────────────────────────────────────┘
```

Figure 17.2. Sample goal sheet.

measured, and, if problems arise, tempers flare, or someone becomes upset, time can be taken to relax or refocus the group. A nice advantage of having free time is that there is the opportunity to take each individual employee aside and discuss issues privately in a nonthreatening environment. Staff members can also take the opportunity to informally discuss pertinent issues with each other. As a facilitator, the practitioner's main responsibility is to keep everyone focused on the issues and to steer them toward desired outcomes.

Training can be time consuming and sometimes frustrating, but the rewards can be tremendous when a program is properly carried out. Studies show that patient load can be increased by 35% for each properly trained optometric technician. Unfor-

tunately, studies also show that nearly half of all employees hired for a given job turn out to have been poor choices. The average length of employment is only 3.6 years. In corporate practices, employee turnover is 25–50% a year.

For these reasons, taking the time to develop the staff into a cohesive, happy team that reflects a competent, cohesive, happy practice will be worth the time and effort invested.

DISMISSING EMPLOYEES

If a practitioner is making a reasonable effort to train and control staff members, the employee who is not able to become an efficient and enthu-

Table 17.3. A Sample Retreat Agenda

Valentine's Day Retreat

9:00	Meet at office. Overview of day's activities.
9:15	Pre-test: "What the Experts Say About Providing Services to Patients."
9:30	Champagne breakfast at Mimi's Cafe.
10:00	Brainstorm activity, "The First 5–10 Minutes of the Patient Visit."
10:30	Brainstorm activity: "Follow Up Your Patients."
11:00	Tour of Dr. Stanley's office.
12:00	Role-playing activity: "How to Say Goodbye to the Patient."
1:00	Lunch at Knotts Berry Farm followed by free time at the amusement park.
4:00	Prioritizing; setting goals and objectives.
5:00	Agenda for next meeting. Adjournment.

Table 17.4. Example of Causes for Dismissal

The following can be cause for immediate dismissal. Any employee dismissed for cause will not be entitled to a minimum notice and will not be entitled to termination vacation pay. This list is not to be construed as inclusive:
- Inefficiency or inability to perform assigned duties
- Excessive absenteeism or tardiness
- Poor personal hygiene
- Dishonesty
- Breach of confidentiality or professional ethics
- Refusal to perform assigned duties
- Theft
- Embezzlement or mishandling of funds

siastic member of the team will know there are problems and will probably resign. Everything should be documented in each employee's file, including the curriculum vitae, résumé, or letter of application sent before employment, the interview notes, results of training programs, progress with training, evaluations, reprimands, warnings, and attendance record.

When it is necessary to dismiss an employee these items should be reviewed with the individual, in a nonconfrontational manner. The good things that the employee has done should be pointed out, so that he or she can see that the evaluation is a balanced one and can understand the achievements and the problems that have been encountered during the course of employment.

Most practices have a probation or trial period for new employees. This is usually 60–90 days. Performance should be carefully monitored during this period. If training is not progressing at an agreed-on schedule, this would be the best time to terminate the employment. Many optometrists are hopeless optimists and assume that, despite a difficult start, things will get better, but often they do not.

Some practices request 2 weeks' notice from an employee when the employee wants to or has to leave employment. It is fair for the employer to offer the same notice. If an employee cannot reasonably contribute to the practice after being informed of termination, the 2 weeks can be used as paid time for the employee to find other employment. This is optional and is not required under the Fair Labor Standards Act.

There are causes for immediate dismissal, and these causes should be included in the employee handbook for each practice. An example is provided in Table 17.4.

When an employee is dismissed, that employee might be eligible for unemployment compensation. Each state has specific eligibility requirements that must be met by a dismissed employee to receive unemployment compensation. If an employee does receive this compensation, the former employer will be required to pay an additional amount of money into the state compensation fund; the amount is based on the number of former employees drawing this compensation.

CONTROLLING STAFF MEMBERS

The controlling aspect of management involves setting standards, measuring performance, and taking corrective actions. To successfully carry out this function with staff, they must first feel that they are a part of the practice.

Mission Statement

The office manual should include a mission statement for the practice. Employees must feel they are a part of the practice, and including them in the mission statement, as well as in the long-term objective of the practice, fulfills this need. This mission statement should be read by all employees (Table 17.5).

Employee Evaluations

Evaluations of all employees should be performed at least once a year. During training periods, evaluations can be provided weekly. These evaluations should be written and made a permanent part of the employee's file. An example employee performance review is provided as Figure 17.3. This format permits the evaluator to address the employee's quality of performance, quantity of responsibilities, and knowledge of the job.

Setting Individual Goals

The use of performance evaluations is the first step in helping employees identify individual goals that will carry out the practice's mission.

The secret to employee development is good communication. Nowhere is this more evident than during a periodic review of the employee's performance. The perceptions of the evaluator can be quite different than those of the employee. How the performance review is conducted can be critical to morale and to the future productivity of the employee.

A good way to begin the first evaluation of an employee is to have the employee complete a self-evaluation survey. Figure 17.3 is one example of a format that could be used. This self-evaluation will provide the evaluator with insights into the employee's perceptions of performance. If these perceptions differ from the evaluator's in many areas, it might be best to choose only a few areas to concentrate on. The evaluator should not forget, however, that 90% of all employees rank themselves in the top 10% in regard to performance.

The evaluator's survey should be reviewed with the employee, including performance scores and the reasons for these scores. Pertinent comments should be written down for future review. Together with the employee, the evaluator should compose goals, a plan to reach these goals, and the consequences that will result if the goals are not reached. After the review, the employee must sign the evaluation and the

Table 17.5. Example Mission Statement

1. To provide our patients with quality eye/vision care, therapy, ophthalmic materials, and contact lenses in a professional, efficient, and friendly setting.
2. To operate as a profitable, secure, and growing optometry practice; to provide maximum care at a fair cost.
3. To be dedicated to providing growth opportunities, a caring environment, and an improved life for all staff members.

plan. This information should be used to increase or decrease employee bonuses. If the desired behavior requires little effort to correct, the time spent for the evaluation and goal setting can serve as a training period for the employee.

Monitoring Implementation of Changes

Sometimes, despite all the preparation, planning, and training, the behaviors sought do not occur. This situation is particularly likely in an office where employees have been following unchanging routines for a long period of time. In this type of office, a daily worksheet can serve as a helpful reminder to encourage employees to change the routine according to recommendations.

On the daily worksheet, the employee must note when the new procedure is employed. Employees should be assured that this extra time will be required only until the new changes become part of their routine. The practitioner might wish to monitor the employees' efforts to incorporate changes into the office routine by using personal observations.

Directing Staff Members

The manner chosen to communicate with employees is referred to as leadership style. Many business authors use the term management style instead, because communications will, unquestionably, affect the entire management process. Generally, there are two extreme types of management style, with most managers falling somewhere in between. The most authoritarian style is the military approach, in which the manager tells the em-

EMPLOYEE PERFORMANCE REVIEW

Name: _____

Today's date: _____

Date hired: _____

Period covered: to _____

Position: _____

Evaluated by: (signature) _____

Please rate the employees in each of the areas below, using the following scale. Your evaluation should reflect an impartial judgment that is based on the entire period covered--not upon isolated incidents.

Outstanding: Employee exhibits consistent, superior ability, far in excess of job requirements.
Very good: Employee exhibits ability above that expected for the position.
Satisfactory: Employee meets the position requirements.
Fair: Employee exhibits ability below job requirements. Some improvement needed.
Unsatisfactory: Employee exhibits ability far below requirements. Much improvement needed.

1. QUALITY:
   a. produces error-free work
   b. handles assignments with thoroughness

2. QUANTITY:
   a. produces an acceptable volume of work
   b. completes tasks promptly

3. JOB KNOWLEDGE:
   a. knows job duties
   b. knows office policies and procedures

4. DEPENDABILITY:
   a. arrives on time
   b. has good attendance record
   c. completes a consistent quantity of work with
   acceptable quality

5. ATTITUDE:
   a. cooperates with associates
   b. maintains pleasant demeanor
   c. conforms to office policies and procedures

6. INITIATIVE:
   a. needs minimal supervision
   b. completes more work than expected

7. APPEARANCE:
   a. dresses according to office standards

8. PERSONAL FACTORS:
   a. concentrates on work rather than personal factors

9. OVERALL PERFORMANCE:
   a. employee's strong points
   b. areas that need strengthening

Figure 17.3. Employee performance review.

ployee what to do and the employee follows the instructions without question. The opposite style is one in which the manager orchestrates situations so that the employee realizes what to do and does it because the employee believes it is in the best interest of the office. Each style has its advantages and disadvantages.

Douglas McGregor calls these management styles theory X and theory Y in his book *The Human Side of Enterprise* (New York: McGraw-

Hill). The two theories are briefly summarized in Table 17.6.

Management style X means that the manager must control everything that goes on in the office and every decision that must be made by employees. The manager must constantly monitor the employees' performances. A specific procedures and policy manual is necessary to direct the staff to handle every situation the way the manager wants it handled.

This management style seems easier because no effort is made to convince the staff to understand or support changes. Their duty and job is simply to carry out orders, not question why. On the other hand, this management style requires more time. The employees must be constantly monitored or they might not provide services correctly because they were not told how to handle a particular situation. The employees will hesitate to act and might, in fact, be ineffective without the manager present. A large policy and procedures manual will be needed; large manuals are difficult to memorize and time consuming to create.

Management style X can be summarized by the statement, "Management is getting people to do things your way." Management style Y is completely different. Staff members participate in the decision making and are allowed to decide how to best handle situations. Office policy and procedures are decided by a group effort, with most input obtained from those providing the services. The manager offers resources and training to help the employees reach their goals for the office.

Initially, this management style seems slow and laborious because meetings must be held, levels of awareness must be raised, and alternatives discussed. The staff must first realize that change is necessary, research the options, and finally agree on the policy to be implemented. Once the policy has been decided, implementation is usually much quicker and easier, because the staff "owns" the changes. They understand the need for change and can adapt the philosophy behind the change to every situation. The employees are able to work independently and are not afraid to offer novel options for consideration. The staff members treat the business as their own, because, in a large sense, it is. This management style can be summarized by the statement, "Management is the ability to let other people have your way."

Table 17.6. Management Styles

Theory X
Assumptions about the average person
    Works as little as possible
    Lacks ambition, dislikes responsibility, prefers to be led
    Inherently self-centered; indifferent to organizational needs
    By nature resistant to change
    Gullible, not very bright
Assumptions about management
    Responsible for organizing staff, equipment, and supplies in the interest of economic ends
    Directs staff efforts, motivates them, and controls their behavior to fit the needs of the organization
    Must persuade, reward, punish, and control staff activities; otherwise staff members would be passive or resistant to organizational needs

Theory Y
Assumptions about the average person
    At least potentially mature
    Trustworthy
    Able to handle responsibility
    Motivated by organizational goals
    Will use self-control and self-direction
Assumptions about management
    Responsible for organizing staff, equipment, and supplies in the interest of economic ends
    Believe it is their responsibility to provide opportunities to develop abilities
    Provides guidance
    Encourages growth
    Removes obstacles
    Arranges the work environment so that employees can achieve their own goals while meeting the goals of the practice

Source: Adapted from D McGregor. The Human Side of Enterprise. New York: McGraw-Hill, 1960.

Which style is best for a given practitioner? One employer might prefer to choose the style that comes most naturally. Another employer might choose the style to which employees respond best. Still another manager might change management styles from one to the other because change is generally more productive than rote routines.

There are arguments that can be made in favor of each rationale.

Selecting a Natural Management Style

Choosing a style that comes naturally requires the least amount of effort on the manager's part. One

Management style questionnaire

The purpose of this exercise is to give you a general idea of your management style. For each statement listed check whether you mostly or completely agree with it or whether you mostly or completely disagree with it.

Respond to all the statements.

Scoring directions follow the questionnaire.

Statement	Mostly or completely agree	Mostly or completely disagree
1. Since patient contact is critical, I try to provide all direct patient services myself.		
2. When I've tried to delegate patient services to an assistant, I've found patients got poorer service.		
3. To assure the right decision is made, I make all the decisions myself.		
4. I expect employees I've hired to learn to do things my way.		
5. I hardly ever hear any complaints from my employees.		
6. The important thing is that employees understand what I want of them.		
7. I assign tasks to whoever is capable of handling them.		
8. There are few employee problems that cannot be solved by better pay.		
9. Employees who insist on making all of their own decisions should open their own business.		
10. It's just not possible for everyone to make a living doing what they enjoy.		
11. The average employee is basically self-centered and indifferent to the goals of my practice.		
12. I allow employees to post humorous sayings about how this office is run, and there are many.		
13. My best technique in dealing with an employee grievance is to assert my leadership in determining what I need to do to correct the situation.		
14. If I let my employees make their own decisions, I will lose control of my practice.		

Figure 17.4. Management style questionnaire. (From American Optometric Association. Practice Enhancement Program II, Professional Enhancement Module, Managing Your Practice Plan, Precourse Workbook. St. Louis: American Optometric Association, 1986. Reprinted with permission.)

means of determining management style is illustrated in Figure 17.4. This exercise provides insight into individual management tendencies.

Selecting a Style to Which Employees Respond

Through experimentation, a manager finds the management style that each employee seems to respond to best. Time and effort can be reduced by predicting the management style that will be most effective in obtaining the best productivity from an employee. To make these predictions, it is helpful to look at the value systems of different groups of people. Managers should not be surprised to observe that an employee's value system is very different from the manager's own value system.

Statement	Mostly or completely agree	Mostly or completely disagree
15. As manager, I am responsible for everything my employees do.		
16. The function of the manager is to set out and enforce clear rules; the function of the employee is to follow them.		
17. Allowing employees to attend optometric conferences and workshops cuts into their working time and may give them ideas to look for work elsewhere or about ideas for equipment or procedures that I can't afford to implement. It will only make them restless.		
18. If individuals are allowed to make their own decisions, they will not be for the good of the office, but for their own benefit.		
19. I enjoy optometry, and I'm unwilling to devote less than my full time to patient care.		
20. I'm in optometry to make a good living by providing quality optometric care. If I let my employees get too independent, I'll lose all my cost controls and jeopardize the profitability of my practice.		

Scoring directions

Now add up the number of your "Mostly or Completely Agree" answers.

If you checked 15 to 20 "agree" answers, you run a very "tight ship." Your style is highly directive, what is called a Theory X management style.

If you checked 7 through 14, your management style includes a number of practices that are consistent with a more participative management style.

If you checked 1 through 6 "agree" responses, your management style is highly participative, and you delegate not so many tasks as you do responsibilities in achieving shared goals. Your management style might be characterized as a Theory Y management style.

 Continue on audiotape

Changing Management Styles

There might be times when a change in management style is needed. Different types of employees, or different types of practice environments, or even staleness in a practice can necessitate a change. When altering management styles, however, the changes should be made readily apparent to all employees. Otherwise, confusion and dissatisfaction can result.

MOTIVATING EMPLOYEES

The information used to predict the response of employees to a management style can also be used to motivate them. There are a number of common factors that motivate individuals in general. By applying Maslow's hierarchy (Figure 17.5) to the profession of optometry, optometrists can learn what will be most effective in motivating employees.

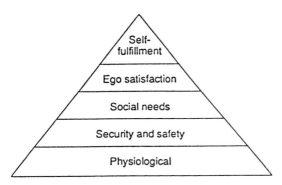

Figure 17.5. Maslow's hierarchy of needs. (Reprinted from AH Maslow. Motivation and Personality. New York: Harper & Row, 1970.)

Physiological Needs

All people have bodily needs such as food, water, rest, exercise, shelter, and protection from the elements. The motivation of staff members is obviously beyond this basic level.

Security and Safety

People require protection against threats, dangers, and deprivation. Many people fear losing their job, benefits such as medical insurance, or an adequate income after retirement. To provide motivation, employers should offer regular performance reviews, with emphasis on feedback that stresses the positive aspects of job security. Updates should be provided on the status of employee benefits and their economic value. Bonus plans or profit-sharing plans can also be offered, contingent on level of performance. Retirement plans can also be provided. The employer should be reassuring when discussing job security and business stability.

Social Needs

People have interpersonal needs, such as belonging, association, acceptance, and giving and receiving friendship and love. Participation in certain activities on behalf of the practice can reinforce these feelings and provide motivation. Attendance at continuing education courses, staff participation in the determination of office policies and procedures, use of staff ideas to improve office functions, membership in various professional organizations and societies, and the periodic use of group functions, such as office retreats and informal staff birthday celebrations, can all achieve this goal.

Ego Satisfaction

People need self-esteem, which comes from self-confidence, independence, and achievement. People also enjoy a sense of reputation, which confers status, recognition, respect, and appreciation. The satisfaction of these needs can greatly improve motivation.

These needs are satisfied by promotions, assignments that provide added responsibilities, participation in the training of new staff members, or evaluations or opportunities in which positive feedback is supplied about performance. Patients should be encouraged to include staff members when offering thanks for services. Employees should be allowed to write or sign memos to other staff members, display an outstanding employee's name in work areas, mention accomplishments in front of patients and peers, and market the employee to patients through the use of biographical sketches, comments on scripts, signs, display of awards and certificates, business cards, and name tags with an office title.

Recognition can be demonstrated by giving flowers, candy, lunches, theater tickets, or other rewards to employees. Saying "thank you" to employees, particularly in public, is effective. So is a letter to the employee, noting a job well done.

Self-Fulfillment

Motivation involves realizing one's own potential, continued self-development, and creativity in its broadest sense. This final area of need is said to come from within. Self-fulfilling employees are motivated through introspection, a recognition of what is important to them. They are able to focus on satisfying their personal needs and require no outside motivation. A manager must provide the resources and the opportunity for employees to reach their fullest potential by using the office as a vehicle to attain self-fulfillment.

Motivating employees must take into account their needs and wishes. The manager must be able to recognize "true" rewards, which differ from individual to individual. When providing a reward, the manager must ask, "Is this reward really what the employee considers something special?"

A motivation plan can accompany a training program. Each opportunity to improve staff performance that is available to an employer can also be used to motivate employees. Retreats, staff meetings, lunch meetings, performance reviews, and opportune moments can all be used to reinforce positive behavior and encourage more of the same. Perhaps the most powerful opportunity of all is the opportune moment when an employee is caught doing something the right way. This moment should be seized, for such acknowledgment builds enthusiasm like nothing else.

Managers have, at their disposal, many strategies with which to motivate employees. Effective managers will utilize as many of these strategies as they can. They will note which strategies work best with individual employees. They will use these strategies to mold the staff into a team that works together to reach the goals of the practice. Management style strategies should be planned and implemented with the same attention that would be given to the planning and conduct of a vision examination. Managers should never forget to set aside sufficient time for administrative duties and responsibilities. If management is properly performed, this time will be enjoyably spent, working with an efficient and enthusiastic office staff.

BIBLIOGRAPHY

American Optometric Association. Practice Enhancement Program II, Professional Enhancement Module, Managing Your Practice Plan, Precourse Workbook. St. Louis: American Optometric Association, 1986.

American Optometric Association. Practice Enhancement Program II, Professional Enhancement Module, Your Marketing Plan Module Two, Precourse Workbook. St. Louis: American Optometric Association, 1986.

American Optometric Association. Practice Enhancement Program, MN 1, Optimize Your Professional Opportunities Through Personal and Professional Goal Setting. St. Louis: American Optometric Association, 1986.

American Optometric Association. Practice Enhancement Program, MN 5, Optimize Your Professional Opportunities Through Effective Office Staff Policies and Procedures. St. Louis: American Optometric Association, 1984.

Baldwin BL, Christensen B, Melton T. Rx for Success. Midwest City, OK: Vision Publications, 1982.

Blanchard K, Johnson S. The One Minute Manager. New York: Berkeley Publishing Group, 1982.

Blanchard K, Lorber R. Putting the One Minute Manager to Work. New York: Berkeley Publishing Group, 1985.

Maslow AH. Motivation and Personality. New York: Harper & Row, 1970;51.

McGregor D. The Human Side of Enterprise. New York: McGraw-Hill, 1960.

Peters TJ, Waterman RH Jr. In Search of Excellence. New York: Harper & Row, 1982;50, 53–54.

Tecker IJ, Tecker GH. "Big boom theory." Assoc Manage 1991;43(1):46–7.

Chapter 18
Patient Communication

Stuart Rothman, Harry Kaplan, and Craig Hisaka

What we got here is a failure to communicate.

—Frank R. Pierson
Cool Hand Luke

Successful health care practitioners find that the way they communicate with patients can be just as important as their clinical proficiency. Modern practitioners will often spend as much time explaining procedures, tests, treatment options, and recommendations as actually examining the patient. This chapter reviews the basic tenets of effective communication, while providing a basis for patient communication in an optometric office setting.

A STANDARD MODEL OF CARE

The classic disease model of health care can be analyzed in six stages:

- The period when the patient is at no risk.
- The period when the patient is at risk due to change in age or environment.
- The period after an agent strikes, during which the patient is in danger of acquiring the disease.
- The period when signs are present.
- The period when symptoms appear and the patient complains.
- The period when disability results.

In the past, health care focused on the last three stages of disease. Patients sought care only when they were in pain and extremely uncomfortable. Because a community's health care practitioners were educated and highly trained, they were respected and often revered. Communication between practitioner and patient was comparable to that between parent and child—the practitioner told the patient what to do; the patient listened and complied. The practitioner's advice was never openly questioned by the patient, who always assumed a passive role. This paternal model of health care persisted for many decades.

Today, the dynamics of health care and of the doctor-patient relationship have changed. Contemporary practitioners are likely to be treating patients of equal education and economic level. Patients are more informed about health and the factors that relate to health. They also understand that health care needs to move beyond a pure disease model of care. Successful patient communication depends on the willingness of practitioner and staff to accept the patient as an equal and to consider the patient a participant in the treatment regimen. Practitioners must also appreciate that a patient who understands diagnoses and treatment options will be a more compliant patient, with the attendant long-term benefits to health that this understanding brings.

A successful practitioner knows the expectations brought to the doctor-patient relationship. The practitioner should enter the relationship expecting to provide the highest level of care. When providing care, the practitioner expects the patient to comply with recommendations and to establish and maintain an open line of dialogue regarding needs, wants, and results. The patient's expectations include being treated with respect, kindness, and compassion, and in a highly ethical and professional manner. Within any relationship, there can be different expectations by both practitioner and patient with each individual encounter. The practitioner who is able to fully understand the expectations of the patient at each encounter will be the one who establishes a long-term relationship with the patient.

THE NEED TO COMMUNICATE EFFECTIVELY

In today's competitive health care environment, patient communication is a key element in the successful delivery of care. The importance of patient communication can be attributed to the following factors:

- Patients are more aware of health care issues and are more knowledgeable about the treatment options available to them.
- There is more competition for health care revenues, and this has led to increases in the advertising of health-related products and treatments.
- Increased specialization in health care has forced patients to triage themselves so that they can see the specialist who best meets their needs.
- Second opinions for major treatment options are expected by practitioners, patients, and insurance companies.
- The risk of liability claims has increased the need for informed consent, requiring patients to understand the risks and benefits of treatment options.
- The increasing automation of tests and procedures has allowed for greater use of technicians and assistants. In the efficient delivery of health care, the practitioner acts as an interpreter of information and has more time to discuss findings, diagnoses, and treatment options.

SETTING THE STAGE FOR EFFECTIVE COMMUNICATIONS

In order for effective patient communication to occur, the practitioner must identify the message or image to be conveyed to patients by the office. This message or image should be communicated to every patient or potential patient at every encounter with the practitioner or staff. It should also be conveyed in every other type of communication that comes out of the office.

The most important messenger that any practitioner will have is the office staff. The staff will be the first contact that a potential patient has with the office. Staff members will also be the first contact the patient has when arriving at the office. Effective patient communications require that the right staff members be hired and that they are trained to communicate properly. Even if an office has a staff manager, it is ultimately the practitioner who must select, train, and monitor staff members.

Telephone Communications

Most patients will have their first contact with an office through the telephone. This first encounter must convey warmth, caring, competence, and efficiency. The staff member responsible for answering the telephone must direct full attention to the person calling and must avoid diversions that convey a negative message. Many practice consultants advise putting a smiling face or humorous saying near the telephone to remind the staff member to convey a positive image to the patient. It is a good idea to have carefully scripted responses to common questions that might be asked in routine telephone conversations. Some practitioners prepare audiotapes of experienced staff members responding to questions, so that they can be used when training new staff members. Telephone communications require that a protocol be observed when responding to callers. Some common requirements are listed in Table 18.1. As optometrists increasingly engage in the treatment of eye disease, it is essential that the person answering the phone be trained to properly triage callers. Staff members must be told what constitutes an emergency or what is urgent, so that prompt and appropriate care is provided.

Communication Through Marketing

Marketing comprises the whole range of efforts that go into building and maintaining a professional practice. To be most effective, the message

Table 18.1. Telephone Etiquette

Do's:
- Answer the telephone with a smile.
- Treat the patient the way you would want yourself or your family to be treated.
- Talk slightly slower than normal conversation and enunciate clearly.
- Offer to call a patient back rather than put the patient on hold for longer than 1 minute.
- Stay as close as possible to the office telephone script.
- Try to reinforce a caring, concerned attitude.
- Remember that the office is there to serve the patient, not the other way around.

Don't's:
- Be abrupt with the patient.
- Rush the patient.
- Continue to put the patient on hold more than once or keep the patient on hold for longer than 30 seconds without checking back in.
- Give professional advice.
- Assume that the patient understands everything about what the office does or the services it provides.

that is communicated must be consistent, fill a need in the community, and be communicated in such a way that patients and prospective patients understand the potential benefits of having this need fulfilled. Specific marketing strategies will be based on the needs of a particular community, but there must be consistency in the message conveyed to the patient. Various themes can be observed in the advertising used by large corporations. These themes range from quality of care to specific product promotions with emphasis on price. Once a marketing niche is established, it becomes difficult to change the image that has been created. Therefore, the initial message needs to be appropriate for the practice.

Communication in the Office

Several factors contribute to effective communication with patients while they are in the office: the appearance of the office, the appearance of practitioner and staff, efforts to alleviate patient apprehension, use of printed materials, and verbal communication.

Office Appearance

Patients expect to be cared for in an office that is clean, neat, uncluttered, and up-to-date. The reception room should be large enough to accommodate several patients without being crowded. The furniture does not need to be of "living room" quality but should not be sterile and impersonal. Refreshments, such as coffee and soft drinks, convey a caring attitude. Patients should be offered a choice of materials to view while they are waiting to be seen. Brochures, pamphlets, books, magazines, and videotapes can be used to entertain and inform patients while they wait.

One of the biggest complaints by patients is the time that must be spent waiting to be seen by practitioners. Patients are expected to arrive at or before their appointment times. They, in turn, expect practitioners to begin the examination within a reasonable period after the scheduled appointment time. No amount of plush furniture, entertainment, or refreshments will negate a 1-hour wait. On days when the office is running well behind schedule, a call to the patient at home or work should be standard procedure.

Patient treatment rooms should convey a feeling of security to the patient. Equipment does not need to be brand new, but it should be in excellent working order and have a modern appearance. While the patient might not know the difference between a phoropter that is 20 years old and one that is new, an examination chair that is worn will be readily apparent.

Patient expectations are usually highest in the dispensary. If the patient has been to or seen a "super optical" showroom, an inevitable comparison will be made. The patient might not expect to see the same number of frames displayed but will expect to see frames arranged in an attractive and tasteful manner. The appearance of the dispensary can be crucial in the patient's decision to purchase eyewear. The image and feeling that the dispensary conveys to the patient will affect the patient's impression of the quality and value of the eyewear being displayed.

Practitioners should set aside a portion of each year's budget for the purchase of new equipment or for the improvement of the office. Existing patients will notice changes that have occurred in the office and will talk about these changes to friends and relatives. This enthusiastic promotion of the practice can help pay for the changes many times over.

Personal Appearance

As competent and as caring as a practitioner might be, the patient will form an impression at the first encounter that can be quite difficult to change if it is negative. This first impression depends as much on the practitioner's appearance as it does on what the practitioner says or does. The office staff can also convey a negative first impression. There are many schools of thought about what constitutes appropriate attire for practitioner and staff. Authority can be conveyed by more formal attire, such as a white clinic jacket or uniforms, but this image can be offset by too much formality. Comfort is important, but practitioner and staff should be dressed in attire that patients are comfortable with as well. Proper attire can vary from one part of the country to another, and even within a relatively small area. What is appropriate for a large city might not be appropriate for a rural community just a few miles away. Appearance can also vary depending on the type of patient seen in the office (e.g., children as compared to adults). Practitioners must take note of all these factors and determine the type of image that is appropriate for the practice and patient population.

Alleviating Patient Apprehension

Many patients come to the office of a health care provider with a sense of apprehension. This feeling is not limited to new patients—it can be held by existing patients as well. New patients are entrusting their health and well-being to an individual they only know by the recommendation of a friend, relative, other practitioner, or preferred provider insurance listing. Aside from the uncertainties these patients might have about this new practitioner, there are the obvious concerns about vision or health that caused them to seek care in the first place. Existing patients share this apprehension, whether they are seeking care for a problem or for a routine examination with no symptoms. Very few people can "be themselves" under these circumstances. Understanding this apprehension can help practitioner and staff make patients feel more at ease, allowing the practitioner to obtain greater insight into the person being treated and generally permitting better treatment to be provided. The patient's openness will also lead to greater willingness on the part of the practitioner to communicate treatment options and will lead to greater understanding of treatment options by the patient.

Calling the patient by name and discussing the patient's hobbies, family, work, and avocational interests help the practitioner and staff relate on a more personal level while also alleviating the patient's apprehension about the office visit.

Use of Printed Materials

Many offices offer printed materials that describe the practice (e.g., a "welcome to the office" brochure), the services that the office provides, new ophthalmic materials available in the dispensary, or the treatment options for various ocular conditions. Representative brochures can be found in Figure 18.1. Printed materials are useful because they provide information even after the patient has left the office. More important, they reinforce, in writing, the information presented verbally during the examination. These brochures can be designed by the practitioner and printed at a modest cost, or they can be purchased from various suppliers such as private companies, contact lens and frame companies, optical laboratories, and professional organizations such as the American Optometric Association.

Videotapes can also be used to disseminate information to patients and, in fact, are enjoying increasing popularity. Tapes can be used for instruction in the office or lent to patients for viewing at home. Subjects include contact lenses, vision training, and treatment options for various conditions. Depending on the subject matter, they can be obtained from private companies or professional organizations.

Verbal Communication

There is no substitute for the face-to-face contact that practitioner and staff have with the patient in the office.

The case history is one of the most important parts of the examination, because it will establish the personal and clinical relationship between prac-

Figure 18.1. Sample printed patient communication brochures. (Reprinted with permission from the American Optometric Association.)

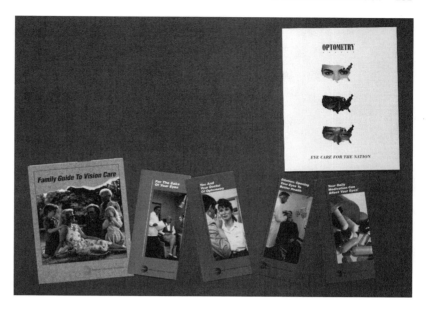

titioner and patient. A good clinician will listen as the patient describes the chief complaint and, as necessary, will help the patient articulate the problem being described. The information conveyed will guide the clinician's examination while ensuring that the clinician addresses the patient's concerns.

Describing the purpose of testing as it is performed will make the patient feel more informed and will enable the patient to become more of a participant in care. It will also educate the patient about the services that are being provided.

The case disposition must address the needs of the patient. A clinician's ability is directly related to his or her capacity to describe how the patient's problem relates to the testing performed and how the treatment prescribed can alleviate the problem. This means talking to the patient in terminology the patient can understand. Effective communication can also involve using demonstration aids so that the patient can better visualize what is being described. Examples of some of these demonstration aids are provided in Figure 18.2. The case disposition might require the practitioner to present the patient with various treatment options and describe the pros and cons of each option. Effective communication means listening as well as talking. The patient should be guided toward the best solution so that the patient

participates in the decision-making process and understands the outcome.

There might be instances when the practitioner has to act like a practitioner of the past and inform the patient of the actions that must be taken. These situations usually will involve direct risk to patient health and well-being, such as sight-threatening diabetic retinopathy. Even in these instances, it is important that the practitioner be able to effectively communicate dangers and risks to the patient to ensure patient compliance.

The issue of informed consent must also be considered in cases that pose a risk of injury. The patient has a right to know the risks, hazards, and likely outcomes of a recommended procedure or treatment and to be informed of the alternatives to that particular test or treatment. Informed consent also requires disclosure when suspicious findings or abnormalities are detected.

The latter obligation is the toughest test of the optometrist's communication skills. For example, a patient with elevated intraocular pressures must be informed of the potential significance of this finding and informed of the specialized testing that must be performed to rule out the possibility of glaucoma. The practitioner must convey the need for testing and the need for long-term follow-up even if the results are negative, so that the

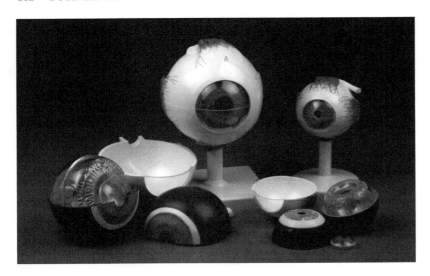

Figure 18.2. Models for explanation of vision problems. (Reprinted with permission from the American Optometric Association.)

patient understands and agrees to periodic assessment for disease.

Communication with Patients After They Leave the Office

Effective patient communication occurs not only when patients are in the office but also after they have left. Patients who encounter a problem, such as with ophthalmic materials, often will not call the office to describe the problem; instead, they simply will not return for further care. They might also tell relatives and friends about their problem. The successful office can prevent such situations from occurring. Problems can be identified by calling patients after services or materials are provided to ensure that they are satisfied. Many offices will conduct periodic patient surveys to obtain feedback about office policies and patient management.

The success of an office in handling patient problems is determined by the attitude of practitioner and staff. The office should regard patient complaints as an opportunity to regain trust and confidence and should convey a positive attitude. The office that handles these problems defensively will further antagonize the patient.

Satisfaction will be determined by the patient's perception that treatment exceeded expectations.

Dissatisfaction occurs when patients perceive that they have not gotten what they expected. Satisfaction can be increased by elevating the patient's perception of treatment or by decreasing the patient's expectations. After the fact—when patients have already been provided with treatment—it is difficult to lower their expectations. Therefore, decreasing patient expectations is not a practical alternative. The most successful strategy is to elevate the perception of treatment. This should be the goal of the office.

Communicating with Special Patient Populations

There are three populations that require special communication techniques: the elderly, persons with disabilities, and children.

The Elderly

The office that communicates well with elderly patients and makes them feel comfortable will invariably do a better job of serving this growing segment of the U.S. population. The elderly population is the group most likely to experience diminished visual performance, and it is important that they be made to understand the age-related visual changes that can occur. More than any other age group, they will be apprehensive about eye health because of the increased prevalence of glaucoma, age-related macu-lopathy, and cataracts among their friends and con-temporaries. They can also be under treatment for systemic conditions that have ocular manifestations, such as diabetes and hypertension. Their under-standing of these conditions might come from what they have learned from friends, relatives, or the media. The key to successful management of these patients is to set realistic expectations. Age-related vision changes are common. The case disposition should describe these changes in terms the patient will understand. Demonstrations, pictures, and videotapes will help elderly patients understand their condition and the visual limitations that can occur.

The practitioner should be aware of any hearing or mobility problems that a patient has before bring-ing the patient into the examination room. Practi-tioner and staff should be especially conscious of talking directly to the patient, not to a caretaker or relative accompanying the patient. Eye contact and clear enunciation are especially important. Elderly patients should not be addressed by first name, es-pecially by practitioners and staff who are younger than the patient.

Elderly patients do not like to feel rushed during an examination. They might have concerns that they will not share with the clinician until they feel com-fortable doing so. The practitioner who is a skilled communicator will be able to guide the patient to the important areas of the case history without mak-ing the patient feel rushed. Unrushed communica-tion should continue throughout the examination to make the patient feel at ease and reassured. Elderly patients with visual problems might not give clear, consistent subjective responses. These responses should be verified for consistency and should be confirmed by objective findings when possible. Clinicians should never forget that subjective re-sponses will become less reliable if patients feel that they are being rushed.

The office staff can be tremendously helpful in making an elderly patient feel welcome and in conveying a caring attitude. Offering the patient a cup of coffee or tea on a cold winter's day, calling a taxi for the patient when the examina-tion is concluded, referring to the patient by name, inquiring about the patient's children and grandchildren, and reinforcing the practitioner's recommendations can go a long way toward cre-ating enthusiasm in elderly patients.

Patients with Disabilities

Many of the communications procedures used for elderly patients are also applicable to patients with disabilities. However, several additional procedures need to be offered. Disabled patients will want to know that the practitioner and staff feel comfortable dealing with them. The office staff needs to convey this attitude to patients when the appointment is made, before the patient ever enters the office. The office policy regarding patients with disabilities should be determined in advance. Nothing destroys confidence more than a receptionist who puts the patient on hold while checking to see if the practi-tioner will see the patient. Practitioners should adopt a policy that is in keeping with legal require-ments. Federal, state, and local laws regulate access to health care offices and providers, and office poli-cies should be consistent with these laws.

The office staff should also be aware of how to handle the office visit by a disabled patient. Care in-volves not only direct communication to the patient but also indirect communication—how to seat the patient during pretesting or how to manage the spe-cial visual requirements and restrictions that influ-ence eyewear selection and dispensing.

Many patients with disabilities will come to the office with a friend, relative, or caretaker but are able to understand and make decisions and should be treated accordingly during testing and case disposition. Practitioner and staff should talk directly to the patient, not to the person accompa-nying the patient. Patients with disabilities should be treated like any other patient in terms of re-spect and equality.

Children

Many practitioners find that the pediatric popula-tion is their most difficult patient group. Children do not respond and act like adults when visiting a health care provider. It should not be forgotten that a child does not make the decision to be examined. This decision has been made for them, and it takes a special ability to get them to cooperate and partici-pate in care. Children have a keen sense of know-ing if a practitioner or staff member feels comfortable with them. They do not like to be ig-nored or talked down to. They want to feel that the practitioner and staff are concerned and interested in them and their lives. They want to be comforted during testing and reassured that they are safe and secure with the care provided by the practitioner and office staff.

The office environment should be inviting to children. A corner area of the reception room can be made into a children's play area with a child-size table and chairs, puzzles, books, and games. All of these items should meet applicable safety standards for children. Some offices will use videotapes to entertain children when they are waiting, though they should be offered only if they can be made unobtrusive to any adult patients who might also be waiting.

Parents might not want to discuss their concerns with the child in the room, requiring that the case history be taken with the parent before the child is brought into the room for examination. Many practitioners do not wear white clinic jackets when examining children, preferring a more informal appearance. The office should be equipped with instrumentation that is specifically designed for children's visual abilities. Objective pretesting can be used to obtain initial information and limit fatigue. Given the limited attention span of children, testing should be performed quickly, with the most important tests, as determined by case history, performed first. Nonthreatening aids like hand puppets and cartoons can be used to maintain visual attention during testing. The practitioner might find it useful to discuss the case disposition with the parent before or after speaking directly to the child.

Using positive reinforcement, behavior modification, and a reward system can help make the practitioner's job easier during testing by making the child more cooperative. It can also leave the child with a positive impression of the experience. Using colorful stickers, toys, or treats can go a long way toward putting a smile on the face of the child as he or she leaves the office.

CONCLUSION

In today's competitive health care marketplace, the office that communicates a caring, compassionate, and competent impression to patients is able to succeed and flourish. More than any other skill, effective communication will attract patients, create a favorable image of practitioner and staff, and moti-

vate patients to return for future care. With effective communication, satisfied patients will become enthusiastic patients. This should be the ultimate goal of any patient encounter.

BIBLIOGRAPHY

Anan B. Understanding the older patient population. Optom Manage 1989;25(11):35–41.

Baldwin BL, Christensen B, Melton JW. Rx for Success. Midwest City, OK: Vision Publications, 1983;105–18.

Baker WJ. Listening will improve your hearing. Optom Manage 1987;23(7):57–61.

Bennett I. Dealing with patient complaints, remakes. Optom Manage 1988;24(2):94.

Bremer A. Caring for older adults. Optom Econ 1991;1(10):14–6.

Brooks DJ. Kid stuff. Optom Econ 1991;1(9):42–5.

Christensen B. Personalities: can you mix and match? Optom Manage 1989;25(12):29–33.

Classé JG. Legal Aspects of Optometry. Stoneham, MA: Butterworth, 1989;295–301.

Fischer BA. Fine tuning the message. Optom Econ 1992;2(1):12–21.

Gailmard NB. Managing the grief patient. Optom Econ 1991;1(8):18–21.

Handler G. Remember the person behind the eyes. Optom Manage 1989;25(2):88–92.

Jameson M, Muhr C. Telephone triage in a primary care practice. Optom Econ 1995;5(1):46–50.

Lee G. Serving hearing impaired patients. Optom Econ 1994;4(11):8–12.

Legerton J. Our two most powerful tools. Optom Econ 1994;4(6):20–2.

Levoy B. Proper etiquette with disabled people. Optom Econ 1992;2(5):41–2.

Lill DJ, Cotham JC, Thomas JC. Listen up. Optom Econ 1991;1(4):24–8.

Marino D. Managing the hearing impaired. Optom Manage 1988;24(10):67–71.

Melton JW, Phillips JH, Plank KE. Answers for success. Optom Econ 1992;2(4):34–6.

Miller PJ, Miller RW. How to manage patients with emotional problems. Optom Manage 1989;25(9):97–100.

Morrison RJ. Quality, caring, and marketing. Optom Econ 1991;1(6):28–31.

Palmer DM. Telephone techniques. Optom Econ 1991; 1(3):18–21.

Persico J. What does your reception area say about you? Optom Manage 1992;27(7):33–8.

Practice Enhancement Program. Optimize Your Professional Opportunities through Patient Communication in Your Practice. Professional Enhancement Monograph, MN 17. St. Louis: American Optometric Association, 1986.

Practice Enhancement Program. Optimize Your Professional

Opportunities through Patient Communication in Your Community. Professional Enhancement Monograph, MN 18. St. Louis: American Optometric Association, 1986.

Schulman E. What patients need to know. Optom Econ 1991;1(9):12–15.

Scipione PA. Capturing and keeping the senior patient. Optom Manage 1989;25(11):24–8.

Sherburne SO. Handling the problem patient. Optom Econ 1991;1(11):25–7.

Stein H. Communication skills: do you rate a ten? Optom Manage 1991;26(1):65.

Stein H. Communication skills, part 2: Opportunities for success. Optom Manage 1991;26(2):59.

Stein H. Dress for success, yes! Optom Manage 1991;26(3):51.

Stein H. Turn complaints into compliments. Optom Manage 1991;26(5):61.

Werner DL. Ethics and the presbyopic patient. Optom Econ 1994;4(3):15–18.

Wright R. The best foot forward. Optom Econ 1991;1(1):46–7.

Zaba J. Catering to the children in your practice. Optom Manage 1989;25(1):80–2.

Chapter 19

Interprofessional Relations

Jack Bridwell, Michael Usdan, and Paul Farkas

*A little sincerity is a dangerous thing, and a great
deal of it is absolutely fatal.*

—Oscar Wilde
The Critic as Artist

Because optometry has become a primary eye care
profession, optometrists increasingly receive referrals from other health care professionals while
steadily providing referrals to these same health
care professionals. A healthy practice will enjoy a
good working relationship with many kinds of
health care providers.

Practitioners should attempt to identify all optometric and nonoptometric referral sources within
the community. Interprofessional referral techniques should also be explored, for they will result
in better patient care and management. Characteristics of resourceful referral partnerships include developing professional relationships, marketing to
target professionals, professional communication
and reporting, professional courtesies, and remem-
brances for referring sources. These characteristics
are the subject of this chapter.

DEVELOPING PROFESSIONAL
REFERRALS

It is a healthy practice that has the confidence of
other professionals who refer patients. These professionals can be other optometrists, other eye care
professionals, practitioners in other fields of health
care, and professionals whose work is not health
care. To develop such a referral base requires a will-

ingness on the part of these professionals to entrust
their patients to the optometrist.

Why Should a Practitioner Refer?

In general, referrals are made from one health care
professional to another if the service needed is beyond the scope of licensure or training of the practitioner making the referral. Legally and ethically,
referral is required when specialized testing or
treatment is needed that cannot be provided by the
referring practitioner.

Certain procedures can be so time consuming
that it is not cost effective for a practitioner to perform them, necessitating that the patient be sent to
a colleague or specialty clinic, even though the referring practitioner is legally allowed to provide
the procedure.

If a practitioner does not possess the specialized
equipment or instrumentation needed to make a diagnosis or provide treatment, the practitioner must refer
the patient so that the appropriate care can be rendered.

Why Don't Practitioners Refer?

Practitioners may choose not to refer for several
reasons. Many times a practitioner enjoys perform-

ing a particular procedure to gain further experience or wants to do the procedure because of the challenge the procedure presents. In a beginning practice that is not yet established, a new practitioner might be motivated to perform a wide range of procedures for economic reasons. Sometimes there is fear that failure to perform certain procedures can result in loss of professional prestige and recognition. Actually, when a patient is referred to a highly qualified individual, the benefit is usually significant and results in an even higher professional regard for the referring practitioner.

There is always the concern that not only the patient but also the patient's family might never return after a referral. In fact, more often than not after a successful referral, the entire family becomes loyal to the referring practitioner. Conscientious practitioners who seek to provide the highest level of care will always gain the respect of patients and their families.

HOW TO ENCOURAGE REFERRAL SOURCES

Optometrists should consider several factors when attempting to develop referral sources. First, skill must be attained in a specific area of practice. A high level of skill is often achieved by limiting practice to a specific specialty, such as contact lenses, low vision, or binocular vision. In such a practice, the optometrist can expect more referrals from primary eye care practitioners. If it is not practical, due to economic considerations, to limit the practice to a specialty area, then patients referred for consultation should be returned to the referring practitioner. Under no circumstances should the consultant provide primary eye care for these patients. A report should be sent to the referring practitioner after testing or treatment has been completed. This report should describe how the patient's problem has been determined and, in clear, concise terms, the results of the treatment or disposition of care.

A new practitioner should be willing to accept difficult cases—difficult cases that are extremely time consuming will often be the first ones that another practitioner refers. These cases might not have a cost-effective result, but success with difficult cases will ultimately provide referrals of patients whose treatment will be more cost effective.

To gain the respect and confidence of referral sources, a new optometrist must gain prestige by obtaining success in a chosen area of practice. An effort should be made to become a diplomate of the American Academy of Optometry in an area of expertise. The academy provides a rather rigorous examination, both written and practical, that must be passed to obtain recognition. Efforts should also be made to publish in professional journals. These publications can be presented to potential referral sources when appropriate. A recognized expert will be asked to lecture at continuing education programs. The greater the number of lectures, the greater the exposure, the more opportunity for receiving referrals from other practitioners.

If specializing, the practitioner should have state-of-the-art, highly specialized instrumentation. If such instrumentation is not available to the average practitioner it provides a rational reason to refer to the "specialist." The specialist must always be available for phone consultation with referring doctors at any time. Sometimes the specialist can be required to offer advice regarding patients not yet referred.

To succeed with difficult patients it is expected that as much time as is required will be spent to fully satisfy the objective of the referral.

Finally, it is essential to send patients back to the referring practitioner. If patients are not returned, further referrals are unlikely.

Marketing to Target Professionals

The many types of health care professionals located in the general area should be identified. Many such professionals are listed in Table 19.1.

Meeting with Local Health Care Professionals

A detailed list of all health care professionals in the area should be developed. A new practitioner should personally visit each of these health care professionals. During the visit, the practitioner should ask if the professional can be used as a referral source for specific problems. The professional will very likely offer to return the favor. A week or two later the practitioner should mail a copy of an office brochure, with a brief cover letter, to the professional.

Table 19.1. Health Care Professionals

1. **Family practice/general practitioners** are truly primary care providers.
2. **Pediatricians** may also be primary care providers.
3. **Dermatologists**, although secondary providers, often see patients who present for primary care and who may require the services of an optometrist when the dermatologist has completed treatment.
4. **Allergists** can be an excellent source of referral because many allergies are eye-related and may create vision problems.
5. **Internists** are similar to family practitioners because many symptoms of problems in internal medicine, such as headaches, are eye- and vision-related.
6. **Cardiopulmonary specialists** can see optometric patients who will need to be comanaged if on certain medications.
7. **Plastic surgeons** frequently require the services of an optometrist for their patients after eye surgery, and specifically, blepharoplasty. Many contact lens problems need treatment following surgery.
8. **Podiatrists** see and treat many elderly patients who also require continuing eye care. They work well with optometrists.
9. **Chiropractors** might see patients who complain of headaches that might fall into the field of ophthalmic care.
10. **Industrial physicians** frequently see patients with injuries, such as foreign body injuries, that benefit from optometric care.
11. **Nurses** are extremely good referral sources because patients who complain of eye strain, headache, and red eyes often seek their advice first. They are respected and trusted by other health care professionals. They are influenced and motivated by quality care. The positions that nurses might fill include:
    - Corporate staff nurses
    - Clinic nurses
    - Hospital nurses
    - School nurses
    - Visiting and licensed vocational nurses

From time to time, articles relating vision to systemic disease can be found in professional journals, medical-pharmaceutical updates, and timely news items. A copy of the article can be sent to the appropriate professional; included should be a brief note indicating that the professional might find the article of interest.

Working with Ophthalmologists

A mutual referral relationship with a local ophthalmologist must include a one-on-one discussion of vision care philosophies, including protocols to be used for the comanagement of specific vision and eye health conditions.

Each practitioner must fully understand and respect the other to establish a successful relationship. For a beginning optometrist, it is helpful to discuss specific referral procedures, such as when to refer, how to make an appointment, what to provide in a referral letter, and when the ophthalmologist will provide written followup after the consultation. When comanagement is necessary, protocols for care should be established and reduced to writing. Table 19.2 provides an example of a comanagement protocol.

For an optometrist to establish a long-term relationship with an ophthalmologist, each practitioner must understand and agree on the other's philosophy of care. For the patient's benefit, there should be no duplication of testing except where absolutely necessary. Information should be freely shared and care coordinated to eliminate duplicative or unnecessary followup.

A similar rapport must be established with a retinal specialist for the management of patients with diabetes, vitreous disorders, and retinal diseases. Inter-referral relationships with neuro-ophthalmologists, oculoplastic specialists, and other ophthalmologists will be less frequent, but the same frank discussions and agreements are needed to ensure strong professional relationships.

Working with Comanagement Centers

Eye care referral and surgical centers have been established nationwide. These centers capitalize on the value of inter-referral relationships. For years, referral was primarily from optometrists to ophthalmologists. Referral and surgical centers have been able to bring ophthalmologists and optometrists together in an as-

Table 19.2. Sample Comanagement Protocol*

CATARACT Post-Op Visit	Procedures	Expecteds
1 day surgeon		Follow-up report
1 week surgeon	BVA, IOP, SLE, refraction	Follow-up report
4 week O.D.	Refraction	Follow-up report
6 week O.D.	BVA, IOP, SLE dilated fundus exam	Follow-up report
9–12 months O.D.	Evaluate capsule	Follow-up report
	Retinal exam	
	IOP check	
Medication tapering protocol—suggested		
1 week	Tobradex qid	
3 weeks	Pred Forte tid tapered by 1 drop/day	
	Each week for 3 weeks as inflammation subsides	

*Contact the comanagement center immediately when patient response is outside normal limits.
Source: Courtesy of Dr. Randall Reichle, Eye Associates of Houston, Houston, TX.

sociation that produces the most efficient health care delivery system for eye care. Each professional practices at the highest level of competency. The initial evaluation and followup are provided by the optometrist, and surgery is performed by the ophthalmologist. Patients referred for care often receive medical and surgical treatment that is beyond the scope of practice for the referring optometrist.

Because information must be freely transferred between the referring practitioner and the comanagement center—often on a timely basis—facsimile transmission is necessary. The use of fax machines permits medical information to be instantly shared by practitioners, allowing diagnostic and treatment decisions to be made on the basis of current data. Use of the facsimile transmission has become state-of-the-art in eye care and should be considered a necessity when working with comanagement centers.

Obtaining Referrals from Optometrists

Because of the expanded scope of optometric practice and the advanced education (such as residency training) available in many areas of optometry, more and more optometrists are now specializing in limited areas of eye care. If an individual practitioner does not provide specialized services, professional ethics and legal standards of care can demand that patients who require specialized services be re-

ferred to the appropriate optometric or other health care specialist.

Examples of specialized practice include pediatrics, low vision, diagnosis of disease, contact lenses, and sports vision.

Pediatric Care

The pediatric specialist will have a practice that is geared toward the young patient, including children's waiting room furniture, pediatric acuity and visual skills assessment charts, up-to-date electronic training equipment, and an unusually large selection of children's eyewear in the dispensary.

The pediatric optometrist offers developmental vision services, as well as treatment for conditions such as strabismus, amblyopia, visually related learning disabilities, and vision perception problems. Today's pediatric optometric specialist might also be well versed in the fitting of infant or newborn eyeglasses. Contact lenses can also be fitted when necessary due to prematurity, surgery, or other related conditions. Pediatric optometrists work closely with teachers, counselors, and family members to ensure that there is continual feedback on any progress achieved in the treatment of the child's condition.

Low Vision

Although there are some "stand alone" low vision clinics, most low vision specialists are located within a facility that provides other vision and eye care services. These optometrists are located in facilities because it is difficult for a low vision practice to be financially self-sustaining. The low vision specialist provides a lengthy examination and uses unique equipment in the evaluation of the visually impaired patient. This equipment usually includes specialized low vision acuity and visual field tests, as well as a large variety of sizes and powers of magnifiers, handheld and spectacle-mounted microscopes and telescopes, lights, and electronic low vision aids such as closed circuit televisions. As the U.S. population ages, referrals for low vision care are sure to grow. The low vision specialist works closely with other optometrists, ophthalmologists, and state agencies that fund low vision care. Low vision care currently is not covered under Medicare or Medicaid, but it can be covered under a state vocational rehabilitation program.

Diagnosis of Disease

In the past, when a medical workup or report was needed by an optometrist, the patient was referred to an internist or specific medical specialist. In many instances, patients were lost after referral— physicians often sent referred patients to an ophthalmologist for followup care and rarely returned them to the optometrist. The optometrist rarely received reports about referred patients or even an acknowledgment of the referral.

The eye care referral center concept was born in the 1980s. Services offered through these referral centers include electrodiagnostic testing, fluorescein angiography, threshold visual field testing, medical care for ocular diseases, treatment of ocular emergencies, and the use of most types of eye surgery. Contact lenses, refractive care, spectacles, low vision aids, and visual training are usually excluded from the care given at these centers.

Since the implementation of these centers, optometrists have been able to participate in the decision-making process for patient care. Most of these centers use an optometrist for the clinic director and a physician for the medical director. Because patients are returned to the referring practitioners, these organizations have ensured that optometrists will play a role in the continuing management and followup of patients. The feedback received from the referral centers also improves

optometrists' education regarding the latest in disease diagnosis and treatment.

Optometric referral centers traditionally offer postgraduate continuing education courses for local and referring practitioners. For local optometrists, these centers will usually provide medical care for patients during periods when the optometrists are out of their offices for sickness, vacation, or emergencies.

Contact Lens Specialists

Most contact lens specialists limit their practices to the fitting and care of contact lens patients. Many work primarily with the "hard to fit" patient. These specialists have the expertise to fit patients with dry eye syndrome, astigmatism, and presbyopia. They have the knowledge and ability to fit unusually shaped and traumatized corneas. Because they are usually on the "cutting edge" of contact lens development, these practitioners often participate in clinical trials of new contact lens materials and solutions.

Sports Vision Specialists

Some optometrists offer sports vision as a subspecialty. Sports vision optometrists provide expertise at all levels of competition, from professional leagues to children's sports. These practitioners detect vision problems affecting athletic performance, prescribe special eyewear for sports and leisure activities, provide training to enhance athletic performance, prescribe protective eyewear to prevent eye injuries, and manage eye injuries suffered during athletic competition. Like the highly competitive athletes they serve, vision care in this field is state of the art, and requires the use of highly specialized equipment and techniques.

PROFESSIONAL COMMUNICATIONS

Optometry's role in health care has expanded significantly, requiring optometrists to describe patient findings and recommend management to other practitioners in the health care field. Optometrists are called on by other health care disciplines to perform specific tests and procedures for patients. Optometrists might offer more services than at any time in the profession's history, but they must rely on others in the health care field to work cooperatively for the benefit of patients. This approach is relatively new to many practitioners who have been in practice for 10 or more years. Emphasis is on personal communications among practitioners—such as letters of referral, consultation and summary reports, and thank you or summary reports for patient referrals.

Letters of Referral

When referring patients to another practitioner or health care facility, certain procedures and protocols should be followed. To ensure that the patient receives the care desired, the appointment for the referral should be made while the patient is in the office. The office to which the patient is referred should be informed of the needs of the patient so that a timely appointment can be scheduled and the appropriate tests performed. A referral letter should be written and sent so that it arrives before the date of the future appointment (Figure 19.1). Timely arrival can require sending the letter by facsimile transmission if a same-day referral is arranged.

A referral letter should describe any or all of the following:

- Patient's name, age, sex
- Date of examination
- Chief complaint and symptoms
- History of past and current eye care
- Pertinent health history, including medications being taken
- Significant tests performed and findings obtained
- Diagnosis and treatment
- Reason for referral
- Date of referral appointment

Copies of any pertinent test results (e.g., visual fields) should be attached.

Consultation and Summary Reports

Consultations for Medicare-eligible patients operate under special rules that have been in effect since 1992. Many of these rules will doubtless be adopted in some format by major medical insurance compa-

nies. Patients might need consultation for one or more reasons:

- Further testing before a definitive diagnosis is made
- Second opinions to confirm diagnosis or treatment
- Suggestions regarding ways to treat or approach the treatment of a specific condition

When a patient is referred for a consultation, the referring practitioner should note the reason for the consultation and request a timely telephone call or written summary report from the practitioner to whom the patient has been referred.

Thank You for Referrals and Summary of Findings

When a patient is referred to an optometrist for treatment, diagnosis, or advice, a summary letter describing test results or recommendations for care should be sent by the optometrist to the referring practitioner or facility as soon as possible. In many instances, a telephone call on the day of the visit can be provided. Words of thanks should be part of the beginning and ending of the call or letter. The summary of testing and results or recommendations should be brief, if possible, and a copy should be retained for the optometrist's file.

A letter should communicate the necessary information in an easy-to-read format. The practitioner should read and check each letter for spelling and accuracy of information before signing. A sample letter is provided in Figure 19.2.

PROFESSIONAL COURTESIES AND EXCHANGE OF SERVICES

There are many ways of handling professional courtesy. Each practitioner should be guided by local and customary practices among health care practitioners in the community.

A common policy is to exchange services only and to exclude costs related to laboratory charges. Under such a policy, an optometrist and the optometrist's family can receive medical and dental care services without cost but must pay for the actual cost of materials such as gold fillings, bridge-

(date)

Dr. M. Dee
1122 Friendly Street
Friendly, TX

Re: Mrs. I.M. Patient

Dear Dr. Dee:

I am referring Mrs. I.M. Patient, a 41-year-old white female seen in our office on April 5th, to you for treatment of diabetic retinopathy.

Mrs. Patient has been treated for diabetes for the past 11 years. She frequently fails to take her oral sulfonylurea, however, and seldom checks her blood glucose level. She reports not having seen her family physician for 18 months.

Examination findings are as follows:

Best visual acuity	OD 20/30-3 OS 20/20-2
Pupils	OD 4 mm R/D3/C3 No APD OS 4 mm R/D3/C3
Versions	Unrestricted
External assessment	Unremarkable
Intraocular pressures	OD 17 mmHg OS 16 mmHg
Fundus examination	Numerous dot and blot hemorrhages extending over four retinal fields in each eye. Hard exudates in and surrounding the macula in each eye, with retinal thickening. There is a hemorrhage in the macula of the right eye. Fundus photography was performed for documentation.
Amsler Grid	Positive OD

Impression: Preproliferative diabetic retinopathy, with clinically significant macular edema.

Mrs. Patient is being referred to you for fluorescein angiography and possible laser treatment. Please let me know if I can be of any further assistance in the care of this pleasant lady.

Sincerely,

Dr. Primary Care

Figure 19.1. Sample referral letter to ophthalmologist.

(date)

Dr. John C. Wright
1234 Aqueous Way
See Port, VA 35434

Re: Patient Tom Jones

Dear Dr. Wright:

Thank you for referring Mr. Jones for low vision care. When he was seen on Jan. 4th, he related his entire visual and physical case history. Your letter explaining his diabetic retinopathy was most helpful. His chief complaint was his recent inability to read fine print.

His vision was evaluated using a complete series of magnifiers and microscopic low visual aids. His best vision result was achieved while using a 4x aspheric hand-held magnifier. He was pleased with his vision (J-1) while using this aid.

Our technician provided complete instructions regarding the use of this aid, and it was dispensed to him today. Mr. Jones was advised to return to your office for your continued care. I appreciate the opportunity to participate with you in his care.

Sincerely yours,

Dr. Low Vision

Figure 19.2. Sample thank you letter for referral.

work, major medical tests, and medical appliances. Physicians, dentists, and other health care professionals (and their families) who are examined by the optometrist would enjoy the same courtesy, paying only for ophthalmic materials and not for services.

Just as frequently, many professionals exchange all the costs of care and treatment that are not reimbursable by third-party insurance carriers.

Successful optometrists will have the opportunity to examine most of the community's health care providers, as well as many nurses and ancillary medical personnel. It is always a rewarding policy to provide 10–20% professional courtesy to as many of the

ancillary personnel as possible, because they appreciate the gesture and they frequently make referrals.

When professional courtesy is offered, the same level of care should be offered as would be provided to a fee-for-service patient.

Developing and Cultivating Professional Relationships Through Common Interests

Generally, people who work or play together develop a common bond of trust and respect. Referrals are inevitable when a personal relationship occurs.

Communities usually offer many opportunities for professionals who share common interests to meet. Professionals possess leadership skills and usually share common interests in education, local government, and community service organizations. They share a civic responsibility to promote growth and excellence in the community. The opportunity to serve in charitable and service organizations is particularly meaningful. Although the primary goal of participation should be "service above self," as the Rotary Club's motto states, participation will nurture friendship as well as a professional association with others who share a civic-minded attitude.

Most professionals will pursue sports, social, or self-improvement activities. Among professionals who share similar interests, friendship is common. Such individuals are often mutually supporting and provide referrals to one another. Friendship becomes the basis for the sharing of care among patients.

Remembrances for Referring Practitioners on Special Occasions

The traditional Christmas or Thanksgiving gift to special referral sources can range from the inexpensive to the elaborate, depending on the extent of the relationship. The most important consideration is a "thank you" for the trust and confidence reposed in the optometrist. A thoughtful letter of appreciation can be as meaningful as, or, in some cases, even more meaningful than the gift. Whatever is given, it is best to be original—the novel gift can be very effective and is more easily remembered. It is also essential to keep track of each year's gift to avoid duplication year after year.

A unique way to thank special referral sources can be used any time of the year—theater tickets or tickets to popular sporting events. Invitations for dinner or cultural events are always appreciated. Social occasions in which spouses or family members participate can further bond the relationship and cultivate strong professional ties.

NON–HEALTH CARE PROFESSIONALS

In general, by developing a superb reputation for expertise, and by developing the credentials of a true specialist, optometrists can become important referral sources for non–health care professionals. Accountants, attorneys, architects, and engineers understand the effort that is required to obtain an advanced degree. They can become excellent patients if they understand and appreciate the quality of optometric education and service. In turn, they should be afforded the respect and consideration that is merited by the years of education and training necessary in their fields of expertise.

BIBLIOGRAPHY

Anonymous. Meeting report: making effective referral decisions. Optician 1987;194(12):14.

Baldwin B, Christensen B, Melton J. Rx for Success. Midwest City, OK: Vision Publications, 1983.

Ball RJ. A positive approach to improved interprofessional relations. Am J Optom Arch Am Acad Optom 1969;46(7):534–8.

Ball RJ, Henderson JW. Interprofessional relations: a solvable dilemma? Sight Sav Rev 1971;41(1):5–8.

Balliett G. Practice Management. New York: McGraw-Hill, 1978.

Bennett I. Bettering O.D.-M.D. referral relationships. Optom Manage 1988;24(12):43–5.

Bennett I. Building a practice the write way. Optom Manage 1983;19(6):63.

Bennett I. Management for the Eyecare Practitioner. Stoneham, MA: Butterworth, 1993.

Brahe NB. 15 Days to a Great New Practice. Appleton, WI: Project D Publications, 1971.

Brumberg JB. Efficient Ethical Private Practice. Dania, FL: Independent Ophthalmic Publishing, 1981.

Byers S, Cornett S. Nurses help lead interprofessional team. Ohio Nurses Rev 1990;65(1):8.

Classé JG. Legal Aspects of Optometry. Stoneham, MA: Butterworth, 1989.

Cohn S. The referral revolution. Optom Manage 1985; 21(11):26–30, 32, 34, 39, 42.

Elmstrom G. Advanced Management for Optometrists. Chicago: Professional Press, 1974.

Farkas P. Build a better contact lens practice. Optom Manage 1981;17(7):53.

Farkas P. Developing a contact lens practice. Contact Lens J 1993; 20(8):15–17.

Farkas P, Kassalow TW, Farkas B. Eight tips to build your contact lens practice. Optom Manage 1985;21(1):68–73.

Farkas P, Kassalow TW, Farkas B. "Extending" your extended wear practice. Optom Manage 1985;21(6):47–55.

Fortner C. Building cooperation with physicians: an interview with Charles Fortner. Am Pharm 1990;30(2):24–6.

Gregg J. The Business of Optometric Practice. New York: Advisory Enterprises, 1980.

Hopping RL. Optometry/ophthalmology interface [editorial]. J Am Optom Assoc 1977;48(1):19–24.

Horder J. Working with general practitioners. Br J Psychiatry 1988;153(10):513–20.

Hubler R. Confident, competent referrals. Optom Econ 1992;2(9):15.

Jackson WE. Family physicians: their referral potential. Optom Manage 1989;25(7):79–84.

Jacobi HP. A Dentist's Flight Manual to Success. Neenah, WI: Project P, 1973.

Kerfoot K. "Managing" professionals: the ultimate contradiction for nurse managers. Nurse Econ 1988;6(6):321–2.

Levoy RP. The $100,000 Practice and How to Build It. Englewood Cliffs, NJ: Prentice-Hall, 1966.

Levoy RP. The Successful Professional Practice. Englewood Cliffs, NJ: Prentice-Hall, 1970.

Mariano C. The case for inter-disciplinary collaboration. Nurse Out 1989;37(6):285–8.

Munson BJ. Doctor to doctor. Optom Econ 1991;1(10):35.

Richter S, Ettinger E. Study of physicians overlooking eye care, New York. AOA News 31(11):1–4.

Roberts BL. Communication between optometrists and physicians in referrals. J Am Optom Assoc 1971;42(1):64–8.

Sachs L. Professional courtesy. Optom Econ 1991;1(11):39–41.

Shaver, DV Jr. Opticianry, optometry, and ophthalmology: an overview. Med Care 1974;12(9):754–65.

Thurburn L, Annunziato T. Modern Optometry—1990; A Practice Management Guide. Houston, TX: Practice Management Associates, 1990.

Wick RE. Interprofessional relations—a case report. J Am Optom Assoc 1968;39(11):1013–14.

Winslow C. Put some muscle in your referral relationships. Rev Optom 1993:130(4):34–6.

Chapter 20

Recall Systems

Craig Hisaka and John Rumpakis

It ain't over 'til it's over.

—Yogi Berra
Comment on 1973
baseball pennant race

The scope of care in optometry has changed significantly over the past few decades. With this change in scope of practice and approach to services, there has been a concomitant change in the purpose and design of recall systems. In the past, the underlying motivation of a recall system was perceived as a strategy to "build a practice." The notion of "goodwill" was associated with recall systems because of the ability of these systems to sustain a practice. There have been several traditional reasons proffered for the use of such systems. A recall system provides an opportunity for the practitioner to get better acquainted with patients through regular interaction. Patients who enjoy a friendly relationship with a practitioner will (it is hoped) be more inclined to adhere to recommendations made by that practitioner. In recall sessions, the optometrist can regularly offer recommendations for preventing eye problems and detect problems unknown to the patients. Recall encourages patients to return for examinations—an important consideration because, frequently, patients will not take the initiative to return, even when they are satisfied with the care and treatment received.

Today, recall systems are also vital because they provide the practitioner with a mechanism to identify and monitor patients who are at risk for or suffer from pathological conditions. Recall serves as a way for the optometrist to keep patients informed of ocular health status and to properly evaluate and treat (when necessary) existing eye conditions. In fact, the concept of recall has been incorporated into the standard of care. Because of modern technology and instrumentation, the expanded scope of optometry, and the responsibilities of a primary care provider, the purpose of recall essentially has been redefined. An inadequate recall system, which results in untimely examination of patients, can result in permanent harm and injury and lead to litigation. Therefore, a successful recall system must be a feature of any practitioner's office. In this chapter, various types of recall systems are described, beginning with the most fundamental consideration—implementation of a system that is compatible with the practitioner's philosophy of care.

PHILOSOPHY OF CARE

The philosophy of the practice often dictates the approach to and the organization of the recall system. The aggressiveness of the system chosen must be acceptable to the practitioner or practice and should not reflect adversely on the professionalism of either.

Methods of Recall

After examination, the practitioner must determine when the patient needs to return for further care. Depending on the patient's status, the appointment could be the next day, week, month, or year. There needs to be a reminder to the patient of the appointment date. The patient needs to be given sufficient notice in advance of the appointment so that it can be changed if necessary, but it should not be so far in advance that the patient will forget. The time frame also needs to be such that, if the patient cancels the appointment, there is adequate time to schedule another patient in the vacated time slot.

There are three basic methods of providing recall to patients: mail, telephone, or a combination of both. (Mail and telephone systems actually tend to use both methods, but for the purposes of this discussion mail and telephone systems are classified as being primarily one of these methods.)

Mail Recall System

The mailing system is traditional and is used by most optometrists and dentists (Figure 20.1). It is probably the easiest system for an office to adopt. Since this approach is nonaggressive, the perception by patients should be favorable. In such a system a card is mailed notifying the patient that it is time for an examination to be scheduled or reminding the patient that a followup appointment has been scheduled. The patient is asked to call the office to make or confirm the appointment.

Because this recall system is passive, the patient response is lower than the other two methods. Also, the costs of printing and mailing makes this system expensive, and it can be time consuming for the staff. The system can be made more personal by using attractive envelopes with picture stamps instead of metered postage, personalized messages generated by computer, and addresses written by hand instead of printed labels.

Telephone Recall System

The telephone recall system allows personal contact with patients. Because it is personalized, it creates a positive perception. However, patients who cannot say "no" when called may fail to appear at the scheduled time, and therefore the "no-show" rate can still be substantial. This method will allow a practitioner to obtain information about why patients have not returned and, if applicable, the rea-

sons why they sought care elsewhere. This valuable information can assist the practitioner in improving the practice.

In implementing a telephone recall system, a staff member is assigned specifically to call patients. If the calls are to remind patients of scheduled appointments, patients to be seen in the morning are called the afternoon before the appointment and patients to be seen in the afternoon are called the morning of the appointment. If the purpose of the calls is to schedule patients for new appointments, calls are usually made in the late afternoon or early evening. If a patient cannot be reached by telephone, a letter or postcard is sent— letters make a better impression and other information can be provided in the letter. If the patient does not respond to the first recall attempt, a 2-year recall process is started. Approximately 1½ years after the last examination, the patient is telephoned and a letter or postcard is sent stating "second reminder." Approximately 2 years after the examination, another recall letter is mailed and a followup telephone call is made. After approximately 28 months, a fourth recall attempt is made by telephone, postcard, or letter. Then, at about 34 months the last telephone call is made, and correspondence stating "final reminder" is sent. If the patient does not respond, the patient's record should be placed in the nonactive file.

Combination Mail and Telephone Systems

As is evident from the preceding discussion, most recall systems use a combination of mail and telephone to contact patients. Usually mail is the means attempted for first contact with the patient, and the telephone is used to confirm that the card or letter was received and that the appointment will be kept or scheduled.

For annual or 2-year recall appointments, a card is sent reminding the patient that it is time to call to schedule an appointment. If the patient does not respond within a certain period of time (usually 1 month), the patient is contacted by telephone to ensure that the card was received and to determine if an appointment can be scheduled. If an appointment is made, the patient is contacted by telephone the afternoon or morning before the appointment as a reminder. Combination mail and telephone systems usually provide a

UAB OPTOMETRY **Primary Care Vision Service**

✓ **A friendly reminder.......**
**at your last visit, we reserved
this time for your next visit**

Day _____   **Date** _____

Time _____

**Please call us at 934-3089 to
confirm that this date and time is convenient !**

Dear
On _____, 19 _____, we had the
pleasure of providing a

☐ Vision Examination

☐ Contact Lens Examination

At that time it was recommended that a re-examination should be
performed in

☐   3 months   ☐   1 year

☐   6 months   ☐   1 1/2 Years

☐   9 months   ☐   2 years

Please call PRIMARY CARE SERV. to make an appointment.
                       934-3089

                                 Thank you,

                                 Resident _____

Resident

Figure 20.1. Sample postcards for mail recall system. (Courtesy of the School of Optometry, University of Alabama at Birmingham, Birmingham, AL. Reproduced with permission.)

Table 20.1. AOA Clinical Practice Guidelines for Examination of Children and Adults

	Examination Interval	
Patient Age	Asymptomatic/Risk-Free	At Risk
Children		
Birth–24 months	By 6 months of age or as recommended	By 6 months
2–5 years	At 3 years of age	At 3 years of age or as recommended
6–17 years	Before first grade and every 2 years thereafter	Annually or as recommended
Adults		
18–40 years	Every 2–3 years	Every 1–2 years or as recommended
41–60 years	Every 2 years	Every 1–2 years or as recommended
≥61 years	Annually	Annually or as recommended

Source: AOA Clinical Practice Guidelines for Comprehensive Adult Eye and Vision Examination and for Pediatric Eye and Vision Examination, 1995–96.

Use of a Preappointment System

With this recall system, an appointment is always scheduled before the patient has left the office, even for examinations 1–2 years in the future. A specific date and time are selected and entered into the appointment book or computer. Two to four weeks before the scheduled date, the patient is called and reminded of the appointment, which can be rescheduled if necessary. If preferred, a card can be sent to the patient approximately 1 month before the scheduled appointment. It contains the date and time of the appointment and asks the patient to call the office to confirm that the patient will be able to come as scheduled. If the patient does not respond to the card by 1–2 weeks before the appointment, a telephone call must be made to confirm the appointment or to schedule a new date and time.

The advantages of preappointing are that the appointment book stays full, avoiding seasonal slow periods, and it is less costly than other methods of recall since it does not necessarily involve printing and mailing expenses. The disadvantages of this method are that it requires careful coordination of effort to ensure that preappointed patients are properly confirmed or rescheduled, and that patients can misinterpret the purpose of preappointing if the system is not properly explained. Patients may perceive this method as aggressive and more attuned to filling appointment slots than providing needed care. If done appropriately, however, the "no show" rate is the lowest for all the recall systems.

Setting a Reasonable Recall Schedule

Recommended guidelines for the examination of children and adults, drawn from the consensus of opinion in the profession, have been established by the American Optometric Association. These clinical practice guidelines generally require different recall periods for asymptomatic individuals who are not at risk than it requires for individuals who are at risk for ocular disease (Table 20.1).

Use of Computers to Facilitate Recall

Using a computer can be as useful, if not imperative, for recall systems as it is for other areas of office management. Every practice should have some type of computer system. Since specific information pertaining to patients can be easily identified by using a database, it is simple for staff members to produce a list of patients due for recall. Also, staff members can measure the effectiveness of the patient recall system by using the computer to create information that can be easily read and interpreted (see Chapter 12).

One of the advantages of computer recall is that mailings can be personalized. Specific messages can be addressed to individual patients, creating a personal touch that assists in the effort to get patients to respond. Computerized recall also works well with preappointment systems, but such a system does require operation by a knowledgeable staff member.

When Patients Ignore Recall Attempts

Patients have a variety of reasons for not responding to recall notices. Common reasons for patients' failure to make recall appointments include shortage of financial resources, satisfaction with vision, perception that the optometrist's fees are not competitive, or dissatisfaction with the optometrist's practice.

The most effective way to determine why a patient has not returned for an appointment is by calling the patient. A telephone call under such circumstances requires the office staff to be tactful. When making such a call, the staff member first inquires about the patient's well-being in general and then explains that a review of the person's file indicates that the patient has not been in the office for a significant period of time, and this has caused some concern. Next, the staff member suggests that the patient come in for an examination. If the patient's response is not positive, the staff member attempts to learn if the patient would like another reminder at a later time. If the patient does not want further communication, the call is ended.

When a patient decides to remain inactive, an exit survey should be sent. Along with the survey, there is a letter stating that the optometrist is looking for ways to improve the delivery of health care and asking that the patient complete the survey anonymously. The survey—concisely written and containing a limited number of multiple choice or true-false questions—elicits responses about the optometrist's fees, location and physical plant, convenience and availability of appointments, professional demeanor, staff, parking and public transportation, services, and selection of eyewear and contact lenses. A self-addressed, stamped envelope is enclosed with the survey for the patient's convenience.

If a patient is being recalled to provide follow-up for an eye problem, and if the patient fails to keep the appointment, the practitioner should have a staff member call the patient to determine why the appointment was not kept and to schedule the patient for a new date and time. If a patient with a problem fails to appear despite repeated efforts to schedule the patient for followup, the practitioner should send the patient a letter (by certified mail, with return receipt requested, if documentation of receipt is necessary). The letter should advise the patient of the necessity for further examination, describe the possible complications that might result if an examination is not performed, and urge the patient to call to schedule an appointment. A copy of the letter should be retained in the patient's file.

CONCLUSION

Patients tend to make appointments when they recognize a vision problem or have some uncertainty about their vision or eyes. Many patients would not return for regularly scheduled examinations without receiving a recall notice. Therefore, a recall system is important, but its effectiveness depends on the practitioner's and the staff's understanding of the system and on the ability of the office to adhere to its procedures. To be successfully implemented, a recall system must not only be appropriately structured but also provide a true benefit to patients. This value to the patient is the most important element of any recall system.

BIBLIOGRAPHY

Bergman L. Winning way with direct mail. Optom Econ 1991;1(5):8.

Crooks CT III. The ultimate recall system. Optom Econ 1991;1(12):34–7.

Freeman D. Recall on line. Optom Econ 1991;1(6):32–7.

Freeman D. Taking the headache out of recall. Optom Manage 1989;25(7):87–92.

Hubler R. Beyond the postcard. Optom Econ 1991;1(12): 12–16.

Levoy RP. The $100,000 Practice and How to Build It. Englewood Cliffs, NJ: Prentice-Hall, 1966;141–9.

Sachs L. Back to the fold: are you making every effort to bring inactive patients home to your practice. Optom Econ 1991;1(5):39–42.

Chapter 21

Ophthalmic Dispensing

Neil B. Gailmard

The engine which drives enterprise is not thrift, but profit.

—John Maynard Keynes
A Treatise on Money

Over the past several decades optical dispensing has not been held in high regard by optometry students. Increasingly, there are more appealing and more challenging areas of specialization within the scope of optometry. It must be remembered, however, that even during these times of primary care, the majority of patients who seek the services of an optometrist do so for the purpose of refractive correction with eyeglasses. Patients do not understand this lack of interest in the mechanics of eyeglasses—any reduced status that dispensing might hold is in the minds of practitioners. To patients, eyeglasses are an important, sometimes vital, aid to vision.

It has long been understood that no matter how expert a practitioner's clinical services might be, the finished pair of glasses that are on the patient's face will be the long-lasting proof of excellent optometric care. Eyeglasses, if they are of high quality, can serve to build an excellent reputation and can become a major referral stimulus for the optometrist. Conversely, glasses that perform poorly and cause problems can be the source of many negative comments by the patient.

If these factors are not enough to encourage the student of practice management to excel in optical dispensing, it should be realized that in most practices the sale of optical materials accounts for about 50% of the gross income. A practice that does not provide dispensing services can usually double its gross income if dispensing is added.

Assuming that optical dispensing and laboratory services are delegated to technicians and assistants, it is almost always financially attractive to provide dispensing. Patients generally prefer the full-service concept of eye care, as evidenced by the fact that most independent practitioners find a very low percentage of patients have their spectacle prescriptions filled by another dispenser. A major benefit of receiving both clinical services and optical materials from one office is that the patient only needs to turn to that office in the event of problems.

The actual duties of the selection and dispensing of eyewear are generally delegated to an optometric technician, frame stylist, or optician. This approach is a sensible one, allowing the optometrist to function at the highest level of skill and to concentrate on the diagnosis and management of eye conditions, while serving as a supervisor with regard to optical dispensing. Many excellent programs exist today for the training of technicians to completely manage and operate an optical dispensary, but the majority of individuals who perform this function are trained on the job.

IMAGE OF THE DISPENSARY

Various styles of optometric practice include dispensaries that convey different images. The form of the dispensary can range from the traditional, spe-

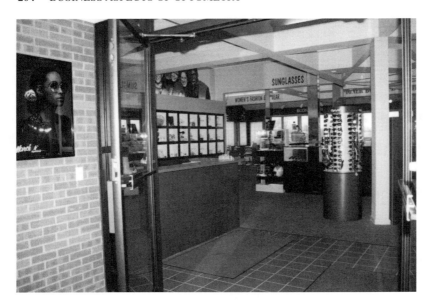

Figure 21.1. Separate optical entrance. (Courtesy of Gailmard Eye Center, Munster, Indiana.)

cialized service available only to the patients of the private practice to the highly retail and commercialized optical superstore. One of the main ways to differentiate between the retail image and the professional image is by the patient's initial impression when entering the office. If the frame showroom area is the first room entered from the outside, the image is largely retail. This design is often found in optometrists' offices where the optical dispensary serves as the reception room or there is no reception room. If the outside entrance opens into a traditional reception area, the impression is one of professional eye care.

A good approach to the separation of the retail and professional aspects of a practice is to have two separate entrances—one of them leading to an optical dispensary and the other one leading to the practitioner's office waiting room (Figure 21.1). This concept does provide some advantages in that it retains the professional image of a health care practitioner while still attracting patients who would like to purchase eyeglasses separately. This arrangement could incorporate the use of a separate business name for the optical dispensary. The name selected could be used in exterior signage and would allow the practitioner to feel more comfortable with the advertising of optical services in the local media. Care should be given to such external marketing, however, to ensure that the public

is being sent the desired message concerning which aspect of care is emphasized as primary and which is deemed to be secondary.

There are obvious advantages and disadvantages to having a separate optical dispensary. In one regard, it should not be allowed to be so separate that there is no connection, visible to the public, between the optometrist and the dispensary. When that connection is broken, so is the loyalty that retains patients and causes them to purchase optical materials from the practice. It can be desirable to have the dispensary still function under the organization of the practice—this will allow for one set of accounting records to be maintained and will also allow the patient to simply write one check for clinical services and eyeglasses.

Having the separate optical dispensary also requires a larger staff. It is important for each entrance to have a receptionist or technician always available to greet patients when they enter. This is not only good etiquette and a custom that is expected by patients in a service-oriented business but is also necessary in the optical dispensary to avoid the problem of shoplifting.

As defined for the purposes of this discussion, optical dispensing includes the following functions:

• Lens design (and selection of options)
• Frame selection and measurements

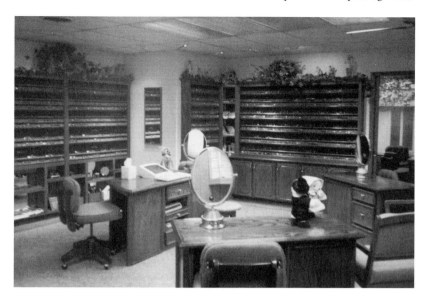

Figure 21.2. Optical dispensary. (Courtesy of Drs. Bob Baldwin, Bobby Christensen, and Russell Laverty, Midwest City, Oklahoma.)

- Ordering and verifying of eyeglasses
- Dispensing and adjusting of eyeglasses
- Maintaining and repairing of eyeglasses

The appearance of the optical dispensary is extremely important to successful operation of the business (Figure 21.2). When a patient enters the optical dispensary, that individual becomes a consumer. Consumers make many subconscious judgments that affect their purchasing habits. The decor and appearance will influence the consumer's decision to purchase a product and even how much the consumer will pay. The optometrist's dispensary has a distinct advantage over other optical dispensaries, because the optometrist has already provided professional and clinical services to the patient and has gained the patient's trust. It is not sufficient to rely solely on this professional relationship, however, for the optical dispensary should appeal to the patient on its own. The optical dispensary must be continuously updated and periodically redecorated with such additions as wallpaper, carpeting, new paint, and new furniture. Patients will judge the entire operation of a practice by what they understand, and they understand retail merchandise displays. While it is a considerable expense, the optical dispensary must be kept modern and tasteful.

Further discussion of the design of the optical dispensary can be found in Chapter 10.

Frame Display Options

It is important to display the inventory of frames in a way that highlights the frames in an impressive manner. There are many options available through professional optical design companies; these companies will fabricate custom frame bars or sell ready-made ones. Frames are often displayed in categories or sections such as men's, women's, and children's groupings. Additional areas can be added, such as sports eyewear and nonprescription sunglasses (Figure 21.3). A decision should be made as to whether the patient is allowed to browse and try frames on, or if they will be seated and frames will be shown one at a time by a technician.

A good merchandising idea is to display more upscale and expensive frames in a different environment. It has been observed that displaying a few very expensive frames will help sales of medium- to high-priced frames because it desensitizes the consumer who might have "sticker shock." Antique furniture can provide an interesting backdrop for a more spread out merchandising effect of individual frames on pedestals. Manufacturers and frame suppliers will supply excellent ideas for merchandising and showcasing their products. Display kits that promote one style of a frame in several colors is appealing in any location in the dispensary. Observing the window displays and accessory displays in

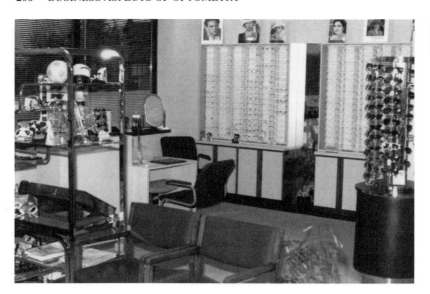

Figure 21.3. Optical dispensary. (Courtesy of Dr. David Hansen, Des Moines, Iowa.)

fine department stores is an excellent way to learn professional display techniques.

Frames can be displayed on glass shelves that allow the frames to sit singly and with temples open. This frame display method tends to make a smaller inventory look larger because it is spread out. The use of frame bars generally places a larger frame inventory into a smaller space.

Dispensing tables should be readily available as a workplace for frames, clinical records, and accessories (Figure 21.4). These dispensing tables will also serve as a counter so that optical measurements can be taken accurately and prescription eyeglass orders can be written up. This table can also be the area where fees are explained and presented to the patient. The dispensing tables, which are used for frame selection, can also double as tables to be used for delivering finished eyeglasses and providing eyewear adjustments. It should be remembered, however, that the use of these tables might be in great demand, and this can make it inconvenient for patients who wish to select a frame if all tables are being used for deliveries and adjustments.

One alternative, if space permits, is to have separate dispensing counters, booths, or small private rooms to deliver and adjust eyewear (Figure 21.5). This specialized delivery and dispensing section also emphasizes the service aspect of dispensing glasses. The basic dispensing tools and

frame warmer can be positioned in a nearby location, preferably with a sink also available. This design allows the patients to see some of the basic adjustments being performed on their eyeglasses and saves the technicians the many steps that must be made to walk back and forth from a separate laboratory.

Lighting is a very important consideration in a dispensary. As experts in visual science, optometrists should display excellent lighting techniques. It is generally noted that skin tones are much more attractive to a person under incandescent lights. However, these lights are quite hot and relatively expensive to operate. The use of track lights or other spotlights can add a pleasing appearance to patients trying on frames and looking at themselves in mirrors. General overall lighting with fluorescent lights is practical in commercial buildings. Indirect fluorescent lighting, where the light is bounced off ceilings or other surfaces, tends to make the light more pleasing. The use of daylight through skylights and windows adds a third type of lighting and can contribute to an attractive blend of all three. One additional consideration in lighting is the use of backlit frame bars. This is an individual decision because, although the frame bars are quite eye appealing when frames are lit from behind, the actual color of a frame is much harder to see when displayed on these frame bars. The frame must

Figure 21.4. Optical boutique area. (Courtesy of Gailmard Eye Center, Munster, Indiana.)

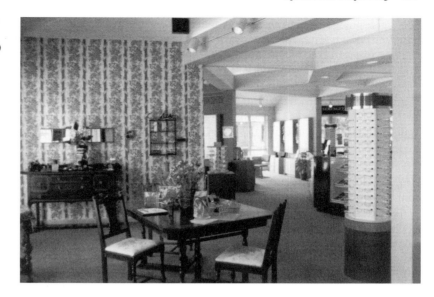

Figure 21.5. Eyeglass adjustment booths. (Courtesy of Gailmard Eye Center, Munster, Indiana.)

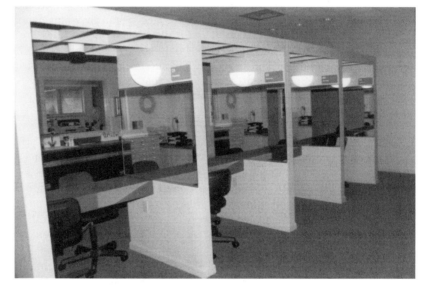

often be removed from the frame bar and viewed in a separate light to actually appreciate the color.

Frame Inventory Management

Ordering and buying frames is described in Chapter 13. The first consideration is the number of frames that should be on display and carried in inventory. This frame number will vary widely, from a range of approximately 500 frames in a very small office to more than 3,000 frames in a typical superoptical environment. The size of the practice, the budget available, and the marketing strategy of the practitioner will dictate the number of frames to carry. The practitioner will need to consider the number of men, women, and children patients so that the appropriate percentage of frames will be carried for each category.

It is possible to display all frames, but some offices will keep an additional stock so that frames can be replaced. Keeping frame boards completely filled with minimum empty spaces makes them more attractive and appealing and also makes it easier to spot potential theft problems. An assistant can check the frame displays every morning and be certain that all empty spots are filled with frames, even if sunglasses or safety frames must be used. It can be an advantage to the large practice to try to use frames from the frame board as much as possible rather than ordering frames to be supplied by the laboratory. This practice has the major benefit of reducing back order problems, which can often occur without the knowledge of the optical staff and delay an order unexpectedly. Additionally, using frames directly off the frame board creates a constant turnover of inventory, which means frames will always be new and not shopworn.

Obviously, the optometrist (or staff members) periodically must meet with frame company sales representatives to buy new frames and replace those that have been sold. This meeting should be arranged by appointment and given due time and consideration since it represents the products that will be shown and dispensed. Frame representatives can provide a valuable service by conducting an inventory of their products and keeping records of what was sold since the last purchase. There will generally be more frame vendors who wish to do business with the optometrist than the optometrist can reasonably manage. It is generally necessary to restrict the number of vendors to those who provide the best products, service, discounts, and return policies.

It can be a good strategy to provide as much business as possible to a limited number of vendors so that the practice becomes an important account to these companies. This important account relationship can result in better buying programs and discounts from the vendor.

The optometrist or staff member who buys frames must stick to a budget and not buy under pressure. The professional sales person is very skilled at selling, and the optometrist must be able to say "no." It is also advisable to try to buy for the entire market of patients and avoid simply purchasing what the buyer personally likes. A wide range of frame prices should be available, and a good mix of frame sizes (large and small), materials (metal and plastic), and styles (conservative and high fash-

ion) should be obtained. Attention must be given to older stock that has not sold; these frames should be returned within the company's return policy. Sales representatives sometimes are not anxious to facilitate returns, so the frame manager must be attentive to this task. Another consideration when buying frames is the use of buying groups, which can help obtain better discounts for an independent practitioner when the number of purchases is small.

Many computer software programs are available for eye care practices, and these programs can provide valuable assistance in inventory management. Computer programs are useful for frames but can also be applicable for uncut ophthalmic lenses and contact lenses. Various printed reports can be generated, and this information can make frame buying more intelligent and scientific. Of course, to obtain excellent data from the computer, considerable effort is required to input the necessary information when new frames are added and when display frames are sold. Each frame must have placed on it an inventory number or bar code, typed in or entered by electronic wand for every transaction (Table 21.1).

Lens Design

Lens design is an aspect of dispensing that is all too often forced into a secondary role even though it is really more important than the selection of the frame. Patients understand the process of frame selection very well, because they try on the frames and look at them and touch them. The lens is not well understood, however, because of the complexities of different types of prescriptions, the placement of optical centers, the use of oversize blanks, the need for antireflection or ultraviolet (UV) coatings, and the various styles of multifocals that can be chosen. It is a good practice to begin the dispensing visit with a discussion of the lenses, before frames are considered, perhaps at an in-office "lens design center." This special area is devoted to samples and demonstration lenses in the form of uncut lens blanks and mockup eyeglasses. Table 21.2 provides some ideas on the kind of information that can be provided.

The process of designing lenses and selecting options simply begins by educating the patient. It is the dispenser's duty to inform each patient of the newest available technologies for ophthalmic lenses. Patients have a right to know what new products are available, and the dispenser should avoid prejudging what the patient will or will not want or can afford. The key to patient education is the use of demonstration items and literature. Nothing can explain different types of bifocals better then having actual eyeglasses made up with different types of bifocals. These items are also perfect when attempting to answer questions such as: "How thick will the edges be in a certain size frame?" or "How does this look with an antireflection coating?" or "How does a lens look when the edges are rolled and polished?" Sample eyeglasses or lens blanks can be provided by the manufacturers at no charge or can be an investment made by the practice.

Lifestyle Dispensing

The educational approach leads to the concept of lifestyle dispensing. This term refers to finding out more about a patient's needs in their daily activities and providing additional pairs of eyeglasses or special lens options to help the patient with those needs. Obviously, this procedure requires more in-depth questioning with regard to patients' occupational and vocational interests. Examples of needs that can be satisfied with lifestyle dispensing include golfing, fishing, special safety glasses for the work environment, or special reading glasses for computers. Some practices will use a printed questionnaire to find out about lifestyle needs, while others simply use a friendly verbal interview.

A side benefit to good lens design is increased optical sales in the form of second pairs, sunglasses, and lens add-on options, but the primary outcome is eyewear that provides optimum visual performance for the patient in his or her daily life. The practitioner's philosophy will determine how much salesmanship should be used during dispensing. One must be careful not to take this technique too far so that it becomes a high-pressure sales tactic that can adversely affect the doctor-patient relationship.

Technicians who serve as frame selection assistants or frame stylists should be trained to assist patients with proper frame sizes and shapes. Frame stylists must be trained to note the lens prescription first so that this information can be considered

Table 21.1. Advantages of Computerized Frame Inventory Management

- Current inventory always available in wholesale or retail dollar amounts and in number of units.
- Inventory reports by frame type, manufacturer, supplier, or model.
- Inventory aging reports: listings of frames, quantity, and date acquired.
- Reports of frames that are on order or at the laboratory.
- History of sales per month by manufacturer or model.
- Reports are of assistance when buying frames, as well as for business and accounting needs and for theft control.

Table 21.2. Lens Design Center Demonstration Items

Uncut lens blanks
1. Grey and brown plastic tints from #1 to #5 for fashion and sunglass
2. Other tint colors including rose #1 and #2 and grey/green sunglass
3. Gradient tint samples
4. Photogrey extra, PhotoSun, and Transitions samples
5. Glass lens coatings for color and mirror
6. High-index plastic vs. CR-39 in same Rx (e.g., −6.00 D.)

Mockup spectacles
1. Right lens rolled and polished, left lens normal, in wire frame
2. Right lens A/R coat, left lens normal
3. Progressive lenses with plano at distance and +1.50 adds
4. Right lens executive bifocal, left lens FT-35
5. Various bifocal and trifocal styles
6. Various high plus and minus powers in different eye size frames

when determining the type of frame to use. Additionally, training in color, style, and the selection of proper shapes for facial features is appropriate. The use of video cameras has become useful in helping patients view themselves while wearing their new eyeglass frames. This technique has some obvious benefits since some patients cannot see well when trying on sample frames that do not contain a lens prescription. Seeing oneself on video also permits angles of view that a mirror does not achieve. The use of a video camera can be somewhat time consuming but, in a high-service practice, does differentiate the practice from the competition.

Frame and Lens Pricing

The most popular method for setting fees for ophthalmic materials is to use a markup system. The amount of markup can vary from two to three times the wholesale cost. Informal surveys should be performed to determine the markup rate for various optical materials in a given area. The marketing philosophy and positioning of the practice will dictate if this practice should be on the high, middle, or low end of the price scale. Prices can be marked on small adhesive stickers that serve to show the patient the cost as the patient tries on the frames. A clever idea is to use a clear label and apply it to the throw-away lens that comes with the frame. Lens prices are generally listed on a printed fee schedule that can be kept near the dispensing tables. This list can show different prices for the different types of lenses—spheres, sphero-cylinders, single vision lenses, bifocals, and progressive addition lenses. Also, various lens options can be listed as add-on prices. A quality, wholesale laboratory's finished lens price list can be used as a guide for determining the patient cost for these options.

An alternative method for the pricing of frames and lenses has been the use of dispensing and prescription fees. These fees represent the profit that would be made on the service aspect of dispensing. When using these methods, optical materials are generally priced at wholesale cost, with a slight add-on margin to allow for operational costs. Dispensing fees and a very low materials fee are often used by third-party companies as an effort to control cost. It has been noted that patients might not accept dispensing fees as easily as they accept a markup on ophthalmic materials.

As part of good dispensing service, the dispenser should be trained to review and explain all fees that are charged for optical materials and, if necessary, the other professional and clinical fees that were charged to the patient at the current visit.

Nonprescription Sunglasses

One area of dispensing that seems to be of growing interest is the provision of nonprescription sunglasses. Optometrists have found the importance of protection against UV radiation to be within the domain of professional services. Even though the majority of nonprescription sunwear purchases are in department and drug stores, there is a market for higher quality sunglasses sold through eye care professionals. A requirement for success in sales of nonprescription sunglasses is a significant investment in inventory (Figure 21.6). The consumer wants selection and variety. Historically, optometrists have not been pleased with sales of nonprescription sunglasses, but this lack of success can be due to the practice of carrying a small inventory of sunglasses by ophthalmic frame companies that are not known by the public. Name brands have great appeal to the public. Promotion to the public might be necessary in the form of media advertising. A natural market for sunglasses is the contact lens population, which has an interest in nonprescription sunwear.

ADVERTISING

The advertising of dispensing services must be performed very carefully so as not to adversely affect the image of a professional practice. The practitioner's "philosophy of practice" should be used to establish the goals of external marketing before any advertising campaign is started. If a practice desires a professional image of the highest quality, advertising should be avoided. If the practice is one in which low-price optical materials are stressed, then advertising is a necessity. The practitioner must consider the position of the practice first and then adopt a promotional campaign that will meet the goals of the practice image. Advertising is a major investment for a practice and speaks loudly to the public about its image. It is best to use advertising agencies for assistance, but this assistance does require a significant budget. Frame manufacturers can provide professional camera-ready advertisements and even cooperative funding for advertising when it is performed within their guidelines.

EYEWEAR DELIVERY

The delivery of finished prescription eyeglasses involves the services of adjustment and fitting. Office policies for the notification of patients and for the dispensing of eyewear should be adopted. Some practices offer dispensing of eyeglasses by appoint-

Figure 21.6. Sunwear display showcase. (Courtesy of Gailmard Eye Center, Munster, Indiana.)

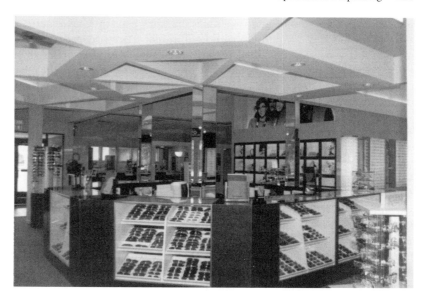

ment only, but this method can result in delays and inconvenience for the patient. If the practice has adequate staff members who can dispense eyeglasses, appointments will not be necessary for this rather brief service. Patients who simply walk in to pick up eyeglasses will generally understand a short wait of 5 minutes or less. Excellent eyeglass dispensing involves:

- Adjustment of the frame to the patient's head to ensure proper fit and comfort
- Instructions to the patient on the use of the new eyeglasses
- A review of the lens options that have been ordered

The technician dispensing the eyeglasses should ask the patient if the type of eyewear being provided has been used before. If it is new to the patient, instructions on adaptation symptoms as well as how to use the eyewear properly can be appropriate. A reading card should be handy, to allow the patient to test nearpoint vision and to learn to use different parts of multifocal lenses. An additional technique that should be included in dispensing is the routine review of special options that can be incorporated into the eyeglasses. Patients forget the purpose of extra options such as antireflection coatings, photogrey tints, scratch-resistant coatings, and

similar items, and the dispenser should use this opportunity for one last review of the options ordered and their purpose. This review can also spark referrals when the patient wears the new glasses and finds the options helpful. Patients should be instructed to return at any time if frame adjustments are needed.

A progressive practice must be aware of the importance of the time taken to fabricate eyeglasses. It is no longer common for 2 weeks to be required to fabricate a pair of glasses, and yet some special lens designs and special frame orders can necessitate a waiting period as long or longer. The important consideration when encountering such orders is to keep the patient informed. It is very important to call the patient if any delay is encountered in the fabrication of new eyeglasses, rather than waiting for the patient to call and ask why the eyeglasses are not ready.

EYEGLASS WARRANTIES

A more consumer-oriented approach is occurring in dispensing, as various marketing strategies are adopted by chain optical stores and private practices. Eyeglass warranties have become popular and generally will extend for 1 year from the date of dispensing. Sometimes an additional charge is required for such a warranty, and sometimes the warranty is provided to all patients at no additional cost. Typically, the eyeglass warranty will repair or replace any broken part of the frame or lenses with a "no-fault" guarantee, so that, no matter how the glasses are broken, a repair or replacement is made.

Sometimes these warranties can have a "one time only" stipulation, while other warranties can be unlimited throughout the year. The eyeglass warranty does remove any potential disagreement about whether the eyeglasses performed adequately, were defective, or were abused by the patient. A separate warranty usually accompanies scratch-resistant plastic lenses and typically provides for replacement at no charge if the lenses scratch within 1 year. These warranties are easy for a practitioner to provide, since both frames and scratch-resistant lenses are usually warrantied by the manufacturer.

MANAGING THE UNHAPPY PATIENT

There will always be a small percentage of patients who are unhappy with their vision or have difficulty with adaptation to new eyeglasses. Additionally, problems will occur where lenses fall out and screws and temples come loose. An office policy should be established for the management of unhappy patients. The best policy is the age-old "customer is always right" approach. Policies should be developed to easily and fairly handle a refund in the event a patient requests one—although solving the problem is a better resolution. All efforts should be made to rectify any problems the patient has as quickly as possible. Generally, job remakes and corrections should be made at no charge to the patient if they occur within a reasonable amount of time. Assistants should allow patients to have access to the prescribing practitioner, usually with a free appointment, if complaints of a visual nature are received.

Additional optical policies can include the use of a payment plan. It is common to accept major credit cards, and this provides an easy way for practices to avoid offering credit to patients. It is common for the office to require a 50% deposit when eyeglasses are ordered, with the balance due at dispensing. Whatever policy is selected, it is vital that patients be informed in advance of what is expected of them. This philosophy can prevent awkward situations, such as instances in which patients arrive to pick up glasses but are not ready to pay. It is difficult to turn patients away or to take back glasses that have just been fitted.

BIBLIOGRAPHY

Allergan, Inc. Pathways in Optometry. Irvine, CA: Allergan, 1992:128–35.

Baldwin BL, Christensen B, Melton J. Rx for Success. Midwest City, OK: Vision Publications, 1983:145–60.

Barnett D. Is your dispensary a sight for sore eyes? Rev Optom 1992;129(9):51–9.

Bennett I. Management for the Eyecare Practitioner. Stoneham, MA: Butterworth, 1993:56–65.

Brooks C, Borish I. System for Ophthalmic Dispensing (2nd ed). Boston: Butterworth-Heinemann, 1996.

Drew R. Professional Ophthalmic Dispensing. Chicago: Professional Press, 1970.

Gailmard NB. How I improved our eyeglass delivery time. Rev Optom 1987;124(5):33.

Gailmard NB. Make your optical dispensary separate—but not too separate. Optom Manage 1982;18(10):21–5.

Gailmard NB. Managing the grief patient. Optom Econ 1991;1(8):18–21.

Gailmard NB. Meet the service challenge. Rev Optom 1989;126(7):23.

Gailmard NB. The Consultant's Corner: a premium lens at a lower premium. Rev Optom 1993;130(3):33.

Guerrein R. Viewpoint: don't dispense with dispensing. Optom Manage 1994;29(2):11.

Kirman B. Keep the right frame sizes on the board. Optom Manage 1994;29(3):46–50.

McMillan PH. Dispensary design trends. Eyecare Bus 1995;9(10):20–4.

Schwartz C. Minimize inventory and maximize return. Rev Optom 1992;129(9):51–9.

Weber J. 101 Dispensing Tips and Procedures. Melville, NY: Marchon Eyewear, 1994.

Winslow C. You can improve your eyeglass service. Rev Optom 1991;128(10):39–42.

Winslow C. Your stylist's biggest frame buying blunders. Rev Optom 1991;128(10):31–4.

Chapter 22

Contact Lens Practice

Paul Farkas and Neil B. Gailmard

If you build it, he will come.

—William P. Kinsella
Shoeless Joe

Contact lens services are among the most common offered by optometrists. The 1995 American Optometric Association Economic Survey found that 98% of optometrists in practice provided contact lens services. For the new graduate, therefore, contact lens services are an essential aspect of care. Whether a practice is new or acquired from another practitioner, an effort will be required to build a contact lens patient base.

In a specialty practice, a significant number of patients are obtained through referral. Methods used to obtain these valuable referrals from other health care providers are covered in Chapter 19. However, practitioners can also build a contact lens practice through marketing efforts directed at existing patients and at the public at large. This chapter describes the various means for developing such a contact lens practice.

OBTAINING NEW CONTACT LENS PATIENTS FROM REFERRALS

There are several obvious means of generating contact lens referrals, including word of mouth from patients, the use of special contact lens techniques and advanced contact lens instrumentation, and through the generation of enthusiasm for contact lenses among lens wearers.

It would seem, on the surface, that patients will refer other patients when they have a suc-

cessful contact lens result. Unfortunately, such is not always the case, because patients who select a professional practitioner expect to obtain good results when a fair fee is paid. It is analogous to someone who, after purchasing an expensive new automobile, expects the vehicle to function; moreover, a buyer would not customarily brag that an expensive new car performs well. Therefore, successful results alone do not create a large referral base. A referral base can be created by a practitioner who has developed special techniques for fitting contact lens patients. These patients will discuss, with anyone who will listen, the special technique that created success. This enthusiasm creates new patients.

Contact lens patients especially like to feel that a practitioner is at the cutting edge of care and that the newest developments are being employed. If a practitioner can obtain the newest instrumentation that helps in the diagnosis and management of contact lens patients—and makes the patient aware that advanced instrumentation is being utilized—this, too, will encourage the patient to inform acquaintances of the advanced state of the practitioner's practice. This information can result in new referrals.

Contact lens patients are more likely to refer other patients when they are enthusiastic contact lens wearers. How does a practitioner create enthusiasm? By reinforcing the patient's perception

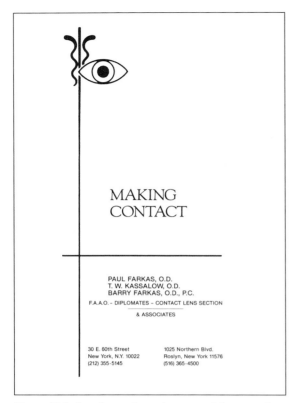

Figure 22.1. Sample newsletter (cover page) for a practitioner providing contact lens care.

that he or she is receiving special care from the best practitioner. There are several ways to create this perception.

Problem Solving

Patients will be enthusiastic if the practitioner has the reputation of being a problem solver. If a patient's difficult problems are solved, the practitioner receives not only patient gratitude but also referrals because of superior expertise.

Supportive Staff

The staff should be excited when a patient succeeds with contact lenses and show concern when a contact lens wearer encounters a problem.

Therefore, it behooves practitioners to train staff members to be sensitive to each patient's needs.

Patient Interaction

When patients are sitting in the reception area, there should be positive conversation about their contact lens experiences. How can this patient interaction occur? First, patients should be introduced to one another by the staff. Assistants can start a conversation indicating, "Oh! Miss Jones had the same problem you had, Mrs. Smith; and, with a bit of perseverance, she was able to solve this problem." At that point, the patients usually will continue the conversation.

In-Office Contact Lens Development from Former Patients

Many primary eye care patients are excellent candidates for contact lens wear. One way to encourage these individuals is by creating a newsletter (Figure 22.1). The newsletter should include the most up-to-date information about contact lenses and about how the office is implementing any new developments. Printed contact lens promotional material should be available in the office and visible to patients waiting to be seen for primary eye care. This material can be printed—in the form of either reprints of articles or brochures supplied by lens manufacturers—or it can be in the form of verbal encouragement by the staff. It is essential, in a contact lens practice, that a significant number of staff members and practitioners wear contact lenses and believe in the product. There is nothing more credible than an enthusiastic staff member who is wearing contact lenses. Staff members should discuss their contact lens experiences in the most positive manner.

In-office referrals are often gained through enthusiastic patient interaction. Primary care patients should be able to meet lens wearers in the office and to hear firsthand about the advantages and benefits of lens wear. In addition, audiovisual aids should be available in the reception area. Answers to commonly asked contact lens questions can be conveniently provided by either a videotape or a laser disc. The video cassette recorder or laser disc player should be operated unobtrusively by a staff member.

Figure 22.2. Yellow Pages advertisement.

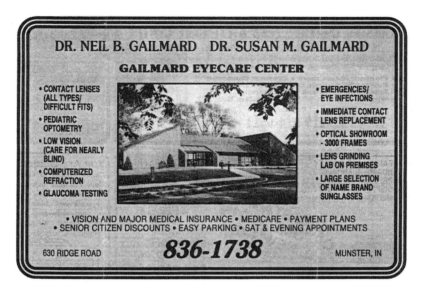

MARKETING

Several different marketing approaches can be taken to build a contact lens practice. The approach chosen should be appropriate for the practice and the image the practitioner wishes to create. Marketing techniques include the use of media and public relations.

Window Marketing

A downstairs location in high-traffic areas can be used to inform the public about certain types of contact lenses and prices. Although this is an inexpensive way to market, it trivializes contact lens care and products. This particular approach can create contact lens price wars and an unprofessional image. It is not recommended.

Media Marketing

Media marketing can take several forms, including radio and television advertising. The advantage of radio and television advertising is that it allows selection of a specific market within a specific age and economic group. The great disad-

vantage, however, is the need for several office locations to make the effort cost effective. In addition, a large number of advertisements are required before patients will react to this particular form of advertising.

Another form of radio and television advertising is the "infomercial." The practitioner can purchase air time for telephone call-in problems or even for a television interview. It allows for an improved professional image, but 30–60 minutes of air time can be extremely expensive and thus beyond the scope of the private practitioner.

Another form of media marketing is display advertising in newspapers. The problem with this particular type of advertising, as with radio and television marketing, is the cost to the single-location practitioner. The expense of this particular type of marketing generally does not adequately pay for itself. It also creates a poor professional image in the eyes of the public.

A popular form of display marketing is Yellow Pages advertising (Figure 22.2). The first practitioner in the area with a large or eye-catching advertisement will probably receive a financial return that will exceed the cost of the advertisement. If there are several practitioners with the same approach, however, they tend to offset each other and to reduce the return to the break-even point (or worse).

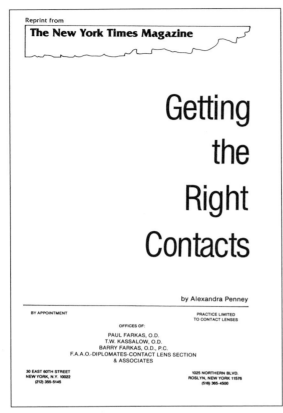

Getting
the
Right
Contacts

by Alexandra Penney

BY APPOINTMENT

PRACTICE LIMITED
TO CONTACT LENSES

OFFICES OF:

PAUL FARKAS, O.D.
T.W. KASSALOW, O.D.
BARRY FARKAS, O.D., P.C.
F.A.A.O.-DIPLOMATES-CONTACT LENS SECTION
& ASSOCIATES

30 EAST 60TH STREET
NEW YORK, N.Y. 10022
(212) 355-5145

1025 NORTHERN BLVD.
ROSLYN, NEW YORK 11576
(516) 365-4500

Figure 22.3. Example article from publication in local media.

Paid Public Relations

A public relations firm will provide advice on the best means of marketing to the public. A sophisticated public relations firm usually recommends a budget that is greater than the average individual practitioner can afford. Optometrists do benefit from professional public relations efforts that are paid for by contact lens companies or interested optometric organizations. This use of a public relations firm puts the practitioner's best image forward in the media, and this benefit can be helpful.

Free Public Relations

Achieving free public relations requires some effort. Radio shows are usually the most available way to promote the practice free of charge. Op-

tometrists are experts in contact lenses, and by communicating with radio stations and informing them of availability, optometrists can be asked to answer contact lens questions on call-in shows. This particular form of marketing is free to practitioners, with the radio station essentially providing an endorsement of the qualifications of the radio expert. Although not many new patients are generated from this form of advertising, it does improve the practitioner's public image. Television interviews also add to prestige but, likewise, do not create a significant increase in new contact lens patients.

The form of free marketing that is most successful in developing a contact lens practice is authorship of articles appearing in well-known magazines or newspapers that are widely read by the practice's patient base. The best choices are fashion magazines or a reputable newspaper (Figure 22.3). In addition to personal practitioner interviews, an article, published in a local newspaper, about new contact lens developments can also create increased contact lens demand. In fact, a popular written article can be saved by a potential patient for future use. With limited time and resources, this approach is favored; however, all of the described approaches can be attempted to achieve the best mix of techniques.

CONTACT LENS ASSISTANTS

Many aspects of contact lens care can be performed cost effectively by a well-trained assistant. Consequently, many duties in contact lens practice are delegated to assistants, including ordering and verification of contact lenses, training of patients in techniques for insertion and removal of lenses, and education of patients in the use of proper lens care regimens. However, assistants must be properly trained, and their scope of responsibilities must be clearly defined.

Training Assistants

There are various ways for an assistant to obtain training. The best means is through formal course work. There are formal training courses for optometric technicians offered at community colleges and at selected colleges of optometry. Although these individuals learn basic skills in a teaching institution, most require on-the-job training to ensure that they conform to the standards of a specific practice. The majority of contact lens assistants are trained in an optometric office. It is easiest to train a contact lens assistant who is presently a contact lens wearer. These individuals are more sensitive to the problems and needs of a potential contact lens patient and have personal experience as a wearer to guide them.

Many times, because of relocation or other circumstance, an individual with an extensive contact lens background can be hired by a practice. Although these individuals understand the basics of contact lens care, it is generally necessary to give them additional on-the-job training to conform to the standards of practice. In fact, all contact lens technicians should be required to attend ophthalmic assistants' courses offered at state and regional educational meetings. Attendance at continuing education courses not only adds new knowledge but also helps keep the assistant motivated and enthusiastic.

Contact lens assistants should know their personal limits and should understand the degree of autonomy allowed to assistants under state law. Any questions of a professional nature concerning the limits of responsibility should be brought to the supervising optometrist for resolution. In many states, trained ophthalmic dispensers can practice contact lens fitting under the direct supervision of an optometrist. In addition, these individuals can act as supervisors to contact lens assistants with less training.

It is possible, by having well-structured office procedures, to empower employees who are contact lens assistants to make some independent decisions. These independent decisions can be outlined in their scope of work and described in the office handbook (see Chapter 16).

Scope of Work

To have a well-run contact lens practice, technicians should have clearly defined responsibilities that are described in writing. The scope of these responsibilities will vary from practice to practice, but basic skills that are generally required include the following:

- Telephone skills are essential. A contact lens technician should be able to answer many procedural contact lens questions by telephone. On occasions when patients do not return for followup care, these contact lens technicians should be trained to call patients and encourage them to return.
- The contact lens technician should be made aware of the philosophy of the office regarding fees and should be able to intelligently negotiate and answer any questions that a potential contact lens patient might have about fees.
- The assistant should understand why a contact lens patient must return for a followup appointment and what procedures will be performed during that visit.
- The contact lens assistant should be trained to understand rigid gas-permeable and hydrogel lenses and should also understand the use of solutions, eye makeup and eye makeup remover, and face creams by contact lens wearers.
- In most states, the contact lens assistant can legally use an automatic refractor, objective/subjective refracting system, keratometer, or lensometer. This use of assistants changes the role of the optometrist from a data collector to a data analyzer and decision maker, decreasing the contact lens practitioner's costs while maintaining professional quality.
- The assistant should understand that questions beyond the scope of his or her expertise should be brought to the attention of the supervising optometrist. By using assistants to their optimum capacity, optometrists can work at their highest level of professional capability in the most cost-effective manner.

CONTACT LENS INVENTORY

For practitioners who fit contact lenses, there is an inevitable need for trial lens sets and a contact lens inventory. A balance must be achieved between the size of the inventory and its cost-effectiveness.

The larger the inventory, the greater the number of options the practitioner can offer to patients. On the other hand, the larger the inventory, the greater the expense of maintaining it. The advantage of maintaining a large inventory—in addition to permitting the patient and the practitioner the maximum choice of product—is the ability to dispense lenses to the patient on the same day the lenses are fitted or needed. Because U.S. citizens live in a society that treasures immediate results, the sooner the patient can receive the lenses, the happier the patient will be. Moreover, there is a great advantage to be realized in terms of quality control. The larger the inventory, the greater the opportunity to replace a lens on the same day.

The disadvantage of a large inventory is that lenses not in use have already been paid for and can constitute a significant expense. The advent of disposable and planned replacement lenses has placed new demands on inventory. This issue should be managed with the "just-in-time" approach, which allows the manufacturer to maintain a large inventory and uses overnight mail and messenger service to replace depleted inventory. Another disadvantage of a large inventory is the problem of obsolescence. It is essential that any arrangements made with a manufacturer include the return of unopened vials for full credit. The final disadvantage of a large inventory is a lack of inventory control. With proper computerization, however, an effort at inventory control can be made.

Practitioners need fitting sets of lenses made by various manufacturers, including different polymers, which allow the broadest range of parameters in hydrogel products. In addition, the contact lens practitioner should select a favorite daily wear, extended wear, and disposable lens, which should be well inventoried. The practitioner should not inventory lenses that are dispensed under different brand names but have the same parameters and polymer.

The inventory should have one favorite daily wear, rigid gas-permeable lens that is inventoried on a consignment basis. The rest of the available rigid gas-permeable lenses should be small fitting sets. It is unnecessary to inventory every type of lens, because required lenses can be received by overnight mail with the "just-in-time" replacement philosophy.

It is inadvisable to try to inventory toric and bifocal lenses since the number of parameters that are available makes stocking these materials extremely expensive. Patients wearing cus-

tom-designed toric lenses, which might take several weeks to produce, should be advised of this fact. In many instances, patients will then decide to keep an unopened backup pair in the event of an emergency.

Every effort should be made to negotiate with contact lens laboratories to persuade them to consign lenses at minimum cost rather than to require outright purchases. The type of arrangement that can be made with a specific laboratory depends on the practitioner's negotiating skills and the volume of contact lens patients.

There is no exact formula for maintaining a contact lens inventory to maximize practitioner efficiency and patient convenience while minimizing inventory expense.

A variety of racks and drawers are designed to store lenses (Figure 22.4). Perhaps the best way to select a storage system is to use photographs of various storage systems found in offices or to visit offices with systems that appear to be preferable.

Reorder Methods for Contact Lenses

There are many reordering systems, but the two basic methods are replacement ordering and computerized systems. An inventory sheet with minimum numbers of lenses will determine when inventory is low, based on a weekly count. More lenses of the most frequently used powers (i.e., −2.00 to −4.00 D) should be maintained in inventory. Using bar codes, a computerized inventory system permits the practitioner to keep current on lenses that need to be reordered.

In most areas, contact lens sales representatives will visit an office, count the number of inventory lenses that have been dispensed, and reorder them for the office. In this way, each time a lens is dispensed another lens of the same parameters is placed back into inventory.

Replacements can also be achieved by having the practitioner or staff order a replacement lens each time a lens is dispensed. The lens is ordered from the laboratory as a "stock lens."

Bar coding and automatic ordering by computer can also be used. Computer systems are now being updated to allow for bar coding that will result in automatic reordering.

Figure 22.4. Example storage system for contact lenses.

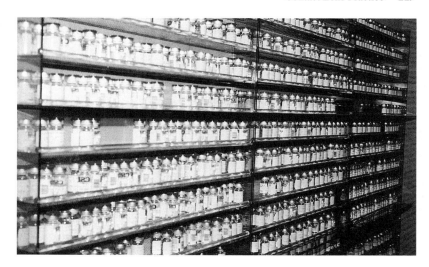

CONTACT LENS FEE STRUCTURE

The contact lens fee structure can be broken down into fees for services and fees for materials. The fee for services is determined by the value of the practitioner's time—this includes the practitioner's charge for services, in addition to base chair cost. Consideration should also be given to the fees charged for contact lens services in the community. Materials charges are based on the cost of lenses. A fee is added to the cost of the lenses to compensate for mailing and handling expenses, which can be as high as two times the cost. The amount to be added will be influenced by the cost to patients of obtaining similar materials in the community.

Replacement lenses are usually covered by some sort of service agreement or exchange policy from the laboratory, and charges are based on these policies. A frequent replacement lens program establishes the cost of office visits and lens replacement as a fixed dollar amount per year and guarantees the patient a certain number of lenses per year. A disposable lens program is like a frequent replacement system—the patient pays a fixed amount per year and receives a certain number of lenses and certain enumerated services. A structured program encourages patients to use the lenses dispensed each year and reduces the tendency of patients to hoard or stockpile supplies of lenses.

REFUND POLICY

Each office should establish a fair adjustment policy for patients who cannot be successfully fit with lenses. The value of such a policy cannot be overemphasized, because it allows an escape clause for both the practitioner and the patient if the fitting does not succeed (Figure 22.5).

The contact lens patient who cannot be successfully fit can be a management problem for the practice. The practitioner can spend an enormous amount of time, effort, and money constantly replacing lenses in the hopes that the fit will succeed. It is often preferable to inform the patient that the fitting was not successful and offer a refund.

Refunds can be made by returning part of the fee for materials, but a more desirable approach is a refund composed of other types of ophthalmic materials (such as sunwear). When a refund is given, the patient should be asked to sign a written release indicating that a refund was received and that the practice is no longer obligated to continue contact lens services.

SERVICE AGREEMENTS

The use of prepaid agreements for contact lens followup care is an extremely valuable management tool (Figure 22.6). These agreements allow

Figure 22.5. Sample office refund policy for patient who cannot be successfully fit with contact lenses.

BY APPOINTMENT

PRACTICE LIMITED
TO CONTACT LENSES

PAUL FARKAS, O.D.
T. W. KASSALOW, O.D.
BARRY FARKAS, O.D., P.C.
F.A.A.O. - DIPLOMATES - CONTACT LENS SECTION

& ASSOCIATES

30 EAST 60TH STREET
NEW YORK, NEW YORK 10022
(212) 355-5145
FAX: (212) 308-3262

1025 NORTHERN BLVD.
ROSLYN, NEW YORK 11576
(516) 365-4500
FAX: (516) 365-6580

You have informed us that you have come to the conclusion that the contact lenses with which we fit you have not performed as you thought they would.

Accordingly, and as we agreed, we are accepting the return of your lenses and are herewith refunding to you $

You have acknowledged to us that you were fully instructed by us as to the use and handling of the lenses, and the necessity for using proper cleaning solutions on the lenses.

You acknowledge to us that you have experienced no adverse reaction or condition from the wearing of the contact lenses, but are just disappointed in their performance. By acceptance of the refund statement, you hereby agree to release us from any further claim in connection with our fitting you with contact lenses.

Sincerely,

Paul Farkas, O.D.
T.W. Kassalow, O.D.
Barry Farkas, O.D.

ACCEPTED AND AGREED:

Signed _____ Patient
Date _____

patients to pay in advance for follow-up visits and to receive solutions and contact lenses at a reduced fee.

The benefits generally include a fixed number of visits per year, while the fees include the cost of the service contract and the charges for lens replacements. In general, the presentation of the service contract should be made at the completion of the initial contact lens fitting procedure. It should be offered by the practitioner and described by the assistants.

A renewal reminder should be sent to the patient 1 month before the expiration of the service agreement (Figure 22.7). A follow-up reminder should be sent to the patient, if there is no renewal of the service agreement, to remind the patient that the service agreement has expired and to allow the patient to compare the costs of lens replacement and office visits with and without a service agreement (Figure 22.8). The reminder should be followed by a telephone call from a staff member, offering to answer questions and asking if the patient would like to renew the agreement.

Practitioners should encourage service agreements to motivate patients to return for care that is prepaid. The practitioner also benefits because contact is maintained with patients and poor habits or ocular problems can be detected. Therefore, contact lens patients should be offered service agreements because it is in their best interest.

Figure 22.6. Sample prepaid service agreement.

> By Appointment
>
> Practice Limited
> To Contact Lenses
>
> **PAUL FARKAS, O.D.**
> **T.W. KASSALOW, O.D.**
> **BARRY FARKAS, O.D., P.C.**
> F.A.A.O. - DIPLOMATES - CONTACT LENS SECTION
>
> ———
>
> AND ASSOCIATES
>
> 30 East 60th Street
> New York, NY 10022
> (212) 355-5145
>
> 1025 Northern Blvd.
> Roslyn, NY 11576
> (516) 365-4500
>
> ## CONTACT LENS SERVICE CONTRACT
>
> This is to certify that_____ has contracted, for a fee of **$150.00**, to receive the following services through: **July 22, 1994.**
>
> 1. Two (2) office visits to maintain optimum performance of your present contact lenses.
>
> 2. Unlimited replacement of contact lenses (of like material) at the following rate:
>
>   **Daily Wear Hydrogel Lenses replaced at $70.00 per lens.**
>
> 3. An office visit within 30 days of dispensing of a lens replacement will be included at no charge while the Service Contract is in effect.
>
> 4. Special visual evaluations outside of normal contact lens follow-up care are not included in this contract. The customary fee for these services will be reduced by 10%.
>
>   Signed: Barry Farkas, O.D.
>   Dated:

CONTACT LENS SOLUTIONS

Most contact lens offices provide complimentary solutions for lens cleaning and sterilization at the time contact lenses are dispensed. After the patient uses up the initial supply, replacement supplies should be sold to the patient to ensure that the patient is continuing to use the recommended solutions.

It is advisable to dispense a 6-months' supply of solutions since, in general, most patients return to the office semiannually. This supply eliminates the need for patients to resort to pharmacies, where a different brand of solution can be obtained—one that might conflict with the best lens care regimen for the particular individual or lens type.

CONTACT LENS FOLLOW-UP CARE

Follow-up care is an inherent aspect of contact lens practice. After the final lens design has been determined, it is appropriate to see the patient for a 1-week and then a 1-month follow-up visit to ensure that the patient is enjoying optimum vision, comfort, and physiologic response. Three-month checkups are required for patients on overnight wear, whether the patient is wearing lenses for 6 consecutive nights or less.

Six-month checkups are recommended for individuals who are daily wear contact lens patients. The followup evaluation can be scheduled by mail

Figure 22.7. Renewal reminder for patients enrolled in a service agreement.

By Appointment

PAUL FARKAS, O.D.
T.W. KASSALOW, O.D.
BARRY FARKAS, O.D., P.C.
F.A.A.O.-DIPLOMATES-CONTACT LENS SECTION

Practice Limited
To Contact Lens

30 East 60th Street
New York, NY 10022
(212) 355-5145

AND ASSOCIATES

1025 Northern Blvd.
Roslyn, NY 11576
(516) 365-4500

Dear   :

On   your Standard Service Contract will expire.* Since
you wear Gas Permeable lenses the **most effective** coverage for you
would be the **STANDARD SERVICE CONTRACT**.

The Standard Service Contract is the most cost-effective approach for
patients like you who require only semi-annual evaluations. If however,
you feel you would like the assurance of knowing that you can use our
service on a more extensive basis without additional cost, you may want
to consider an Extended Care Service Agreement.

Below is an outline of the lens replacement costs and office visit fees
with and without a Service Contract. We hope that you are enjoying your
contact lenses and we look forward to seeing you for your next routine
examination which is due to take place in September of this year.

If you have any specific questions regarding your individual circumstances
please feel free to communicate with us.

Upon deciding which approach is best for your specific needs, please
complete the enclosed envelope and return it to our office. For your
convenience please consider using your MasterCard, Visa or American
Express card.

The Standard Service Contract:
Annual Fee: $150.00   3 Office Visits at NO Charge.
                                 $75.00 per replacement lens.
                                 10% reduction on additional services.

The Extended Care Service Agreement:
Annual Fee: $230.00   UNLIMITED Office Visits at NO Charge.
                                 $55.00 per replacement lens.
                                 20% reduction on additional services.

No Coverage: $115.00 per office visit.
                                 $130.00 per replacement lens.

Sincerely,
Drs. Farkas & Kassalow
FIRST REMINDER

(Figure 22.9) or, if the practice has a telephone recall program, through a personal telephone call. Many practitioners feel that the best approach is to preappoint these patients for the 6-month checkup at the conclusion of the fitting period and to call them 1 week in advance of the appointment to remind them of the scheduled date and time.

The approach that is most efficient for a particular practice is the approach that should be followed; however, a routine follow-up evaluation system is absolutely necessary for the patient's continued contact lens comfort and safety.

If the patient does not respond to the initial 6-month checkup reminder, a letter should be sent to the patient at the 1-year point, indicating that the contact lenses might have aged to such an extent that they could be creating a problem (Figure 22.10). If the patient does not respond to this 1-year letter, a telephone call at 15–18 months is strongly advised. At that point, the caller can explain to the patient the reason that the lenses should be evaluated. Many times this call elicits additional information, usually that the patient has discontinued wearing lenses or has selected the services of another practitioner. In either case, the patient's record should be brought up to date and further action should be taken. If a patient does not respond to the telephone call, a strongly worded letter at 2 years is advisable. If there is still no response, a "final" letter placing the patient on inactive status should be mailed (Figure 22.11).

Figure 22.8. Reminder notice for patients failing to renew membership in the agreement.

By Appointment

PAUL FARKAS,   O.D.
T.W. KASSALOW, O.D.
BARRY FARKAS, O.D., P.C.
F.A.A.O.-DIPLOMATES-CONTACT LENS SECTION

Practice Limited
To Contact Lens

30 East 60th Street
New York, NY 10022
(212) 355-5145

AND ASSOCIATES

1025 Northern Blvd.
Roslyn, NY 11576
(516) 365-4500

Dear   :

On   your **Standard Service Contract** expired. We have not as yet received a response from you regarding the reinstatement of it. Our Service Agreements are designed to allow you to receive the quality follow-up care which is essential for continued safe and effective contact lens wear in the most cost-effective manner. The services provided include:

*Periodic evaluations to maintain proper comfort and vision.
*Guaranteed quality assurance of all lenses replaced [within 30 days of receiving the new lens(es)].
*Special cleaning of lenses when needed.
*Refit to updated contact lens materials at significantly reduced fees.
*Special visual services in addition to normal contact lens care at reduced rates.

If we do not hear from you within 30 days of the expiration date stated above, your Service Contract will have lapsed and you will be on a per visit basis. If at some future time you wish to take advantage of our Service Contract you may do so only after an office visit, lens inspection and a 30-day waiting period from the date of your remittance.

If non-renewal was an oversight, please complete the enclosed envelope and return it with a remittance to avoid interruption of your service. Below is an outline of the lens replacement costs and office visit fees with and without a Service Contract to help you decide which course of action to take.

The Standard Service Contract:
Annual Fee: $150.00

3 Office Visits at NO Charge.
$105.00 per replacement lens.
10% reduction on additional services.

The Extended Care Service Agreement:
Annual Fee: $230.00

UNLIMITED Office Visits at NO Charge.
$75.00 per replacement lens.
20% reduction on additional services.

No Coverage:

$115.00 per office visit.
$160.00 per replacement lens.

Sincerely,
Drs. Farkas & Kassalow

FINAL NOTICE - IMMEDIATE ACTION REQUIRED

Many health insurance carriers do cover a significant portion of the cost of your eye evaluations up to the cost of your Service Agreement. Reimbursement forms are available on request during your office visit.

CONCLUSION

This chapter summarizes how to develop a contact lens practice from within an existing patient base as well as how to efficiently administer a contact lens practice for optimum benefit to patients. The techniques described are used in successful contact lens practices throughout the United States. Although not every approach is suitable for every practice, most of these suggestions should be helpful to any practitioner, whether the practitioner fits contact lenses on a full-time basis or occasionally as part of a primary care practice.

Figure 22.9. Postcard reminder for patients scheduled for a 6-month follow-up examination.

Figure 22.10. One-year reminder of missed 6-month appointment.

Figure 22.11. Letter placing the patient on inactive status.

BY APPOINTMENT

PRACTICE LIMITED
TO CONTACT LENSES

PAUL FARKAS, O.D.
T. W. KASSALOW, O.D.
BARRY FARKAS, O.D., P.C.
F.A.A.O. · DIPLOMATES · CONTACT LENS SECTION

& ASSOCIATES

30 EAST 60TH STREET
NEW YORK, NEW YORK 10022
(212) 355-5145
FAX: (212) 308-3262

1025 NORTHERN BLVD.
ROSLYN, NEW YORK 11576
(516) 365-4500
FAX: (516) 365-6580

Dear :

I am sorry to learn that you have discontinued wearing your contact lenses.

As soon as time permits, I hope you will have the opportunity to make an appointment so that we may evaluate the reasons for your discontinuing lens wear. There are many new products which could eliminate any minor difficulties you experienced in the past. Enclosed please find a newsletter which I hope you will find informative.

We shall place your record card in our Inactive File, for the time being, and no further communications will be forwarded to you. But a note as a reminder-- routine eye health evaluations including glaucoma tests and dilated examinations are extremely important. Please make sure you are receiving routine examinations either through our office or the doctor's office of your choosing.

If we may be of any future service, please feel free to communicate with us at any time.

Sincerely,

Drs. Farkas, Kassalow & Assoc.

/dg

BIBLIOGRAPHY

Anan BS. In search of...the ideal contact lens inventory. Optom Manage 1986;22(4):48–9, 53–6.

Bennett I. Management for the Eyecare Practitioner. Stoneham, MA: Butterworth, 1993.

Farkas P. Build a better contact lens practice. Optom Manage 1981;17(7):53–7.

Farkas P. The cause and cure of the harem syndrome. Optom Manage 1976;12(4):115–27.

Farkas P. Developing a contact lens practice. Contact Lens J 1993;20(8):15–7.

Farkas P. How to find the perfect aide. Optom Manage 1974; 10(9):18–21.

Farkas P. A rational refund policy. Contact Lens J 1992; 20(2):23.

Farkas P. Road rules for contact lens referrals. Optom Manage 1972;8(3):37–41.

Farkas P. Setting ground rules. Optom Econ 1993; 3(2):40–1.

Farkas P, Kassalow TW. Employer-employee relationships in an optometric practice. J Am Optom Assoc 1973;44(1):71–4.

Farkas P, Kassalow TW, Farkas B. "Extending" your extended wear practice. Optom Manage 1985;21(6):47–55.

Gailmard NB. Disposable contact lens management. Optom Manage 1989;25(5):73–6.

Gailmard NB. How to succeed with specialty lenses. Optom Manage 1992;28(9):33–4.

Gailmard NB. Soft lens inventory for practice growth. Optom Manage 1982;18(2):69–73.

Gailmard NB. Soft toric lens inventories. Optom Econ 1992;2(3):34–6.

Kassalow TW, Farkas P, Farkas B. Eight tips to build your contact lens practice. Optom Manage 1985;21(1):68–73.

Koetting R. Marketing, Managing, and Contact Lenses. Stoneham, MA: Butterworth-Heinemann, 1992.

Lee J. Take command of lens replacement inventories. Optom Manage 1993;28(6):44–7.

McLaughlin R. RGP fitting from inventory vs. custom fitting lenses. Contact Lens Spectrum 1990;5(2):11.

Winslow C. A bigger contact lens dispensary can build your practice. Rev Optom 1991; 128(11):39–44.

Part IV
Financial Aspects of Practice

Chapter 23

Fees and Accounting Systems

John G. Classé and Donald H. Lakin

Money makes the world go around.

—Fred Ebb
Cabaret

Before the publication of Charles Percival's enlightening work, *Medical Ethics*, in 1803, physicians routinely charged for services based on the ability of patients to pay rather than on a fixed fee schedule. His ideas on the ethics of payment for services profoundly influenced medicine in America. In time these ideas came to represent the prevailing point of view—that each patient should be charged the same amount for the same service.

Optometry has followed a similar evolutionary process in the setting of fees. Practitioners working in commercial environments at the start of the twentieth century were subjected to "free examination" promotions by the businesses employing them, and it was common practice to "charge for glasses" in a lump sum rather than to separate fees into amounts for services and for materials. Gradually, the use of fee schedules and the separation of fees for services from materials by professional optometrists affected the profession, causing the value of services to be given greater emphasis. Even so, a survey of practitioner attitudes conducted by the American Optometric Association in 1966 found that optometrists:

- Lacked confidence in fee schedules
- Could not effectively answer questions asked by patients about fees

- Felt fees were inconsistent from one group of services to another
- Considered fees to have no rational relationship to the cost of services and materials
- Believed these inconsistencies were widespread throughout the profession

Third-party reimbursement, principally by government, has also affected the optometry profession. Through Medicare and Medicaid, fees were established for services rendered to the elderly and to indigent children and adults. For other individuals, private insurance plans that offered reimbursement for examinations and, to a lesser degree, for ophthalmic materials, established the fees. The effect of these programs was to change the traditional mode of payment from patient to practitioner, inserting a third party into the process, and to take the ability to set fees out of the hands of practitioners.

Medicare, in particular, has wielded considerable influence on fee schedules. After the Medicare "parity" amendment was enacted by the U.S. Congress in 1986, optometrists examining Medicare-eligible patients were able to receive reimbursement for services—within the scope of licensure—that led to the diagnosis or treatment of disease. Reimbursement levels were established by determining a fee "profile" for the optometrist's area of practice. The fees charged by all the practitioners in the area were used to establish this profile, and reimbursement levels were set at 70% of the mean fee. Optometrists who charged more than the 70% level were limited to this amount, but optometrists who charged less than the 70% level received the lesser amount. However, fees charged to Medicare patients for services could not be more than the fees charged to patients under 65 years of age for these same services. As a result, fees for services received a considerable amount of revision for patients of all ages.

Charges for ophthalmic materials have been less subjected to regulation, because few insurance plans provide complete reimbursement for spectacles or contact lenses, offering instead a partial payment or credit toward purchase. The difference is paid by the patient. Under Medicare, the only ophthalmic materials for which reimbursement will be provided are the initial spectacles or contact lenses used for the correction of aphakia or pseudophakia. The setting of charges for ophthalmic materials has been an ongoing problem for optometry, one that is confounded by the ethical obligation to separate charges for services from those for materials.

Ethically, a professional has the responsibility to inform patients of the charges for care and how they were determined. Abuses such as "free" examinations hid the practitioner's fee for services in the charge for spectacles, and "bait and switch" tactics lured patients to practitioners for the purpose of selling eyewear at high markup rather than the inexpensive eyewear advertised. Even worse, "rebates" paid to a prescribing practitioner for ophthalmic materials sold by a dispenser kept the patient from realizing the practitioner's financial incentive to "steer" the patient to that particular dispenser. These and other unsavory practices led to a demand for reform within optometry and to passage of practice rules that emphasized the obligation to set uniform fees, to separate charges for materials from fees for services, and to avoid economic discrimination in patient care.

Within this historical context, contemporary practitioners still struggle to determine the amount to charge for services, the proper pricing of ophthalmic materials, the fair apportionment of charges between services and materials, and the ethical presentation of fees to patients. The most fundamental

of these problems, particularly for a beginning practitioner, is determining a fee schedule.

DETERMINING A FEE SCHEDULE

The determination of a fee schedule must be divided into two parts: setting fees for services and establishing charges for ophthalmic materials. Because optometrists not only provide vision services but also dispense a product, two different methods of setting the fee schedule must be used. As recounted, in the past the services of the optometrist were frequently undervalued, often amounting to less than the chair cost (i.e., the cost per patient of keeping the office open and operating), while the price of the materials was increased two- to four-fold for purposes of sale, so that a reasonable profit could be realized. In addition, the fee for both examination and spectacles was presented as one charge, usually being described as "the cost of the glasses." Much of the effort to promote professionalism during the past few decades has been directed toward the elimination of the "single charge" concept. This effort has been aided by the Federal Trade Commission's "Eyeglasses Rules," which granted to patients an unfettered right to the spectacle prescription, allowing them to take the prescription from an optometrist charging a low fee for services to a less expensive dispenser. Aid was also received from Medicare "parity" legislation, because its fee "profiles" for services caused optometrists charging lower fees than those described on the profile to recognize that their services were undervalued. The result of this reconsideration was an increase in the relative value of professional services and a devaluation of the charge for ophthalmic materials. As a result, the emphasis today is on fees for services.

Fees for Services

Although fees for services have become the key consideration in optometric reimbursement, the ability of optometrists to establish a reasonable return for their professional skill has been significantly influenced by the steady emergence of vision care as an insurance benefit. Because of the success of managed care programs such as health maintenance organizations (HMOs) and preferred provider organizations (PPOs), and because of the dictates of companies providing vision care benefits to workers, fees for services have been increasingly determined not by practitioners but by these entities. If many workers enrolled in an insurance program are the patients of an optometrist or would likely become the patients of an optometrist, the reimbursement offered by the insurer must be accepted by the optometrist or these patients will be lost. The fee paid by the insurer is often well below the optometrist's usual and customary fee, but it is accepted by the optometrist in return for the prospect of serving a sizeable population of patients. The optometrist's autonomy over fee setting is lost in such an arrangement, but the ramifications extend beyond fees to include ethical concerns, such as the time to be allocated for examination. Since the optometrist receives less compensation for each examination, there is a natural tendency to attempt to increase the number of examinations within the same unit of time. Such a development can result in less thorough examinations, to the potential detriment of patients. This effect is certainly not what patients had in mind when they joined an insurance program.

The determination of fees to be charged for services is complicated, therefore, by the erosion of the traditional payment philosophy of health care—in which the practitioner set the fee to be paid, and the payment was received directly from the patient. The intrusion of third parties—government and the insurance industry—has created a complication, in which the fee to be received by the practitioner is most often set and paid by the third party. As a result, true "fee for service" is rapidly diminishing as the most common payment mechanism for optometric health care services.

Given these developments, when optometrists do establish fees to be charged for professional services, several factors must be considered: the optometrist's "chair cost," the fees for like services charged by other practitioners in the community, the fees paid by third parties (most notably in the Medicare program) for like services, and the optometrist's determination of the value of individual experience, skill, and knowledge.

Determining "Chair Cost"

The "chair cost" is the expense incurred by the optometrist to perform examinations, usually expressed as an hourly amount. If an optometrist determines the overhead costs for patient examinations and divides this amount by the time spent performing these examinations, the cost of services can be calculated (see Chapter 28). If the hourly fee derived from patient fees is less than this figure, the optometrist is operating at a loss. An optometrist must know the "chair cost," because it exerts an obvious effect on the fee to be charged for services. The examination fee must be at least this amount, or the optometrist will not be able to operate an economically viable practice. The "chair cost" therefore represents a minimum fee for services below which the optometrist cannot operate the practice (or at least cannot continue to operate the practice at its current level).

Comparison with Other Practitioners

Within the group of optometrists in any community there is a range of fee schedules from which a minimum, a maximum, and a mean charge can be derived. A new practitioner, entering a community to start a practice, should be familiar with this range of fees and should consider them when attempting to establish the fee schedule for the new practice. In general, it is preferable to be neither the lowest nor the highest in such a situation. For an established practitioner, seeking to alter fees, this information is also valuable and should be considered during the decision-making process, along with the other factors previously enumerated. It can also be useful to determine the fee schedules for ophthalmologists in the community, particularly if optometrists work with them. This information allows the fee schedule that is finally chosen to fit within the economic boundaries of the community's ophthalmic marketplace, and for the practitioner to understand where within that marketplace the fees might rank.

Fees Paid by Third Parties

A practitioner cannot determine fees for services without being cognizant of the fee schedules established by third parties such as government and insurance companies. Because of the growing use of

Table 23.1. Office and Other Outpatient Services for Medicare[a]

Sub-category	History	Exam	Medical Decision-Making	Counseling	Coordination of Care	Nature of Presenting Problem	Time[b]
New patient							
	All three components required						
99201	Problem focused	Problem focused	Straight-forward	Contributory	Contributory	Self limited or minor	10 min
99202	Expanded problem focused	Expanded problem focused	Straight-forward	Contributory	Contributory	Low to moderate severity	20 min
99203	Detailed	Detailed	Low complexity	Contributory	Contributory	Moderate severity	30 min
99204	Comprehensive	Comprehensive	Moderate complexity	Contributory	Contributory	Moderate to high severity	45 min
99205	Comprehensive	Comprehensive	High complexity	Contributory	Contributory	Moderate to high severity	60 min
Established patient							
99211	Requires physician's supervision only					Minimal	5 min
	2 of 3 components required						
99212	Problem focused	Problem focused	Straight-forward	Contributory	Contributory	Self limited or minor	10 min
99213	Expanded problem focused	Expanded problem focused	Low complexity	Contributory	Contributory	Low to moderate severity	15 min
99214	Detailed	Detailed	Moderate complexity	Contributory	Contributory	Moderate to high severity	25 min
99215	Comprehensive	Comprehensive	High complexity	Contributory	Contributory	Moderate to high severity	40 min

Shaded areas = required.
[a]Counseling/coordination of care must be documented in record. Please refer to CPT definitions/guidelines.
[b]Time is only pertinent in determining the level of service when it constitutes more than 50% of the face-to-face physician encounter.
Source: Procedure codes and definitions are copyrighted by the American Medical Association.

optometric services by Medicare-eligible patients, the influence of government reimbursement schedules is obvious. Practitioners cannot charge more for the same service to patients who are not Medicare-eligible than to patients who are Medicare-eligible, so the reimbursement allowed to Medicare providers must be considered when establishing a fee schedule or when changing fees. It is particularly important to determine the skill level required for the service. Because of the requirements of Medicare, the fee to be charged must reflect the skill exercised during the examination. As a result, fee schedules are organized to reflect these differences, not only for Medicare patients but also for patients of all ages

(Table 23.1). A discussion of different levels of service is given elsewhere (see Chapter 26).

Individual Experience, Skill, and Knowledge

Every practitioner should consider individual capacity when setting fees. Generally speaking, as a practitioner grows in experience and skill, fees are adjusted to reflect the knowledge acquired in these years of practice. This individual factor should be tempered, however, by the economic realities of the ophthalmic marketplace, the prevailing fees in the community, and the other considerations previously described.

An optometrist must evaluate all these factors when deciding on a fee schedule for services or the alteration of an existing fee schedule. A different set of influences is exerted on the decision making necessary to determine the charges for ophthalmic materials.

PRICING OF OPHTHALMIC MATERIALS

Historically, ophthalmic materials have been supplied not only by optometrists but also by opticians, optical companies, and other retail establishments. Because of this wealth of competition, it is wise for optometrists to be familiar with the pricing strategies used in the marketing of goods and services. Marketing is the process of studying the wants and needs of a target population and satisfying those needs with quality goods and services at competitive prices (see Chapter 29). Once a specific need has been identified, the marketing process involves four factors:

- Designing a product that satisfies the need
- Placing the product where people will purchase it
- Promoting the product
- Setting a price for the product

These four factors are interdependent in terms of both real and perceived value to the consumer. For the optometrist, the "need" that has been identified is quality vision and eye health care, including ophthalmic materials. To satisfy the need for ophthalmic materials, optometrists offer a quality "product"—the determination of the prescription and the fitting and dispensing of eyewear from a single source. The optometrist's dispensary serves as the place where the eyewear can be purchased. To ensure that patients are aware of the availability of these services and materials, they are marketed both to existing patients and the public. The pricing of the ophthalmic materials is based on three fundamental business strategies:

- Neutral pricing—the price is based on the product's value to the average consumer, so that the price equals the worth of the product.
- Skim pricing—the price is set to obtain the highest participation from the segment of the

market that is insensitive to price, so that the price is higher than the product's value to the average consumer.
- Penetration pricing—the price is set at a low level to obtain and hold a large share of the price-sensitive segment of the market, so that the price is lower than the product's value to the average consumer.

In the ophthalmic marketplace all three strategies are used. In the discussion of fees for services, a neutral strategy was presented, with consideration given to the cost of delivering services, the external influence of third-party payers, and the perception of value that is based on individual skill and knowledge. A skimming strategy can be found in the pricing of new surgical techniques such as posterior chamber intraocular lens implantation, radial keratotomy, and photorefractive keratectomy. Services for refractive care have long been subjected to penetration pricing, to the extent that even "free" examinations have been offered to capture and hold market share.

Because of the great variety of competitors and strategies within eye care, it cannot be said that there is one best way to price ophthalmic materials. Each practitioner has to assess the patient population, the location, and the competition in the marketplace. Even so, it should be emphasized that the pricing of ophthalmic materials is not to be determined by the low prices inherent in penetration strategies. The dispensing of ophthalmic materials in a professional office is quite different from the retail sale of eyewear in an optical shop. Patients appreciate the unified quality service that can be obtained in a professional office and expect a consistent value—not the lowest value—for the materials purchased.

When establishing a neutral strategy the optometrist must assess the cost of purchasing and maintaining an inventory of frames; the expense involved in the use of staff members for the selection, dispensing, and repair of eyewear; and the proportionate cost of operating an in-office dispensary. To offset these expenses, the practitioner should consider the contribution to profit that can be made by the sale of frames and lenses. Using this approach, a practitioner can determine a "cost per unit" for eyewear, much in the same manner that "chair cost" was calculated for professional services. The amount calculated becomes the minimum markup to be added to the cost of the ophthalmic materials. This amount is often referred to as a "materials service fee"; under some insurance plans this amount must be used for the pricing of ophthalmic materials. Because the costs of maintaining an inventory of frames (and providing related services) increases with more expensive materials, the markup for ophthalmic materials is usually two to two and a half times the cost of the materials. Ophthalmic lenses are usually priced in the same manner. If discounted materials costs are required by some vision care plans, this factor must be built into the materials service fee charged by the practice.

The price of ophthalmic materials must be organized and presented in a coherent way to patients. Spectacle frames, ophthalmic lenses, and contact lenses must be categorized in some practical manner and charges must be set for each category. For ophthalmic lenses, the results are typically described on a fee schedule, which lists the various categories and charges to be applied. Spectacle frames are priced on an individual basis, and the price is often attached to the frame with a small sticker or other means of identifying differences.

Contact lenses have become a very competitive part of the ophthalmic materials market. There has been a gradual decrease in the markup for lenses and an accompanying increase in the professional fees charged for fitting and followup. Disposable lenses are usually priced at one to one and a half times their cost, while other lenses are usually priced at two times their cost. Prepaid service agreements and planned lens replacement programs have been used to support the cost of providing services and materials to contact lens wearers. These approaches also join the pricing of services and materials for the convenience of the patient.

In response to consumer demands for faster delivery of spectacles by ophthalmic providers, many optometrists have obtained in-office equipment to edge and dye lenses or apply lens coatings. The purchase price of this equipment, the cost of operation and maintenance, the value of the time expended by employees to operate it, and other factors must be considered by the optometrist in setting the charge to patients for edging, tinting, and coating services. The prevailing charges for these services in the community must also be considered. These ancillary services can be an impor-

tant source of income and can add to patient satisfaction by reducing the amount of time needed to provide eyewear after examination.

Fees for services and materials can also be influenced by the method of payment chosen by the patient.

METHODS OF PAYMENT

Payment can be immediate or deferred. The usual methods of immediate payment are cash, check, or credit card. If cash is paid, the optometrist receives full value for the amount charged. If a check is used, the same result is usually obtained, but a small percentage of patients will have insufficient funds in their checking account. The optometrist will be required to spend time and, occasionally, money in an effort to collect the amount owed. The result is less than full value for the amount charged. Credit cards allow payment to be received, but at a discount. The credit card companies customarily receive 1–4% of the amount charged on the card for insuring payment, and, thus, the optometrist will not receive full value for the services rendered.

If payment is deferred, it is because the payment is to be made by a third party or credit has been extended to the patient. In both situations, the optometrist will not receive full value for the amount billed. Third-party claims for reimbursement are subject to approval by the third party before payment; often reimbursement is delayed or payment is disallowed. If the claim is denied, the optometrist can turn to the patient for payment, but the collection of the amount due is achieved in less than 100% of cases. The same is obviously true of situations in which credit is extended to patients. Even though billing and collections efforts can be employed, some payments inevitably will not be received. Again, the end result is less than complete payment for the amount charged.

Optometrists must consider carefully the method of payment to be permitted (particularly the credit policy to be used), attend scrupulously to the billing requirements of third parties providing vision and eye care benefits, and organize workable procedures for the collection of accounts receivable. The setting of fees and their method of payment are intimately related and cannot be separated.

One other essential consideration is the accounting system used to document the charges made and payments received for services and materials.

Accounting Systems

The ideal accounting system is simple and accurate and requires little time to use. Unfortunately, no system available today meets these requirements. The traditional system is known as the "pegboard" (named for the pegged binder that holds the system's documents in exact alignment). The pegboard system uses one-entry bookkeeping, which is preferable to the old system of ledger books and patient accounts that required financial information to be transferred from one to the other. The pegboard system allows all financial records to be completed at one writing, reducing the likelihood of error. However, today the trend is away from pegboard systems in favor of the use of computers for financial accounting. Computers can be used to bill patients and track accounts with great efficiency and accuracy. Software programs can be purchased that will permit individual payment schedules to be set for patients, calculate interest on unpaid accounts, and provide preprinted receipts to be mailed to the practice with payment. Tracking of accounts payable can also be efficiently performed by the computer, as can the financial productivity of the office. This versatility gives the computer an edge over traditional methods of financial recordkeeping.

Pegboard

There are four components of the pegboard system: day sheet, patient transaction slip, patient statement card, and deposit slip. These documents are arranged in a binder so that a single entry on the day sheet can, at the same time, make entries on the other three documents. Each component of the pegboard system has a specific function.

Day Sheet. The name of the patient is entered on the day sheet, which is divided into columns; this configuration allows the services rendered, the fees charged, the payment received, and the balance due to be entered as one transaction. Each patient is listed chronologically, and the financial informa-

tion for each patient is updated at every visit. As the information is transcribed on the day sheet, it is automatically transferred to the patient transaction slip. The fee paid by the patient and the balance outstanding are similarly entered and transferred to the other documents. A deposit slip is provided to maintain an itemized list of cash payments made by patients. At the end of each day, the day sheet can be totaled—both for payments received and for accounts receivable.

Patient Transaction Slip. The patient transaction slip is an itemized bill that lists the services received by the patient and the payment made by the patient on the date of examination. Procedure codes are printed on the bill so that the services rendered can be identified. Since the payment made (or balance due) is transcribed onto the slip, it also serves as a receipt for the patient. If desired, future appointments can also be noted on the slip.

Patient Statement Card. A patient statement card is maintained for each patient, with a chronological listing of the dates of examination, fees charged, and payment received. This card can list each member of a family individually, or all members of the family can be listed together, whichever the practitioner desires. With the visit of each patient or family member, the card is updated simultaneously as entries are made on the day sheet. If needed, it can be copied and mailed to patients as a monthly bill for accounts outstanding or provided to patients as a summary for tax purposes.

Deposit Slip. As cash payments are entered on the day sheet, they can also be copied onto a deposit slip. Not only is time saved, but an itemized list of deposits is maintained for use as needed.

Because all entries are achieved with one writing, the likelihood of mistakes is reduced. The pegboard system also allows for daily, weekly, or monthly financial information to be collected for analysis and use, and it maintains a running summary of accounts receivable. The pegboard system has begun to be replaced, however, by computerized systems—which are more expensive, more complicated, and often more time consuming but offer greater opportunity for collection and analysis of information.

Computer

Personal computers are used by the majority of optometrists in private practice. Software programs have been designed for use in optometric offices and offer many features that provide time-saving steps in the scheduling of appointments, recording of patient information, tracking of orders for ophthalmic materials, entering and analysis of financial records, completion and submission of insurance claims, and preparation of communications with patients.

Scheduling Appointments. Computers allow appointments to be easily scheduled or rescheduled, with a set of related information (such as telephone numbers) that allow for patients to be contacted by mail or telephone to verify appointment dates and times. Appointment entries can usually be linked to the recall system and to computerized billing for services and materials.

Recording Patient Data. Some software systems permit "paperless" records to be maintained. To provide security for entries, some systems prevent changes from being made to the record after the passage of a certain period of time (to prevent alteration or destruction of data). The computer will print the information on a specialized form or a personalized letter or transfer it electronically to another computer. Computers can also be linked to instruments such as automatic refractors and lensometers to record patient data automatically.

Ophthalmic Materials. Computer programs can send orders for lenses and frames to optical laboratories, track the status of orders, keep track of frame and lens inventories, track frame and lens usage, use bar code scanning, and perform helpful analyses of ophthalmic materials costs and usage.

Financial Records. Software programs can be used to perform a variety of financial management functions, including the completion of day sheets, statements for patients, deposit slips for payments, bills, and accounts receivable. They can even prepare the checks for employees, maintain payroll accounts, and issue annual W-2 forms for employees.

Insurance Claims. There are programs that enable forms to be completed and printed for various health insurance plans, including the HCFA 1500 form (used for most medical insurance plans and Medicare) and the form for Vision Service Plan (VSP).

Communications with Patients. Cards and letters can be printed through computerized programs that generate recall notices, service agreements for contact lens patients, referral letters, thank you letters, and vision analyses. Computer programs allow these communications to be personalized, making them more effective with patients.

It is this versatility that makes computer programs favored over other means of data management. Regardless of the system used, the opportunity always exists for manipulation of the system by a dishonest employee and for loss of funds through embezzlement. No system is foolproof, and it is appropriate for practitioners to take steps to improve their own familiarity with the system, which at the same time discourages dishonesty on the part of an employee.

INSPECTION AND EVALUATION OF FINANCIAL RECORDS

There are several steps that a practitioner should take to reduce the likelihood of loss from embezzlement. One is to obtain insurance protection. Although employees who handle substantial amounts of money can be bonded (guaranteeing reimbursement to the employer by the bonding company), the experience that employees must go through to obtain the bond usually makes it a less desirable alternative to insurance coverage. The optometrist purchases a rider as part of professional liability insurance protection, usually at a nominal fee.

Employees should be hired only after references have been verified and questioned. Employees who manage money should be informed that their work will be checked periodically. If possible, more than one employee should be assigned to bookkeeping tasks. Vigilance on the part of the practitioner can be an important deterrent to this unfortunate, but too often encountered, downside of practice.

CONCLUSION

Although the setting of fees for services and of charges for materials is a personal act that must be performed by the individual practitioner, considerable influence is exerted by outside factors. The fees charged by competitors, the economic status of the community, and the practitioner's skill, experience, and knowledge are among the factors exerting that influence. The greatest influence on professional fees is the trend toward increasing use of third-party reimbursement plans.

The reimbursement "parity" achieved by optometrists under Medicare was a great legislative achievement for the profession. Still, it significantly changed the economic relationship between optometrists and their patients and changed even the manner in which optometrists regard the issue of charging for services. Added to the influence of Medicare is the growing use of vision care plans and the utilization of optometrists as providers under eye health plans, which have substituted insurance reimbursement for the traditional method of payment. Despite these changes, the earnings of optometrists continue to rise, and patient loads continue to increase, offering a suggestion that the profession is adapting well to these changes in health care reimbursement mechanisms.

BIBLIOGRAPHY

American Medical Association. Physicians Current Procedural Terminology (4th ed) (CPT–4). Chicago: American Medical Association, 1995.

American Optometric Association. Codes for Optometry (3rd ed). St. Louis: American Optometric Association, 1995.

American Optometric Association. Handbook for Assistants. St. Louis: American Optometric Association, 1989.

American Optometric Association. Manual on Completion of Insurance Claim Forms (4th ed). St. Louis: American Optometric Association, 1994.

American Optometric Association. An Optometrist's Guide to Managed Care. St. Louis: American Optometric Association, 1992.

Barresi BJ, Brooks RE. Full-scope optometry meets managed care. Optom Econ 1994;4(6):10–13.

Beebe K, Hoffer D. Give insurers the slip. Optom Manage 1992;27(3):43–6.

Cleinman A. How to guard your margin. Optom Manage 1993;28(5):17–20.

Coleman DL. Watch for these booby traps in managed care contracts. Optom Econ 1994;4(7):14–7.

Consultant's Corner. Cracking the codes: how to use CPT–4 codes to get prompt payment. Rev Optom 1995;132(3):33.

Elmstrom G. Advanced Management Strategies for Optometrists. Chicago: Professional Press, 1982.

Everett S. Don't undercharge for medical services. Rev Optom 1991;128(12):25.

Hayes J. The fearless way to raise fees. Optom Manage 1991;26(6):14–20.

Hayes J. How to guarantee a higher net. Optom Manage 1993;28(1):16.

Irving F. Are your fees in line? Optom Manage 1993;28(10):22–5.

Lahr J. A no-nonsense guide to third-party plans. Optom Manage 1991;26(10):29–32.

Lee J. Set your fees for a fair profit. Optom Manage 1993;28(9):26–9.

Lookabaugh R. Double your patient-pleasing power. Optom Manage 1992;27(3):16–20.

Maino DM. Personal finance programs tell you where it all went. Rev Optom 1993;130(11):25–7.

Muellerleile J. Fix your prices without price fixing. Optom Econ 1994;4(3):19–22.

Shuldiner R. Total recall. Optom Manage 1991;26(9):14–22.

Tlachac CA. Fees for difficult fits. Optom Econ 1994;4(6):24–7.

Chapter 24

Credit and Collections

John G. Classé

Ah, take the Cash and let the Credit go.

—Edward Fitzgerald
The Rubaiyat of Omar Khayyam

Even for practitioners on the cash system, it is inevitable that billing of patients will be required, and for the majority of practitioners, collection of accounts receivable is a constant problem, one directly related to the necessity of billing for fees. The time, labor, and money expended on billing and collection efforts can be considerable, particularly in practices that do not have a well-organized and coordinated system. If billing and collections practices are inadequate, a financial loss will be incurred, one that could have been prevented if proper planning and procedures had been instituted. For these reasons, it is important for practitioners to consider the related issues of billing and collections, which can be divided into three topics: payment for services, methods of billing, and methods of collection. All of these issues should be considered and decided on by the practitioner before beginning a billing and collections program.

This discussion concerns only the billing and collection of fees for service—it does not describe the remediation of disputes with third-party providers, such as insurance companies and government agencies. For the collection of debts from third parties, practitioners must consult individual dispute settlement guidelines.

PAYMENT FOR SERVICES

There are five basic methods of payment. Practitioners might be required to use many of these methods or relatively few, depending on the services offered and the preferences of the practitioner.

1. *The advance payment method.* This method requires that payment be made before services are rendered or materials are obtained. The most common example is the prepaid service agreement for contact lens patients, in which the fee is paid at the start of the covered period of services.

2. *The step payments method.* This method permits the patient to make serial payments as services or materials are received. An example would be planned replacement of contact lenses, in which periodic replacement of lenses is a program feature.

3. *The traditional deposit and balance method.* This method requires the patient to pay a percentage of the amount due after services have been rendered and to pay the balance when ophthalmic materials are received. An example would be to require payment of 50% of the services and spectacles cost after the examination, with the remainder due when the spectacles are received.

4. *The credit and billing method.* In this method, no payment is required and credit is extended to the patient; billing is used to obtain payment of the amount credited. For example, the patient is billed for the cost of the examination and ophthalmic materials with no payment required until the bill is received.

5. *The installment method.* This method requires payment in stated amounts or over a fixed period of time. An example would be to allow payment in three fixed installments over 3 months.

Of all these methods, only the first and second do not result in the extension of credit to the patient. The third, deposit and balance, has been relied on by optometrists because the deposit can be used to cover the cost of ophthalmic materials, thereby preventing financial loss to the optometrist if the patient fails to pay the balance. The last two methods are true credit transactions, because they do not obligate the patient to make payment until after services and materials have been received. Billing of the patient is necessary to collect the amount due. If credit and billing is used, it has been determined that approximately 70% of patients will pay on receipt of the first statement, approximately 25% will require extra billings or special arrangements, and the remaining 5% cannot or will not pay. In a well-run practice, the percentage of unpaid accounts should not exceed 3–5% of the patients billed.

The billing of patients requires that a statement be prepared and mailed. If the pegboard system of accounting is used, the amount due is entered on the daily ledger. It can be transferred to the patient's individual statement at the time the unpaid balance is entered, then mailed to the patient for payment. If a computerized system is used, the amount due can be posted in the patient's file, for transfer to a statement at the time of billing. Under both systems, it is relatively easy for these accounts receivable to be monitored.

The unpaid accounts control sheet lists the patient accounts that are 30, 60, 90, and 120 days in arrears. It not only permits the practitioner to keep track of the accounts that remain unpaid and the period of time that they have been due but also allows in-office collection efforts to be documented. These efforts must be organized by the practitioner in a manner that is in keeping with the practitioner's philosophy toward collections.

If billing is to be used, collections will become necessary. If bills remain unpaid beyond a reasonable period, the practitioner must decide if an effort will be made to collect the amount due and, if such an effort is instituted, whether the practitioner will collect the account or will allow a third party to serve as the collection agent. This decision is an important one and must be given due consideration by the practitioner, because it will dictate the manner in which the office is organized to initiate collections efforts. It will also have ramifications outside the office, for the method chosen by the practitioner for the collection of unpaid accounts can adversely affect the practitioner's reputation if it is poorly done. It is advisable to discuss methods of collection with other practitioners before instituting a policy and to seek legal counsel so that ill-advised policies or efforts will not be incorporated into the practice's procedures.

LEGAL CONSIDERATIONS

Several legal issues are important when credit is extended to patients. First, the decision to deny credit to an individual is regulated by federal law. Second, the Truth-in-Lending Act can be imposed on certain credit practices. Third, the collection of unpaid fees by collections agencies and attorneys is subject to both federal and state regulation. This latter factor has significant ramifications for the optometrist employing an agency or attorney.

Extending Credit

Equal Credit Opportunity

If an optometrist extends credit to patients, it must be awarded on a nondiscriminatory basis. Credit cannot be refused because of a patient's race, color, religion, national origin, sex, marital status, age, or because the patient is on public assistance. If an optometrist refuses credit to a patient, the proper basis for the denial should be documented. Violation of this federal law is punishable by both civil and criminal penalties.

Truth-in-Lending

Practitioners who permit credit, and subsequently bill patients for amounts due, should be careful to structure the billing program to avoid the voluminous disclosure and reporting requirements of truth-in-lending. This federal law, which is applicable in all jurisdictions, requires creditors to provide certain information when extending credit to individuals, even when the creditor is a health care professional such as an optometrist. To fall under the obligations of truth-in-lending merely requires an optometrist to apply a finance charge to unpaid accounts or to structure payment from patients in more than four installments (not including a down payment). To avoid the complications of truth-in-lending, therefore, an optometrist should not use finance charges and should allow patients to either make payments in four installments or should allow payments to be made by the patient on an unstructured basis (i.e., not on a fixed schedule). Civil and criminal penalties are possible for violation of this act.

Fair Debt Collections

Federal law regulates the collections practices of collection agencies and attorneys-at-law. In-office collections efforts by an optometrist to collect unpaid fees are not subject to federal requirements. All states have enacted statutes that regulate the harassment of debtors, however, and the collections efforts of optometrists would be subject to these laws.

Because of legal regulations, the awarding of credit and the collection of unpaid fees should be carefully organized and scrupulously managed. The first step in structuring a practice to meet these demands is to prepare a written contract for services.

Contracts for Services. To prevent misunderstanding between practitioner and patient and to provide a legal basis for the resolution of disputes with patients over the payment of fees for services and materials, a printed contract should be used. This form should contain three parts: a section requesting certain patient information, a section devoted to the practitioner's payment policy, and a statement concerning collections efforts (Figure 24.1).

PATIENT INFORMATION. The patient's name, birthdate, address, workplace, and other basic information should be requested, as should vital information concerning the patient's spouse.

PAYMENT POLICY. The method of payment chosen by the practitioner (e.g., deposit and balance) should be described, as should the manner in which payment can be tendered by the patient (e.g., cash, check, credit card).

COLLECTIONS POLICY. If the practitioner has decided to collect unpaid accounts, information should be provided to the patient concerning the method of collection. It is also essential to notify the patient that if an attorney's services are required or if it is necessary to resort to small claims court, the patient will be required to pay the attorney's fees and the court costs in addition to paying the amount due or ordered by the court. Only if this language is included in the agreement can the practitioner collect the full amount due and have legal and court costs borne by the patient.

This contract is signed by the patient and retained in the patient's record of care. If legal action becomes necessary, the contract can be used as evidence of the agreement between the parties. The patient contract should be updated at each annual examination to ensure that the patient information is current and to provide documentation of the agreement.

If a patient does not pay as agreed and collections become necessary, the usual resort of practitioners is an in-office collections effort that involves the use of letters. Telephone collections efforts should not be attempted because of the vulnerability of such efforts to charges that they constitute harassment under state laws regulating debt collections. A three-letter sequence is the preferable means of encouraging payment, with the first letter serving as a reminder that payment has not been received (Figure 24.2), the second letter requesting that contact be made with the office to arrange payment (Figure 24.3), and the third letter asserting that alternative action is imminent unless payment or an explanation is forthcoming (Figure 24.4). These letters are generally sent out after the bill has been unpaid for 30, 60, and 90 days, respectively.

If payment is not received despite these in-office efforts, the practitioner must decide whether to pursue the matter further or to dismiss the claim as a bad debt. If the practitioner is on the cash system of accounting, the bad debt cannot be claimed as a tax deduction; if the practitioner is on the accrual system, it can be written off because it has already been claimed as income. If the practitioner decides to pursue the collections effort, there are two alternatives available—collect it in small claims court or turn it over to an attorney or collections agency for further disposition.

Methods of Collection. If an optometrist is in a community that has a small claims court and is

Optometry Eye Group

111 Main Street
Anytown, US 12345

PATIENT INFORMATION

PATIENT'S NAME _____ BIRTHDATE ___/___/___ AGE ____

HOME ADDRESS _____ CITY _____ STATE _____ ZIP _____

IF PATIENT IS A CHILD, SHOW PARENT'S NAME _____ HOME PHONE _____

Provide the following information for the RESPONSIBLE party:

NAME OF PERSON RESPONSIBLE FOR THIS ACCOUNT _____

ADDRESS _____ CITY _____ STATE _____

SOC SEC # ___/___/___ EMPLOYED BY _____ BUSINESS PHONE _____

SPOUSE'S NAME _____ EMPLOYED BY _____ BUSINESS PHONE _____

IN CASE OF EMERGENCY, NOTIFY _____ PHONE _____

STATEMENT OF FINANCIAL POLICY

As a service to you, this office offers several means of payment for the services and materials that you may require:

- It is customary to pay the examination fee at the time of the examination.
- 50% of the cost of spectacles and contact lenses must be paid when ordered, and the balance when dispensed.
- Payment for follow-up examinations is required at each visit.

To ensure that we understand how you wish your account to be handled, please check the payment plan that you prefer and sign in the place indicated. If you have any questions, please ask the receptionist before you make your choice.

[] CASH   [] PERSONAL CHECK   [] CREDIT CARD (select one)   __ American Express
                                                                           __ Discover
                                                                           __ Mastercard
                                                                           __ Visa

The doctor, at the doctor's discretion, may place an UNPAID account with an attorney for collection. In the event the account is referred to an attorney for collection of unpaid charges, the patient or person responsible for the account agrees to pay an attorney's fee, court costs, and any other reasonable costs of collection.

DATE _____ SIGNATURE OF RESPONSIBLE PARTY _____

Figure 24.1. Sample contract for services.

Figure 24.2. Sample "first letter" for in-office collections.

Optometry Eye Group

111 Main Street
Anytown, US 12345

Date

Mr. Unpaid Account
123 Central Avenue
Anytown, US 12345

Dear Mr. Account:

We have not heard from you with regard to our recent statement concerning your account with this office.

If the enclosed account is in error, please contact us so that we may make the appropriate adjustment.

If it is correct, we would enjoy hearing from you soon.

Sincerely,

Accounts Manager

AM/ab
Enclosure

---

willing to invest the time and effort involved to file, process, and collect a legal claim, then small claims court is a viable option. If the optometrist wishes to turn the matter over to a third party, an attorney or a collection agency should be consulted. The choice is the practitioner's, based on individual preferences and attitudes. Each option has its own strengths and weaknesses.

SMALL CLAIMS COURT. Small claims court, which settles disputes involving no more than a few thousand dollars, does not require an attorney, uses relatively informal rules, and is not expensive. The procedures of these courts vary somewhat from community to community, but the general requirements are to file a complaint, allege a legal cause of action (i.e., breach of contract), and pay a filing fee. The address of the defendant must be known so that the complaint can be served. (If the optometrist's contract specifies that the patient is responsible for the costs of collection, an attorney can be hired to file the claim and collect the debt, with the attorney's fees charged to the patient.) A date and time will be set for the trial, which is held before a judge. At the trial, strict rules of evidence are not followed, but the optometrist will need documentation of the examination, services rendered, and reasonable fees charged. Once this evidence is presented, the defendant can offer a defense. After the presentation of evidence is completed, the judge issues a ruling. If it favors the optometrist, the defendant will be ordered to pay a judgment and court costs. If the defendant pays the judgment, the matter is concluded.

Although the defendant has the right to appeal the judgment to a trial court, the amount of money in question virtually always precludes this alterna-

Optometry Eye Group

111 Main Street
Anytown, US 12345

Date

Mr. Unpaid Account
123 Central Avenue
Anytown, US 12345

Dear Mr. Account:

We are disappointed in the fact that we have not received a response to the letter and statement mailed to you last month.

However, we are aware that unexpected developments can make it difficult to meet financial obligations from time to time.

Please consider how you wish to take care of the enclosed statement of account, and contact this office within the next few days so that we may discuss this matter with you.

Sincerely,

Accounts Manager

AM/ab
Enclosure

Figure 24.3. Sample "second letter" for in-office collections.

tive. If the defendant does not pay the judgment within a reasonable period, the optometrist can obtain an order from the court—allowing the judgment to be satisfied by the seizure and sale of the defendant's assets, the taking of money from the defendant's bank account, or periodic payment from the defendant's salary.

Occasionally, a defendant will not answer the complaint or appear in court. At the time set for trial the optometrist can ask the judge to award a default judgment. After a certain period the judgment will be deemed final, and the optometrist will be able to seek the remedies described above for the satisfaction of the judgment.

COLLECTIONS ATTORNEY. An attorney hired to manage the collection of unpaid accounts should be instructed by the optometrist in the methods to be used. For example, an optometrist might not want the attorney to file suit, or might not be willing to have the patient's assets sold to satisfy a judgment awarded in small claims court. The practitioner should establish the bounds of the attorney's efforts. If an attorney is to be used, however, it is advisable to require patients to sign a written contract and to include the clause requiring payment of attorneys' fees and courts costs if legal action must be instituted against the patient to collect the amount owed. The reason for this language is that a collections attorney will charge the optometrist 33–50% of the amount collected for professional services. If the clause is used, the optometrist can collect the full amount owed, and the patient will pay for the attorney and other legal costs of collection.

Figure 24.4. Sample "third letter" for in-office collections.

Optometry Eye Group

111 Main Street
Anytown, US 12345

Date

Mr. Unpaid Account
123 Central Avenue
Anytown, US 12345

Dear Mr. Account:

In our previous efforts to contact you concerning your overdue account, we have evidently failed to make it clear that this is a matter requiring your immediate attention.

Much to our regret, unless we hear from you about the enclosed statement, we will be compelled to take an alternative course of action.

Please contact this office immediately so that we may resolve this matter.

Sincerely,

Accounts Manager

AM/ab
Enclosure

COLLECTIONS AGENCY. Before a collections agency is hired to collect overdue fees, the optometrist should evaluate the reputation of the agency and assess the collections efforts that it employs. Collections agencies are subject to federal and state laws that regulate debt collections practices, and aggressive or dubious collections practices could result in undesirable ramifications, ranging from injury to the optometrist's reputation to legal action involving the optometrist. The optometrist should be comfortable with the collection agency's practices, for they will represent the optometrist in the community.

A second consideration is payment of the collections agency. The preferred method of payment is based on the debts actually collected—the usual fee is 33–50% of the amount collected for the op-

tometrist. The less desirable method is one in which the optometrist is charged for collections efforts, whether successful or not. This situation can become very expensive, with little return, and should be avoided. The optometrist should have a clear understanding of how the agency will charge for its services before entering into a contract for collections.

CONCLUSION

If an optometrist chooses to provide credit to patients, billing and collections are an integral part of the process and must be planned for. The optometrist must determine:

- The type of payment plan to use

- How to keep track of the accounts receivable
- How to prepare and use a written contract for patient services
- The philosophy of the office with respect to collections
- In-office billing procedures (including "past due" letters)
- How past due accounts will be collected

In making these decisions, the optometrist should consult with other practitioners, practice management advisors, and legal counsel to ensure that efforts are legal, tasteful, and within the bounds of professional conduct.

BIBLIOGRAPHY

Consumer Credit Protection Act, 15 USC §1601 et seq.
Equal Credit Opportunity Act, 15 USC §1691 et seq.
Fair Credit Reporting Act, 15 USC §1681 et seq.
Fair Debt Collection Practices Act, 15 USC §1692 et seq.
Regulation Z, Truth-in-Lending, 12 CFR §226.2.
Truth-in-Lending Act 102(a), 12 CFR §226.

Chapter 25

Managed Care and Third-Party Reimbursement

Roger D. Kamen, David L. Park, and Craig Hisaka

Oh, I get by with a little help from my friends.

—John Lennon and Paul McCartney
With a Little Help from My Friends

During this century the financing of health care in the United States has changed drastically. In the early part of the century, patients paid their health care providers directly "out of pocket." There was little, if any, involvement of employers or government in paying the fees. Providers set fees, and patients paid them.

In the mid-twentieth century, due to the impetus of unions, employers began to offer health insurance to employees as a low-cost alternative to salary increases. Insurance companies, which had handled traditional life and property insurance, began offering health coverage. Health insurance programs were modeled after the casualty insurance these companies were accustomed to handling. The type of insurance was an indemnity plan, used to protect against catastrophic loss. Health insurance assumed this same indemnity format, at a very low cost to employers.

The federal government in 1965 became a major player in financing health care with the introduction of Medicare and Medicaid (see Chapter 26). Health insurance became more comprehensive as employers and the federal government added additional benefits for their employees. Over time the low-cost health benefit became a high-cost item. This high cost became burdensome for businesses competing in a global market and a federal government struggling with sizable deficits.

In an attempt to counter the spiraling cost of health care, the United States turned to managed care. This chapter explores third-party reimbursement in this context. Managed care has become widespread throughout the country and is still growing rapidly. It is imperative that providers understand managed care in order to function and flourish in the U.S. health care environment.

HEALTH CARE PLANS

Third-party reimbursement occurs when someone other than the patient pays directly for the health care provided. (Patients pay indirectly in the form of premiums, taxes, and benefits.) Managed care is a health care system that controls the use, cost, and quality of care. It includes both the delivery and financing of health care.

There are various types of health care plans, including traditional indemnity insurance, health maintenance organizations (HMOs), preferred provider organizations (PPOs), and service plans. In the past, particularly during the period of spiraling increases in health care costs (in the 1970s and continuing into the early 1990s), traditional indemnity insurance was the primary health care plan. In this system, providers are actually rewarded financially for performing more and more procedures for patients. There are no controls on cost or use. As long as the patient has a medical problem, the services are covered. One can see how this system promotes increased health care costs.

In this environment, managed care blossomed. HMOs and PPOs are the major types of managed care systems.

Health Maintenance Organizations

HMOs incorporate the delivery and financing of health care. Traditionally, HMOs offered a prepaid system to deliver care to an enrolled group at a predetermined rate; this is known as per member per month (PMPM) rate. It covers all services provided to the member (patient). Currently there are five types of HMOs:

- Staff—the HMO owns the facility, and the providers are employees.
- Group—the HMO contracts with one medical group for member services.
- Network—the HMO contracts with more than one medical group to provide services at various locations.
- Independent practice association (IPA)—the HMO contracts with a provider association, a network of providers who work in their own personal offices.
- Point of service (POS)—a hybrid HMO that allows members the option of going outside the HMO for a particular needed service, but at higher personal cost. The POS HMO has overcome the main complaint of HMO members— the inability to go outside the HMO for care when the member believes it is in his or her best interest.

Preferred Provider Organizations

The second type of managed care organization is a PPO. A PPO is a network of select providers (panel) operating under utilization management and negotiated fee schedules. Patients might use nonpanel providers, but at a higher personal cost.

A type of PPO is the specialty PPO, which consists of one specialty or type of provider. Many vision plans are examples of specialty PPOs.

Service plans can be part of a managed care organization. Service plans pay providers set fees for covered services but might or might not involve utilization management and quality control. A provision of the plan is that the provider must accept the fee schedule as payment in full (i.e., no balance billing).

As managed care has evolved, the distinctions among the various systems has become blurred. Traditional indemnity insurance has added utilization management and is more appropriately labeled managed indemnity. PPOs and HMOs have taken on common features, some of which include permitting patients access to outside providers (at higher personal cost), utilization management, and the passing of financial risk to the provider. The provider needs to look closely at the plan organization and not just at the label or classification of the health plan to determine its actual status.

Currently, health plans are turning to an integrated system of health care delivery. This system involves the integration of many types of providers or a hospital/provider network. Integration allows for greater cost reduction, better efficiency, and more convenience for patients. Examples of integration include:

- Independent practice association
- Group practice without walls
- Group practice
- Physician hospital organization

Optometrists can be included in these networks, joining with ophthalmologists and other physicians to offer the convenience of "one-stop" health care.

COMPENSATION METHODS

Health care plans reimburse for patient care through different methods. It is essential for the provider to understand how the plan reimburses for services. Examples of compensation methods include fee for service, discounted fee for service, fee allowance schedule, relative value scale, and capitation.

Fee for Service

Under fee for service, providers are compensated for services rendered. Compensation is determined by a "usual and customary" fee. Usual and customary compensation is based on the provider's fee record as it equates to that of different providers in the region. The "usual fee" is the standard fee that is charged by the provider for a given procedure to private paying patients. Usual fees are determined by the provider and are on record with the health care plan as the provider's fee profile.

"Customary fees" for each particular procedure are set by the health care plan. The health care plan determines the customary fee as a percentile of the usual fees charged by providers in the same general area (e.g., ninetieth percentile).

Under fee-for-service programs, providers are paid the actual amount of their usual fees, if those fees fall within the range of customary fees. If the provider charges more than the customary fee, the provider will be paid only the customary fee (in essence, writing off the difference). On the other hand, if the provider charges less than the customary fee, the provider will be paid at the usual fee. Under discounted fee for service, providers receive their usual and customary fee, minus a certain discount (e.g., 25%).

Fee Allowance Schedule (Fee Schedule)

Under a fee allowance schedule, providers are compensated based on a schedule of fees for each procedure. The fee schedule is not correlated to the provider's usual and customary fees.

Relative Value Scale

Under a relative value scale, each procedure (described by a current procedural terminology [CPT] code) is assigned, by the health care plan, a relative value that indicates the "value" of the procedure. For example, the intermediate eye examination, new patient (92002) can be assigned a relative value of 1.1; whereas a comprehensive eye examination, new patient (92004) can be assigned a relative value of 1.7. Reimbursed amounts are determined by multiplying the relative value of the procedure by a predetermined negotiated number (the multiplier). If the multiplier is $30, then the reimbursement for the above relative values would be $33 for 92002 and $51 for 92004. Medicare uses a form of this

method called a resource-based relative value scale (see Chapter 26).

Capitation

Capitation is a prepayment program that pays the provider a fixed amount for each member (patient) per month. The amount paid covers all provided health care services for the member regardless of the number of visits or the associated cost of the services. If the patient is healthy and requires little service, then the provider is in a positive financial status. On the other hand, if the patient is sickly and requires many services, the provider might be in a negative financial status. It is assumed that the overall mix of members will result in a positive income status for the provider. With the capitation method, the provider assumes financial risk for the patient.

Optometrists participate in health care plans that might use any of the above compensation methods. In fact, the optometrist deals with patients who can have two kinds of insurance—vision and medical.

MEDICAL OR VISION INSURANCE

A confusing issue for many patients, and for some optometrists, is the case of a patient with separate vision and medical plans.

Vision Insurance

Coverage usually provides for basic periodic vision examinations, ophthalmic lenses, eyeglass frames, and contact lenses. Vision claim forms can request information about vision examination procedures performed, refractive diagnosis, visual acuities, lens prescription details, and frame data.

Medical Insurance

Coverage is limited to medical services and supplies. Medical necessity is needed to bill major medical plans for services and supplies rendered. A medical diagnosis has to be included on the claim form to substantiate medical necessity. Ex-

Table 25.1. Example Medical Diagnosis

Code	Description
367	Disorders of refraction and accommodation
367.2	Astigmatism
367.22	Irregular astigmatism
370	Keratitis
370.2	Superficial keratitis without conjunctivitis
370.22	Macular keratitis

Table 25.2. Sample "Includes" and "Excludes" for Diagnostic Coding

372.04	Pseudomembranous conjunctivitis
Includes	Membranous conjunctivitis
Excludes	Diphtheretic conjunctivitis (032.281)

amples of medical diagnoses include headaches, hypertensive retinopathy, blepharitis, glaucoma, and conjunctivitis.

The optometrist must first decide which plan (vision or medical) to bill for services rendered. This decision is based on the diagnosis. If the diagnosis is refractive, the vision plan, not the medical plan, should be billed. However, if there is a medical diagnosis, the medical plan should be billed. For the patient with both medical and refractive diagnoses, the reason for the patient's visit should be the determining factor in billing the appropriate plan. If the reason for the visit was medical in nature, the major medical plan should be billed. If the chief complaint for the visit was refractive in nature, the vision plan should be billed.

Vision plans lack uniformity and standardization in claim forms and submitting requirements. Most plans have their own unique claim forms with unique codes (if any) for procedures. This diversity makes it very difficult for the optometrist to process vision claims efficiently and makes office computer systems less effective in the billing process.

Medical insurance has become more standardized, and there is uniformity of claim forms, with

most major medical plans using the HCFA 1500 form. Additionally, over time various systems have been developed to improve the efficiency of handling third-party claims. These improvements include diagnostic and procedural codes.

Diagnostic Codes

To indicate diagnoses and diseases for third-party reimbursement, the *International Classification of Diseases (9th edition) Clinical Modification* (ICD-9-CM) system (Washington, DC: U.S. Department of Health and Human Services, 1995) must be used. The ICD system is required by the United States Public Health Services and the Health Care Financing Administration (Medicare and Medicaid Programs), and most medical third-party programs. Codes are published in two volumes; one provides a tabular list and the other provides an alphabetical list.

For each patient, the code should be used that is appropriate for the diagnosis, whether it is visual or medical in nature.

The number of digits for each code varies from 3 to 5. The more digits, the more specific the diagnosis. Three-digit codes are the basic subdivision of the disease classification. Four-digit codes are a subdivision of the primary three-digit codes. Five-digit codes are the most precise and specific of the subdivisions. Examples of three-, four- and five-digit vision and medical codes are provided in Table 25.1.

ICD codes and titles are all listed in bold type. "Includes" are notes that additionally clarify or give samples of the contents of the category. "Excludes," which are printed in italics, list items that are not included in this code and must be coded elsewhere. An example of "includes" and "excludes" can be found in Table 25.2.

Codes should be as specific as possible, and the five-digit category should be used whenever obtainable. If there are no further subdivisions, four- and three-digit codes can be used. "Includes" and "excludes" need to be monitored and evaluated as they relate to billing procedures. A diagnosis code should not be used if the diagnosis is uncertain or supported only by intuition or suspicion. In this case, signs or symptoms should be used to describe the condition. The practitioner should only code to the level of certainty.

Procedural Codes

The American Medical Association has published a book containing medical and visual diagnostic procedures and treatment service codes. The book is titled *Current Procedural Terminology (4th edition) (CPT-4)* (Chicago: American Medical Association, 1995). These codes are used to report to third parties the services provided to patients regarding the examination, diagnosis, treatment, and patient management plans. The CPT-4 has been adapted by HCFA for use in Medicare programs and by most other third-party programs. Examples of CPT-4 codes are provided in Table 25.3.

Format of the Terminology. CPT procedure terminology has been developed as a stand-alone description of medical procedures. Stand-alone descriptions are self-contained and ready to use.

Some of the procedures in CPT are not printed in their entirety, however. They refer to the common portion of the procedure listed in the preceding entry. For example, in Table 25.4 it can be seen that Code 92226 is not printed in its entirety and refers back to Code 92225, which is termed an "add-on" description. Add-on entries are used to conserve space.

Modifiers. A modifier provides the ability to report that a procedure or service has been altered by some specific circumstance but has not changed in its definition or code. When there is something unusual about a procedure, the appropriate modifier should be used to report the change. Modifiers are found in Appendix A of the CPT. Examples of modifiers can be found in Table 25.5.

The modifier is listed on the claim form next to the procedure code. Space is allowed to explain further unusual circumstances. An example of a procedure code with modifier is also included in Table 25.5.

Evaluation and Management Service. Evaluation and management (E/M) service codes are used to report the length and type of care provided to the patient. E/M codes are broken down into major categories that describe the location where the service was provided (e.g., practitioner's of-

Table 25.3. Example Medical Procedures Codes

Code	Procedures
99201	Office or outpatient visit for the evaluation and management of a new patient that requires three key components: a problem-focused history, a problem-focused exam, and straightforward medical decision making
92081	Visual field examination, unilateral or bilateral, with interpretation and report; limited examination (e.g., tangent screen, arc perimeter on single stimulus level automated test)

Table 25.4. Example "Add On" Procedural Code

Code	Procedure
92225	Ophthalmoscopy, extended with retinal drawing (e.g., for retinal detachment, melanoma), with interpretation and report; initial
92226	Subsequent

Table 25.5. Example Procedural Modifiers

Code	Modifier	Procedure
–	-50	Bilateral procedure
–	-51	Multiple procedure
–	-52	Reduced services
92283	-51	Color vision examination, extended, e.g., anomaloscope or equivalent (including Farnsworth-Munsell 100 Hue test and Edridge-Green color perception lantern test)

fice, hospital, nursing facility, emergency room). These categories are further broken down into subcategories (e.g., new or established patient for the office setting).

It is important to stress that these codes cannot be determined before the patient's visit, nor can they be assigned by the office staff. Only after providing the care to the patient can the practitioner determine the proper level for the service rendered. The purpose of this coding system is to accurately reflect (and identify for reimbursement)

Table 25.6. Sample E/M Codes

New patient
  99201
  99202
  99203
  99204
  99205
Established patient
  99211
  99212
  99213
  99214
  99215

Table 25.7. Types of History, Examination, and Medical Decision Making

History
  Problem focused
  Expanded problem focused
  Detailed
  Comprehensive
Examination
  Problem focused
  Expanded problem focused
  Detailed
  Comprehensive
Medical decision making
  Straightforward
  Low complexity
  Moderate complexity
  High complexity

the nature of the services the practitioner has provided the patient. The higher the level of service, the greater the reimbursement.

Most of the care provided by optometrists is in the office setting. Codes available for the office setting are divided into two subgroups: new patient or established patient. An established patient is one who has been seen in the practice within the preceding 3 years. There are five levels of codes (Table 25.6).

The selection of the proper level is based on seven components: history, examination, medical decision making, counseling, coordination of care, nature of presenting problem, and time. Of the seven components, three are particularly impor-

tant: history, examination, and medical decision making. These three key components normally determine the proper level of service provided. The CPT-4 book specifically describes these three key components and divides each into four types (Table 25.7). The CPT manual discusses the specific description and documentation requirements for each type of history, examination, and medical decision making.

Table 25.8 illustrates the key component requirements for each level of service. For a new patient, all three key components must meet or exceed the requirements for a particular level of E/M code. For an established patient (one seen in the practice within the last 3 years), two of the three key components must meet or exceed the requirements for a particular level of service. For example, the proper E/M level is 99213 if it is determined that, for an established patient, the key components are as follows:

• History—problem focused
• Examination—expanded problem focused
• Medical decision making—low complexity

These codes only cover the evaluation and management of the patient and do not include independent diagnostic and treatment procedures, if clinically indicated (e.g., visual fields—99081). Both the E/M code and the independent procedure code should be reported on the claim form, along with the proper diagnosis.

General Ophthalmologic Service Codes. In addition to the E/M codes, there are four codes that cover general ophthalmologic services:

• 92002—intermediate medical examination, new patient
• 92012—intermediate medical examination, established patient
• 92004—comprehensive medical examination, new patient
• 92014—comprehensive medical examination, established patient

Intermediate and comprehensive ophthalmologic services constitute integrated services, which do not permit medical diagnostic evaluations to be separated from the examining techniques used. Itemiza-

Table 25.8. Sample Examination Codes

Code	History	Exam	Decision Making
New patients (three components required)			
99201	Problem focused	Problem focused	Straightforward
99202	Expanded problem focused	Expanded problem focused	Straightforward
99203	Detailed	Detailed	Low complexity
99204	Comprehensive	Comprehensive	Moderate complexity
99205	Comprehensive	Comprehensive	High complexity
Established patients (two components required)*			
99211	Physical supervision only	–	–
99212	Problem focused	Problem focused	Straightforward
99213	Expanded problem focused	Expanded problem focused	Low complexity
99214	Detailed	Detailed	Moderate complexity
99215	Comprehensive	Comprehensive	High complexity

*Two of the three components must meet or exceed the requirements for a particular level of service.

tion of service components such as slit lamp examination, keratometry, ophthalmoscopy, retinoscopy, tonometry, and oculomotor evaluation are not applicable. If a complete eye examination was performed as described by these codes, the appropriate code could be used. The office examination E/M codes can be used as necessary to provide reimbursement for other levels of care.

Because the CPT codes are frequently modified, the American Medical Association annually publishes an updated book containing the newest procedure codes. Each update contains hundreds of changes, and it is important to use the most current edition. Improper coding will cause delays in reimbursement and can result in the claim being paid at a lower level.

The American Optometric Association publishes *Codes for Optometry* (St. Louis: American Optometric Association, 1995). This manual consists of four parts:

- Procedural codes (CPT-4)
- Diagnostic codes (ICD-9-CM)
- Codes for materials (HCPCS)
- Pharmaceutical codes (AHFS)

This manual reprints the appropriate information for the optometrist and displays it in an easy-to-use format. The manual is updated annually by the AOA.

COST SHARING

One aspect of third-party reimbursement is cost control through cost sharing. To achieve this goal, third-party health plans use two important concepts: deductibles and copayments.

Deductible

A deductible is a specified sum that the beneficiary must pay toward the cost of care before the benefits of the health plan go into effect. Deductible amounts can range from zero to $2,000, with $100–300 common. Deductibles might be required for each individual covered by the plan or for the family. If a patient has not paid the deductible, the provider should collect the deductible from the patient at the end of the examination. This is a complicated process, because many patients do not know whether they have paid their deductible. The provider's office will often have to call the plan to obtain this information.

Copayment

A copayment is the patient's share of cost for covered materials and services. It is usually set as a fixed

Table 25.9. Example Copayment

Procedure: Gonioscopy (90020)
  Total charge = $35.00
  Insurance coverage (80%) = $28.00
  Patient portion (20%) = $7.00

dollar amount per visit. Another term, coinsurance, is used to describe a sharing of cost when the amount is a percentage of the covered materials and services. Common major medical insurance plans are termed 80/20 plans. After the patient has met the deductible, the plan pays 80% of covered services and the patient is responsible for the remaining 20%. An example of an 80/20 payment can be found in Table 25.9.

Other cost-sharing measures include maximums and exclusions.

Maximums

Health care plans can stipulate a maximum amount paid for a given year or for a lifetime. For example, Medicare pays a set maximum for an eyeglass frame, once in a lifetime (one for each eye), for a patient with a diagnosis of pseudophakia.

Exclusions

Health plans can exclude payment for certain services and materials. Examples of exclusions include:

- Pre-existing conditions
- Cosmetic contact lenses
- Orthoptics

Individual plan provisions will have to be consulted to determine the requirements for a particular patient.

CLAIM FORM

The most widely used claim form is the HCFA-1500 (Figure 25.1), which is used in billing for medical conditions. Like most claim forms, it has two primary information sections. Patient and subscriber information is found on the top half of the form in sections 1–13. Physician information is recorded on the bottom half of the form in sections 14–33.

Sections 1–13 can be completed by insurance staff after the information has been reported by the patient on the registration form. It is important to have the patient sign line 13, regarding release of information. Information about the patient's diagnosis and treatment is confidential and can be released only with the patient's permission. The patient's signature on line 12 gives the practitioner authorization to disclose details regarding medical or vision care to the insurance company.

Item 13 provides an assignment of benefits and should be signed by the patient if the practitioner prefers to collect benefits from the insurance company directly. The patient's signature authorizes the insurance company to pay allowable benefits directly to the practitioner. If the patient does not sign box 13, the insurance payment will go directly to the patient.

If benefits are assigned to the practitioner, financial settlements of the patient's share (deductibles, copayments) of the costs are usually made at the end of the visit. If benefits are not assigned to the practitioner, financial arrangements are made for the total fee to be paid directly by the patient. When benefits are not assigned, it is as if the patient had no insurance. Then the patient pays the practitioner directly for the materials and services.

Signature on File

It is important to have patients review and sign statements authorizing release of information and payment of benefits on a patient registration form. The registration form should have wording similar to that found in boxes 12 and 13 of the HCFA-1500 form. If the patient is not available to sign an insurance claim form, it is permissible to type "signature on file," since that authorization is provided on the registration form.

Physician Information

Items 14–33 are to be completed by office personnel. Most of the boxes are self-explanatory,

APPROVED OMB-0938-0008

PLEASE
DO NOT
STAPLE
IN THIS
AREA

CARRIER

| PICA | | | | | | | **HEALTH INSURANCE CLAIM FORM** | PICA | |

| 1. MEDICARE | MEDICAID | CHAMPUS | CHAMPVA | GROUP HEALTH PLAN | FECA BLK LUNG | OTHER | 1a. INSURED'S I.D. NUMBER | (FOR PROGRAM IN ITEM 1) |

[X] (Medicare #)   (Medicaid #)   (Sponsor's SSN)   (VA File #)   (SSN or ID)   (SSN)   (ID)   12345678A

2. PATIENT'S NAME (Last Name, First Name, Middle Initial)
VISION JOSEPH A

3. PATIENT'S BIRTH DATE   MM 01 | DD 02 | YY 31   SEX   M [X]   F [ ]

4. INSURED'S NAME (Last Name, First Name, Middle Initial)

5. PATIENT'S ADDRESS (No., Street)
2020 REFRACTION LANE

6. PATIENT RELATIONSHIP TO INSURED   Self [ ] Spouse [ ] Child [ ] Other [ ]

7. INSURED'S ADDRESS (No., Street)

CITY **ANYTOWN**   STATE **MI**

8. PATIENT STATUS   Single [ ]   Married [ ]   Other [ ]

CITY   STATE

ZIP CODE **49000**   TELEPHONE (Include Area Code) **(616)5551221**

Employed [ ]   Full-Time Student [ ]   Part-Time Student [ ]

ZIP CODE   TELEPHONE (INCLUDE AREA CODE) ( )

9. OTHER INSURED'S NAME (Last Name, First Name, Middle Initial)

10. IS PATIENT'S CONDITION RELATED TO:

11. INSURED'S POLICY GROUP OR FECA NUMBER
NONE

a. OTHER INSURED'S POLICY OR GROUP NUMBER

a. EMPLOYMENT? (CURRENT OR PREVIOUS)   YES [ ]   NO [X]

a. INSURED'S DATE OF BIRTH MM | DD | YY   SEX M [ ] F [ ]

b. OTHER INSURED'S DATE OF BIRTH MM | DD | YY   SEX M [ ] F [ ]

b. AUTO ACCIDENT?   PLACE (State)   YES [ ]   NO [X]

b. EMPLOYER'S NAME OR SCHOOL NAME

c. EMPLOYER'S NAME OR SCHOOL NAME

c. OTHER ACCIDENT?   YES [ ]   NO [X]

c. INSURANCE PLAN NAME OR PROGRAM NAME

d. INSURANCE PLAN NAME OR PROGRAM NAME

10d. RESERVED FOR LOCAL USE

d. IS THERE ANOTHER HEALTH BENEFIT PLAN?   YES [ ]   NO [ ]   *If yes*, return to and complete item 9 a-d.

READ BACK OF FORM BEFORE COMPLETING & SIGNING THIS FORM.

12. PATIENT'S OR AUTHORIZED PERSON'S SIGNATURE I authorize the release of any medical or other information necessary to process this claim. I also request payment of government benefits either to myself or to the party who accepts assignment below.

SIGNED **SIGNATURE ON FILE**   DATE

13. INSURED'S OR AUTHORIZED PERSON'S SIGNATURE I authorize payment of medical benefits to the undersigned physician or supplier for services described below.

SIGNED **SIGNATURE ON FILE**

14. DATE OF CURRENT: MM | DD | YY   ILLNESS (First symptom) OR INJURY (Accident) OR PREGNANCY(LMP)

15. IF PATIENT HAS HAD SAME OR SIMILAR ILLNESS. GIVE FIRST DATE MM | DD | YY

16. DATES PATIENT UNABLE TO WORK IN CURRENT OCCUPATION FROM MM | DD | YY TO MM | DD | YY

17. NAME OF REFERRING PHYSICIAN OR OTHER SOURCE

17a. I.D. NUMBER OF REFERRING PHYSICIAN

18. HOSPITALIZATION DATES RELATED TO CURRENT SERVICES FROM MM | DD | YY TO MM | DD | YY

19. RESERVED FOR LOCAL USE

20. OUTSIDE LAB?   YES [ ] NO [ ] $ CHARGES

21. DIAGNOSIS OR NATURE OF ILLNESS OR INJURY. (RELATE ITEMS 1,2,3 OR 4 TO ITEM 24E BY LINE)
1. **373 . 02**   3. ___ . ___
2. ___ . ___   4. ___ . ___

22. MEDICAID RESUBMISSION CODE   ORIGINAL REF. NO.

23. PRIOR AUTHORIZATION NUMBER

24. A DATE(S) OF SERVICE From MM DD YY To MM DD YY	B Place of Service	C Type of Service	D PROCEDURES, SERVICES, OR SUPPLIES (Explain Unusual Circumstances) CPT/HCPCS	MODIFIER	E DIAGNOSIS CODE	F $ CHARGES	G DAYS OR UNITS	H EPSDT Family Plan	I EMG	J COB	K RESERVED FOR LOCAL USE
11 30 95 11 30 95	11		99213		1	28 00	001				013
11 30 95 11 30 95	11		92015		1	10 00	001				013

25. FEDERAL TAX I.D. NUMBER   SSN [ ] EIN [X]

26. PATIENT'S ACCOUNT NO. **531**

27. ACCEPT ASSIGNMENT? (For govt. claims, see back) YES [X]   NO [ ]

28. TOTAL CHARGE $ **38** 00

29. AMOUNT PAID $

30. BALANCE DUE $

31. SIGNATURE OF PHYSICIAN OR SUPPLIER INCLUDING DEGREES OR CREDENTIALS (I certify that the statements on the reverse apply to this bill and are made a part thereof.)
Jim Smith OD
SIGNED   DATE **12/1/95**

32. NAME AND ADDRESS OF FACILITY WHERE SERVICES WERE RENDERED (If other than home or office)

33. PHYSICIAN'S, SUPPLIER'S BILLING NAME, ADDRESS, ZIP CODE & PHONE # **6165552020**
SMITH JIM OD
455 BROOK AVE
HAPPY MI 49307
PIN#   GRP# **0E123456789**

(APPROVED BY AMA COUNCIL ON MEDICAL SERVICE 8/88)   **PLEASE PRINT OR TYPE**

FORM HCFA-1500 (12-90)
FORM OWCP-1500   FORM RRB-1500
#19423 – #29423 – Medical Arts Press
Use with Envelope #14145 (gummed) or #14146 (self-seal)

Mfd. by Medical Arts Press
Call toll-free: 1-800-328-2179

PATIENT AND INSURED INFORMATION

PHYSICIAN OR SUPPLIER INFORMATION

Figure 25.1. Sample HCFA-1500 form.

and additional instructions can be found in the provider manuals for each health plan. Line 21 requires a diagnosis listed by ICD code—carried out to two decimal points if possible. The first diagnosis listed should be chiefly responsible for the patient's visit that day. This should be followed by additional codes describing any current co-existing conditions.

Box 24D requires a (CPT) procedure or (HCPCS) material code. Box 24E should list the diagnosis (referenced by line number), that corresponds to the billing procedure or materials.

Item 24B requires a code for place of service. "Place of service" refers to the practitioner's office, hospital, nursing home, and so forth. Type of service (item 24C) refers to medical care, surgery, consultation, or other service. A sample form with completed information can be found in Figure 25.1.

PROCESSING PROCEDURES FOR CLAIMS

Because of the current environment of managed care, practitioners first need to determine if care can be provided to the patient. Many health care delivery systems use a closed network or panel of providers (e.g., HMOs and PPOs). If the practitioner is not a member of the panel, the practitioner may not provide the care. Even if the provider is a member of the panel, there still can be utilization requirements and controls, including a primary care physician as a gatekeeper who authorizes all care. The provider needs to understand the structure and organization of the health plan.

If the practitioner determines that care can be provided, several issues must still be addressed, including eligibility, patient information, processing steps, and computerization of claims.

Eligibility

The provider needs to determine if a patient is entitled to benefits under the health plan or the vision plan. A patient can be eligible for a vision examination only once every year. If it has been 11 months since the last vision examination, the plan might not pay for the visit.

It is important to verify that spouses and children are covered under the plan. If questions arise regarding eligibility, it is best to call the plan to determine who is eligible for services and materials. Most plans have authorization cards that provide a telephone number to verify coverage. It is prudent to verify coverage before substantial fees are charged because payment can be lost if there is a misunderstanding.

Patient Information

Information is needed to provide details about plan beneficiaries and the plan that supplies reimbursement. It is best to obtain patient information on a registration form (Figure 25.2). This information must be correct and complete because a claim will be rejected without proper facts. If information is incorrect, the claim will be returned for correction. Payment will be delayed, and extra work will be created.

Processing Steps

As patients schedule appointments, the receptionist should request that all insurance forms, identification cards, and benefits information be brought to the appointment. With so many different carriers and policy provisions, it is helpful to have trained staff review and explain coverage to patients.

When the patient arrives, the registration form should be completed and the patient's identification card should be reviewed to confirm coverage. It is wise to photocopy the identification card for the patient's record and for future reference.

The patient should be informed of the benefits, deductibles, and coinsurance. At the end of the visit, the patient's share of the services and material fees should be collected.

Claims should be mailed or electronically transferred to the plan at a suitable time. Unprocessed claims represent money owed to the practice. All claims should be complete and legible. A copy of the claim should be kept in a "claims pending" file for review until payment is received.

PATIENT REGISTRATION FORM

PLEASE COMPLETE THE FOLLOWING INFORMATION SO THAT YOUR VISION RECORD WILL BE COMPLETE. ALL INFORMATION IS NECESSARY.

NAME_____
    FIRST   MIDDLE   LAST

ADDRESS_____
    NUMBER AND STREET   CITY   ZIP

HOME PHONE (   )_____, WORK PHONE (   )_____

SOCIAL SECURITY NUMBER_____

BIRTHDATE_____. SEX ( ) MALE ( ) FEMALE

DRIVER'S LICENSE NUMBER_____

REFERRED BY_____

OCCUPATION_____

NAME OF EMPLOYER_____

WORK ADDRESS_____

ARE YOU COVERED BY MEDICARE?   ( ) YES   ( ) NO
ARE YOU COVERED BY Medi-Caid?   ( ) YES   ( ) NO

  ARE YOU ENROLLED IN AN HMO SUCH AS KAISER, FHP, CIGNA OR OTHERS?
                    ( ) YES   ( ) NO

VISION INSURANCE COMPANY_____

MEDICAL INSURANCE COMPANY_____

NOTIFY IN CASE OF EMERGENCY_____

RELATIONSHIP_____TELEPHONE NUMBER_____

I consent to optometric evaluation and treatment by Dr. _____

_____
                (signature)

I authorize the release of any medical information necessary to process my insurance claims. I also request payment of my insurance benefits to Dr. _____

_____
                (signature)

Figure 25.2. Sample patient registration form.

If claims have not been paid within 4 weeks, it is advisable to call the carrier to determine if a problem exists. If a claim is returned because of an error, corrections should be made and the claim should be resubmitted in a timely manner. Many carriers can deny claims if they are not submitted within a specified period.

Computerization of Claims

Many of the computer software packages for office management include the ability to complete claim forms such as the HCFA-1500. The computer templates match the claim form, and the information can automatically be transferred. It is important to enter the correct diagnosis, procedures, fees, patient insurance information, and any additional information required.

"Electronic claims submission" refers to the ability to send claims to the insurance company through telephone lines. The office's computer links with the carrier's computer through a modem, and information is downloaded to the carrier. Sending claims by modem speeds up processing time by eliminating the need to mail the claim. It also reduces errors since the data does not have to be reentered by the carrier into the computer. Payment is often faster because of the time saved in processing claims. It is anticipated that, in the future, electronic transfer might be required by some third-party payers, such as Medicare.

CONCLUSION

Health care financing is in a state of flux. The pace of change is exponential, with no sign of slowing down. All practitioners need to understand the basics of managed care and third-party reimbursement. Managed care is spreading throughout the country, and no region or area will escape. The knowledgeable practitioner will likely flourish in this environment, while the uninformed practitioner will likely struggle and perhaps not survive.

BIBLIOGRAPHY

American Medical Association. Physicians' Current Procedural Terminology (CPT-4). Chicago: American Medical Association, 1995.

American Optometric Association. Codes for Optometry. St. Louis: American Optometric Association, 1995.

American Optometric Association. Manual on Completion of Insurance Claim Forms (4th ed.) St. Louis: American Optometric Association, 1994.

American Optometric Association. An Optometrist's Guide to Managed Care. St. Louis: American Optometric Association, 1992.

Barresi B, Brooks R. Full scope optometry meets managed care. Optom Econ 1994;4(6):10–13.

Boland P. Making Managed Health Care Work, A Practical Guide to Strategies and Solutions. Gaithersburg, MD: Aspen, 1993.

Coleman D. Watch for these booby traps in managed care contracts. Optom Econ 1994;4(7):14–7.

Fischer B. Managed care in practice: Vision Services Plan of Florida. Optom Econ 1994;4(8):19–21.

Kongstvedt PR. Essentials of Managed Health Care. Gaithersburg, MD: Aspen, 1995.

Krefman A (ed). Managed care and contracting. A primer for the practicing optometrist. Optom Today 1994;(Suppl); 2(9):1–30.

Newcomb RD, Marshall EC. Public Health and Community Optometry (2nd ed). Stoneham, MA: Butterworth, 1990.

Rosenthal J, Soroka M. Managed Vision Benefits. Brookfield, WI: International Foundation of Employee Benefit Plans, 1995.

Chapter 26

Medicare and Medicaid

Roger D. Kamen, David L. Park, Thomas Sandler, and W. Howard McAlister

You can be young without money but you can't be old without it.

—Tennessee Williams
Cat on a Hot Tin Roof

The government executes and finances numerous third-party insurance plans that include optometric participation. These plans include programs such as Medicare, Medicaid, CHAMPUS, the Veterans Administration, the Department of Defense, the Public Health Service, health departments, Vocational Rehabilitation, the Developmental Disabilities Program, and Maternal, Child Health, and Crippled Children's Services. This chapter focuses on the two most commonly used programs—Medicare and Medicaid.

Although this chapter describes government as a third-party financier, it is important to understand that much overlap exists between government (or public sector) and private sector (nongovernment) programs. For example, health maintenance organizations (HMOs) are private sector programs with significant government involvement, especially with regard to grants. Medicare and Medicaid are government programs managed, in many states, by private insurance companies.

MEDICARE

The Medicare program was authorized by the U.S. Congress in 1965 as Title XVIII of the Social Security Act. Medicare originally provided hospital and medical insurance benefits to persons age 65 and older. Over the years, Medicare has increased the program to include care for people under age 65 who are blind, or disabled, or who suffer from chronic renal disease.

Medicare benefits include basic hospital insurance (Part A) and medical insurance for physicians' services (Part B). Part A is financed by universal compulsory contributions. Part B is obtainable on an elective basis. It is half-financed by the government and half-financed by premium payments from the enrollees.

Eligibility

The Social Security Administration determines who is eligible for Medicare. To be eligible for Part B, the person must be one of the following:

- 65 years old or older
- Under age 65, with permanent kidney inadequacy
- Under age 65 and permanently disabled

The Social Security Administration issues a card to all patients entitled to Medicare benefits. To determine if a patient is eligible for medical benefits (Part B), it is necessary to review the patient's Medicare card. The card identifies the Medicare recipient and contains the following details:

- Name
- Medicare health insurance claim number
- Enrollee's signature
- Date of entitlement
- Kind of benefits for which the beneficiary is entitled under the Medicare policy (Part A, Part B, or both)

It is critical to check the Medicare card at least once a year. Medicare numbers and suffixes can change according to the beneficiary's record of entitlement. Changes are particularly significant in the case of marriage or remarriage.

On claim forms, the name and health insurance claim numbers (HICNs) should be entered exactly as shown on the Medicare card. All claim forms are transmitted to one of nine host sites, where records regarding Medicare eligibility and deductible status are kept. Any mistake in entering the name and HICN on the Medicare Request for Payment form (HCFA-1500) will cause the claim to be rejected because it will not agree with the Social Security register.

Claim Submission

Medicare requires the use of the HCFA-1500 claim form (Figure 26.1) for the submission of paper claims. The claim form is available in a single sheet, two-part snapout, and a two-part computer pin-feed continuous form. Optometrists are responsible for purchasing their own claim forms, which can be obtained through the U.S. Government Printing Office or through commercial outlets. Commercial forms must contain the information required by HCFA on both the front and back of the form. The current version (12/90) has been in use since 1992. Claim forms must be printed in "drop-out red." (See Chapter 25 for information on completing the form.)

Diagnostic Codes

All Medicare providers must use the Health Care Financing Administration Common Procedure Coding System (HCPCS) Levels I, II, and III procedures codes for claim submission.

Level I codes are the procedures contained in the *Current Procedural Terminology, 4th edition* (CPT-

4), which is revised periodically (Chicago: American Medical Association, 1995) (see Chapter 25 for a description of these codes).

Level II codes are national alphanumeric codes that supplement the CPT-4 codes. These five-digit codes include services such as audiology, physical therapy, and vision care, and supplies such as drugs and durable medical equipment (including frames, lenses, contact lenses, and prosthetic devices). The codes start with a letter (A through V) and are followed by four numbers.

Level III codes are local codes assigned by the local carrier for Medicare. These codes cover procedures not included in the first two levels. The codes begin with a letter (W through Z) followed by four numbers.

Time Limits for Filing Medicare Claims

Claims must be filed by the end of the calendar year following the year in which services are provided. Services provided during the last 3 months of the calendar year are considered, for billing purposes, to be provided in the next calendar year. An example of applying the time limits is provided in Table 26.1.

Covered Services

Eye examinations by an optometrist (or physician) for the purpose of determining or changing the prescription for eyeglasses or contact lenses are not covered under Medicare. Eye examinations are covered:

- When performed in conjunction with the fitting and prescribing of postsurgical lenses when the lens of the eye has been removed (aphakia or pseudophakia). (Refractive services are excluded from coverage, even with the diagnosis of aphakia or pseudophakia.)
- When performed for a medical condition, diagnosis, sign, or symptom.

Therefore, eyeglasses or contact lenses that are required to replace a lens removed as a result of intraocular surgery or to replace congenitally missing lenses are covered benefits. Corneal bandage contact lenses are a covered benefit when used as a

PLEASE
DO NOT
STAPLE
IN THIS
AREA

CARRIER →

| | PICA | | | | | | **HEALTH INSURANCE CLAIM FORM** | | PICA | |

1. MEDICARE (Medicare #) [X] **MEDICAID** (Medicaid #) **CHAMPUS** (Sponsor's SSN) **CHAMPVA** (VA File #) **GROUP HEALTH PLAN** (SSN or ID) **FECA BLK LUNG** (SSN) **OTHER** (ID)

1a. INSURED'S I.D. NUMBER (FOR PROGRAM IN ITEM 1)
12345678A

2. PATIENT'S NAME (Last Name, First Name, Middle Initial)
Vision Joseph A

3. PATIENT'S BIRTH DATE   MM 01 DD 02 YY 31   **SEX** M [X] F [ ]

4. INSURED'S NAME (Last Name, First Name, Middle Initial)

5. PATIENT'S ADDRESS (No., Street)
2020 Refraction Lane

6. PATIENT RELATIONSHIP TO INSURED Self [ ] Spouse [ ] Child [ ] Other [ ]

7. INSURED'S ADDRESS (No., Street)

CITY Anytown   **STATE** MI

8. PATIENT STATUS Single [ ] Married [ ] Other [ ]

CITY   **STATE**

ZIP CODE 49000   **TELEPHONE (Include Area Code)** ( )

Employed [ ] Full-Time Student [ ] Part-Time Student [ ]

ZIP CODE   **TELEPHONE (INCLUDE AREA CODE)** ( )

9. OTHER INSURED'S NAME (Last Name, First Name, Middle Initial)

10. IS PATIENT'S CONDITION RELATED TO:

11. INSURED'S POLICY GROUP OR FECA NUMBER
None

a. OTHER INSURED'S POLICY OR GROUP NUMBER

a. EMPLOYMENT? (CURRENT OR PREVIOUS) YES [ ] NO [X]

a. INSURED'S DATE OF BIRTH MM DD YY   **SEX** M [ ] F [ ]

b. OTHER INSURED'S DATE OF BIRTH MM DD YY   SEX M [ ] F [ ]

b. AUTO ACCIDENT? YES [ ] NO [X]   PLACE (State)

b. EMPLOYER'S NAME OR SCHOOL NAME

c. EMPLOYER'S NAME OR SCHOOL NAME

c. OTHER ACCIDENT? YES [ ] NO [X]

c. INSURANCE PLAN NAME OR PROGRAM NAME

d. INSURANCE PLAN NAME OR PROGRAM NAME

10d. RESERVED FOR LOCAL USE

d. IS THERE ANOTHER HEALTH BENEFIT PLAN? YES [ ] NO [ ] *If yes*, return to and complete item 9 a-d.

READ BACK OF FORM BEFORE COMPLETING & SIGNING THIS FORM.
12. PATIENT'S OR AUTHORIZED PERSON'S SIGNATURE I authorize the release of any medical or other information necessary to process this claim. I also request payment of government benefits either to myself or to the party who accepts assignment below.

SIGNED Signature on File   DATE 9/1/96

13. INSURED'S OR AUTHORIZED PERSON'S SIGNATURE I authorize payment of medical benefits to the undersigned physician or supplier for services described below.

SIGNED Signature on File

14. DATE OF CURRENT: MM DD YY ◄ **ILLNESS (First symptom) OR INJURY (Accident) OR PREGNANCY(LMP)**

15. IF PATIENT HAS HAD SAME OR SIMILAR ILLNESS. GIVE FIRST DATE MM DD YY

16. DATES PATIENT UNABLE TO WORK IN CURRENT OCCUPATION FROM MM DD YY TO MM DD YY

17. NAME OF REFERRING PHYSICIAN OR OTHER SOURCE

17a. I.D. NUMBER OF REFERRING PHYSICIAN

18. HOSPITALIZATION DATES RELATED TO CURRENT SERVICES FROM MM DD YY TO MM DD YY

19. RESERVED FOR LOCAL USE

20. OUTSIDE LAB? YES [ ] NO [ ] $ CHARGES

21. DIAGNOSIS OR NATURE OF ILLNESS OR INJURY. (RELATE ITEMS 1,2,3 OR 4 TO ITEM 24E BY LINE)
1. 250 .50   3. ___ . ___
2. ___ . ___   4. ___ . ___

22. MEDICAID RESUBMISSION CODE   ORIGINAL REF. NO.

23. PRIOR AUTHORIZATION NUMBER

| 24. A. DATE(S) OF SERVICE | | | | | | B. Place of Service | C. Type of Service | D. PROCEDURES, SERVICES, OR SUPPLIES (Explain Unusual Circumstances) CPT/HCPCS   MODIFIER | E. DIAGNOSIS CODE | F. $ CHARGES | | G. DAYS OR UNITS | H. EPSDT Family Plan | I. EMG | J. COB | K. RESERVED FOR LOCAL USE |
From MM	DD	YY	To MM	DD	YY											
9	1	96	9	1	96	11	3	99245	1	175	00	001				013

25. FEDERAL TAX I.D. NUMBER SSN [ ] EIN [X]
123-45-6789

26. PATIENT'S ACCOUNT NO.
531

27. ACCEPT ASSIGNMENT? (For govt. claims, see back) YES [X] NO [ ]

28. TOTAL CHARGE $ 175 00

29. AMOUNT PAID $

30. BALANCE DUE $

31. SIGNATURE OF PHYSICIAN OR SUPPLIER INCLUDING DEGREES OR CREDENTIALS (I certify that the statements on the reverse apply to this bill and are made a part thereof.)
SIGNED John O'Dee OD   DATE 9/1/91

32. NAME AND ADDRESS OF FACILITY WHERE SERVICES WERE RENDERED (If other than home or office)

33. PHYSICIAN'S, SUPPLIER'S BILLING NAME, ADDRESS, ZIP CODE & PHONE # 616-555-2020
O'Dee John OD
2020 Vision Street
Insight MI 49000   PIN#   GRP# OE 123-45-6789

(APPROVED BY AMA COUNCIL ON MEDICAL SERVICE 8/88)   **PLEASE PRINT OR TYPE**   FORM HCFA-1500 (12-90) FORM OWCP-1500   FORM RRB-1500

PATIENT AND INSURED INFORMATION

PHYSICIAN OR SUPPLIER INFORMATION

Figure 26.1. Sample HCFA-1500 form used for billing a Medicare claim.

Table 26.1. Time Limits for Filing Medicare Claims

Date of Service	Claim Must Be Submitted By
Jan. 1, 1995, through Sept. 30, 1995	Dec. 31, 1996
Oct. 1, 1995, through Sept. 30, 1996	Dec. 31, 1997
Oct. 1, 1996, through Sept. 30, 1997	Dec. 31, 1998

moist bandage to aid corneal healing, relieve pain, reduce erosion, and improve vision.

Independent procedures are covered benefits when billed with an appropriate diagnosis. A sampling of independent procedures includes gonioscopy, extended ophthalmoscopy, external photography, retinal photography, color vision testing, contrast sensitivity testing, ultrasonography, and electrodiagnostic testing.

Claim Payment

Every Medicare carrier is charged with processing claims in accordance with Medicare regulations. No payment may be made for any items or services that are not reasonable or necessary for the diagnosis or treatment of an illness or injury.

During each calendar year a $100 deductible must be satisfied before payment can be made. Bills for services are applied toward the deductible on the basis of incurred medical expenses. The deductible is applied to the approved charge. Noncovered services do not count toward the deductible.

Expenses are allocated to the deductible in the order in which the bills are received by Medicare. Enrollees must satisfy the deductible—regardless of when during the calendar year they became eligible—before they can receive any medical benefits.

After the Part B deductible has been satisfied, Medicare reimburses 80% of the approved charge incurred during the calendar year. The remaining 20% is the responsibility of the patient, as coinsurance.

For services rendered on or after January 1, 1992, Medicare payments are based on physician payment reform (PPR). The payment methodology reform contains three major elements:

- National fee schedule—for dates of service on or after January 1, 1992, reimbursement for

physician services is based on a fee schedule. The fee schedule is based on a resource-based, relative value scale adjusted by geographic cost differences.
- Medicare volume performance standard (MVPS)—MVPS is a mechanism for limiting growth in Medicare Part B expenditures.
- Beneficiary protection—under PPR, the new limiting charge caps the amount nonparticipating physicians may bill Medicare patients above the fee schedule.

The fee schedule is a relative value scale (described in Chapter 25) that is resource-based. A relative value unit is assigned to each procedure and is based on the relative amount of provider work (time and intensity), overhead expenses, and malpractice expense for the procedure. This unit value (adjusted for geographic location) is then multiplied by a conversion factor (multiplier) to obtain the reimbursement amount.

Medicare Assignment Agreement

Under Medicare law, the physician who accepts assignment also accepts the carrier's allowable (approved) charge as the full charge. Medicare will reimburse 80% of this allowable amount if the deductible has been met. The beneficiary is responsible to the physician for the remaining 20%. The beneficiary is also responsible for any portion of the unmet deductible and the full charge for services not covered by Medicare.

For services covered under the assignment agreement, the physician cannot bill the patient the difference between the allowable amount and the actual charge. Medicare law also requires that on an assigned claim, the physician must make an effort to collect from the beneficiary any deductible amount as well as the coinsurance. Repeated, willful violations of the assignment agreement can result in fines of $2,000, up to 6 months' imprisonment, or both.

Participating or Nonparticipating Provider

Providers are either participating (par) or nonparticipating (non-par). The par provider must accept assignment for all covered services on all claims. The non-par provider can accept assignment on a claim-by-claim basis. There are incentives given to providers to become par providers. Examples of these incentives include:

- Reimbursement that is 5% higher than non-par providers
- A listing in the directory of providers
- Exemption from limiting charges
- Direct payments (reimbursement) from Medicare
- "One stop" billing for Medigap coverage

Even if the non-par provider accepts assignment, reimbursement will be based on a 5% lower fee schedule. If a non-par provider does not accept assignment, the charge for the procedure is subject to a limiting charge. This charge is the maximum amount the non-par provider is allowed to bill the patient. Currently this amount is 115% of the non-par fee schedule amount.

The Medicare carrier issues an Explanation of Medicare Benefits (EOMB) as the final step in the processing of a Medicare claim. The EOMB is sent to the beneficiary. A copy is not provided to the physician if assignment was not accepted. When assignment is accepted, the original EOMB is sent to the physician, and the beneficiary also receives a copy. If benefits cannot be paid for a claim, or if all the benefits are applied to the deductible, the EOMB will still be issued advising the beneficiary and the physician of the disposition of the claim.

The EOMB gives detailed information on the action taken on the claim. It shows the name of the physician, dates of service, amount billed, amount approved, and total payable amount. It will also provide the beneficiary with the current deductible status.

For assigned claims, Medicare uses the Remittance Notice for settlement of assigned Medicare claims. The check sent to the provider often includes payment for several patients. This helps reduce paperwork. Claims are processed on a weekly basis. If there is no reimbursable amount due on the summary statement, the statement is still issued, and it provides detailed information on every claim listed. Each claim line shows the date of service, type and place of service, procedure code, amount billed, and amount approved for payment.

MEDIGAP AND CROSSOVER CLAIMS

Medigap is a private, supplemental insurance that is used to fill the "gaps" in Medicare benefits—in particular the 20% coinsurance. Only par providers can take advantage of the single claim submission to Medicare and the Medigap company. With single-claim submission, neither the provider nor the beneficiary needs to file a secondary claim. After the Medicare carrier finishes processing the Medicare benefit, a payment record is sent to the Medigap carrier for the payment of supplemental insurance benefits.

Crossover claims involve an automated process in which Medicare sends an electronic EOMB to the supplemental insurance carrier. This service applies to both par and non-par providers. The crossover carriers have a contract (fee per claim) to receive this information for their insurees. Medicare and Medicaid crossover claims are an example of this process.

A Medicare and Medicaid crossover claim is a claim for services covered under two separate programs. Crossover claims must contain covered Medicare services provided to a Medicare patient who is also eligible under the state Medicaid program. Benefits are paid by both programs on the basis of a single claim. The claim is first submitted to the Medicare carrier and then transferred, or crossed over, to the Medicaid program.

Medicare determines the approved charge for the service, which is established if an annual deductible has been met and pays 80% of the approved charge. Medicaid considers payment of any unmet deductible and of the remaining 20% of the approved charge.

Medicare and Medicaid crossover claims must clearly identify that the patient is covered by Medicaid in order for the claim to be crossed over. Many claims do not cross over because the provider does not indicate that the patient is covered under the Medicaid program. The patient should be identified on the HCFA-1500 form as covered by Medicaid, and a copy of the Medicaid identification card, proof of eligibility label, or eligibility number should be included (Figure 26.2).

For claims to cross over, the provider must accept assignment and the assignment must be

APPROVED OMB-0938-0008

HEALTH INSURANCE CLAIM FORM

PLEASE DO NOT STAPLE IN THIS AREA

CARRIER

PICA | | | PICA | | |

1. MEDICARE	MEDICAID	CHAMPUS	CHAMPVA	GROUP HEALTH PLAN	FECA BLK LUNG	OTHER	1a. INSURED'S I.D. NUMBER (FOR PROGRAM IN ITEM 1)
[X] (Medicare #)	(Medicaid #)	(Sponsor's SSN)	(VA File #)	(SSN or ID)	(SSN)	(ID)	12345678A

2. PATIENT'S NAME (Last Name, First Name, Middle Initial)	3. PATIENT'S BIRTH DATE		SEX	4. INSURED'S NAME (Last Name, First Name, Middle Initial)
Vision Joseph A	MM 01	DD 02 YY 31	M [X] F	

5. PATIENT'S ADDRESS (No., Street)	6. PATIENT RELATIONSHIP TO INSURED	7. INSURED'S ADDRESS (No., Street)
2020 Refraction Lane	Self [ ] Spouse [ ] Child [ ] Other [ ]	

CITY	STATE	8. PATIENT STATUS	CITY	STATE
Anytown	MI	Single [ ] Married [ ] Other [ ]		

ZIP CODE	TELEPHONE (Include Area Code)		ZIP CODE	TELEPHONE (INCLUDE AREA CODE)
49000	(616) 555-1212	Employed [ ] Full-Time Student [ ] Part-Time Student [ ]		( )

9. OTHER INSURED'S NAME (Last Name, First Name, Middle Initial)	10. IS PATIENT'S CONDITION RELATED TO:	11. INSURED'S POLICY GROUP OR FECA NUMBER
		None

a. OTHER INSURED'S POLICY OR GROUP NUMBER	a. EMPLOYMENT? (CURRENT OR PREVIOUS)	a. INSURED'S DATE OF BIRTH	SEX
Medicaid 45678910	[ ] YES [X] NO	MM DD YY	M [ ] F [ ]

b. OTHER INSURED'S DATE OF BIRTH	SEX	b. AUTO ACCIDENT? PLACE (State)	b. EMPLOYER'S NAME OR SCHOOL NAME
MM DD YY	M [ ] F [ ]	[ ] YES [X] NO	

c. EMPLOYER'S NAME OR SCHOOL NAME	c. OTHER ACCIDENT?	c. INSURANCE PLAN NAME OR PROGRAM NAME
	[ ] YES [X] NO	

d. INSURANCE PLAN NAME OR PROGRAM NAME	10d. RESERVED FOR LOCAL USE	d. IS THERE ANOTHER HEALTH BENEFIT PLAN?
	MCD	[ ] YES [ ] NO If yes, return to and complete item 9 a-d.

READ BACK OF FORM BEFORE COMPLETING & SIGNING THIS FORM.

12. PATIENT'S OR AUTHORIZED PERSON'S SIGNATURE I authorize the release of any medical or other information necessary to process this claim. I also request payment of government benefits either to myself or to the party who accepts assignment below.

SIGNED Signature of File   DATE 9/1/96

13. INSURED'S OR AUTHORIZED PERSON'S SIGNATURE I authorize payment of medical benefits to the undersigned physician or supplier for services described below.

SIGNED Signature on File

14. DATE OF CURRENT: ILLNESS (First symptom) OR INJURY (Accident) OR PREGNANCY(LMP) MM DD YY	15. IF PATIENT HAS HAD SAME OR SIMILAR ILLNESS. GIVE FIRST DATE MM DD YY	16. DATES PATIENT UNABLE TO WORK IN CURRENT OCCUPATION MM DD YY MM DD YY FROM TO

17. NAME OF REFERRING PHYSICIAN OR OTHER SOURCE	17a. I.D. NUMBER OF REFERRING PHYSICIAN	18. HOSPITALIZATION DATES RELATED TO CURRENT SERVICES MM DD YY MM DD YY FROM TO

19. RESERVED FOR LOCAL USE	20. OUTSIDE LAB? $ CHARGES [ ] YES [ ] NO

21. DIAGNOSIS OR NATURE OF ILLNESS OR INJURY. (RELATE ITEMS 1,2,3 OR 4 TO ITEM 24E BY LINE)

1. 373 . 02   3. ___ . ___

2. ___ . ___   4. ___ . ___

22. MEDICAID RESUBMISSION CODE ORIGINAL REF. NO.

23. PRIOR AUTHORIZATION NUMBER

24. A. DATE(S) OF SERVICE						B. Place of Service	C. Type of Service	D. PROCEDURES, SERVICES, OR SUPPLIES (Explain Unusual Circumstances) CPT/HCPCS MODIFIER	E. DIAGNOSIS CODE	F. $ CHARGES		G. DAYS OR UNITS	H. EPSDT Family Plan	I. EMG	J. COB	K. RESERVED FOR LOCAL USE
From MM	DD	YY	To MM	DD	YY											
9	1	96	9	1	96	11		99213	1	28	00	001				013
9	1	96	9	1	96	11		92015	1	10	00	001				013

25. FEDERAL TAX I.D. NUMBER SSN EIN	26. PATIENT'S ACCOUNT NO.	27. ACCEPT ASSIGNMENT? (For govt. claims, see back)	28. TOTAL CHARGE	29. AMOUNT PAID	30. BALANCE DUE
123-45-6789 [ ] [X]	531	[X] YES [ ] NO	$ 38 00	$	$

31. SIGNATURE OF PHYSICIAN OR SUPPLIER INCLUDING DEGREES OR CREDENTIALS (I certify that the statements on the reverse apply to this bill and are made a part thereof.)	32. NAME AND ADDRESS OF FACILITY WHERE SERVICES WERE RENDERED (If other than home or office)	33. PHYSICIAN'S, SUPPLIER'S BILLING NAME, ADDRESS, ZIP CODE & PHONE # 616-555-2020
SIGNED John O'Dee OD DATE 9/1/96		O'Dee John OD 2020 Vision Street Insight MI 49000 OE 123-45-6789 PIN# GRP#

(APPROVED BY AMA COUNCIL ON MEDICAL SERVICE 8/88)

PLEASE PRINT OR TYPE

FORM HCFA-1500 (12-90)
FORM OWCP-1500   FORM RRB-1500
#19423 – #29423 – Medical Arts Press
Use with Envelope #14145 (gummed) or #14146 (self-seal)

Mfd. by Medical Arts Press
Call toll-free: 1-800-328-2179

PATIENT AND INSURED INFORMATION

PHYSICIAN OR SUPPLIER INFORMATION

Figure 26.2. Sample HCFA-1500 form used for billing a crossover claim.

checked on the claim form. The claim must include positive identification of the patient's Medicaid eligibility. The claim must have paid at least one covered item or must have applied at least one covered item on the claim to the patient's deductible.

Medicare and Medicaid crossover claims should be submitted to the Medicare carrier on the customary HCFA-1500 claim form. Separate billing to the Medicare carrier and to the Medicaid carrier is required when services included on the crossover claim do not automatically transfer for payment. For example, dual billing requirements for eyewear might be required.

Services that are denied or not covered under Medicare, but that are Medicaid benefits, will not automatically cross over. These services can be billed to the Medicaid program. For example, eyeglasses for a patient who has not had cataract surgery is a noncovered service under Medicare. If the patient is eligible for Medicaid, the eyeglasses should be billed to the Medicaid program. If the provider did not know that the patient was eligible for Medicaid at the time of Medicare billing, the billing will not cross over. The Medicare EOMB should be attached to a Medicaid form to bill for deductible and coinsurance amounts that did not cross over.

Services and supplies not covered by Medicare, but payable by Medicaid, should be billed separately to the Medicaid program, indicating they are not Medicare-covered services. These services can be billed directly to the Medicaid program.

MEDICARE AND MANAGED CARE

Managed care is expanding into the Medicare program because the federal government hopes to control the high cost of health care for Medicare patients. The Tax Equity and Fiscal Responsibility Act of 1982 (TEFRA), implemented in 1985, provided the means for managed care to become involved with Medicare. Since then, other laws have strengthened the ties between managed care organizations and Medicare.

Currently there are three basic types of managed care contracts with the government for Medicare: risk contracts, cost contracts, and Medicare demonstration programs.

Risk Contracts

Federally qualified HMOs and competition medical plans (CMPs) contract with Medicare on a prepaid basis to provide covered services to eligible patients under risk contracts.

Cost Contracts

Federally qualified HMOs and health care prepayment plans (HCPPs) contract with Medicare to provide covered services on a cost recovery basis. This contract is less advantageous to Medicare than risk contracts.

Medicare Demonstration Programs

Currently, there are two Medicare demonstration programs:

- Medicare insured group (MIG)—an entity (corporation or union) contracts with Medicare to provide both the Medicare benefits and supplemental coverage for the beneficiary.
- Medicare select—Medicare supplemental insurance carriers are allowed to offer a preferred provider organization (PPO) for basic Medicare coverage and supplemental benefits.

All of these programs are optional for the Medicare beneficiary. However, there are some advantages for patients to forego the fee-for-service Medicare plan in favor of these managed care plans. Possible incentives include the waiving of the 20% coinsurance and the use of additional benefits not normally covered by Medicare (e.g., prescription drugs).

FRAUD AND ABUSE

Abuse refers to practices by Medicare providers that are not consistent with accepted sound medical, business, or fiscal practices. Examples include:

- Excessive charges for services or supplies
- Claims for services that are not medically necessary

• Breach of assignment agreements
• Exceeding the limiting charges
• Submission of bills to Medicare instead of to the primary insurer
• Routine waiver of copayment and deductible

Fraud is an intentional deception by the provider that results in some unauthorized benefit to the provider. Examples include:

• Billing for services not provided
• Altering claim forms to obtain a higher payment amount
• Soliciting, offering, or receiving a kickback
• Claims for noncovered services billed as covered services

The Medicare carrier is responsible for identifying and investigating incidents of suspected fraud or abuse. These cases can then be referred to the Office of the Inspector General for further investigation and possible criminal, civil, or administrative sanctions.

MEDICAID

Medicaid is a joint federal-state program that provides funding of health care for the poor. Title XIX, an amendment of the Social Security Act known as Medicaid, became effective January 1, 1966. Although Medicaid operates under federal guidelines, it is administered by individual states. Funding is provided by both federal and state governments.

Each state develops a single comprehensive medical care program. Twenty-one services are permissible under the federal act. States are given broad authority in the determination of eligibility requirements and covered services, but federal guidelines require the inclusion of the following seven services in any plan:

• Inpatient hospital services
• Outpatient hospital services
• Laboratory and x-ray services
• Skilled nursing home services
• Physician's services
• Home health services
• Early and periodic screening, diagnosis, and treatment (EPSDT)

The other services are optional and can be included if the state desires. Vision care is an optional service. Nevertheless, a 1992 survey conducted by the American Optometric Association found that optometrists were used to provide periodic vision examinations to Medicaid-eligible individuals in all states but that significant variations existed among the states in covered services. The survey reported that:

• In 11 states, the approval of gatekeepers or prior approval from the Medicaid carrier is needed before contact lenses, low vision therapy, and vision therapy can be provided.
• In 13 states, contact lenses, low vision devices, and vision therapy cannot be provided.
• In 12 states, spectacles cannot be provided to adults.
• Significant limits exist in all states with respect to spectacle lenses and frames. Restrictions include the cost of ophthalmic materials, the dioptric changes in prescriptions needed before eyewear can be changed, and the limited availability of frame styles.
• EPSDT screenings are typically performed by optometrists or nurses. There are only three states where physicians are used for vision screenings.
• Reimbursement in the vast majority of states is based on a fixed fee schedule. CPT-4 codes are used in all but nine of the states.

The screenings, required by EPSDT for eligible individuals under age 21, must include vision testing. If vision deficits are discovered during the screening, the patient must be referred for diagnosis and treatment, at Medicaid's expense. In this manner eye examinations, eye appliances, visual therapy, and other visual treatments can be covered in a state that does not offer vision care services.

Billing Information

Because of the great variance that exists from state to state, it is not possible to address the issue of billing in any detail. The 1992 AOA survey found that fees for vision examinations under Medicaid ranged from $16 to $55. Individual state vision care provider manuals must be consulted for information on billing.

MEDICAID AND MANAGED CARE

Medicaid program costs have significantly increased for the state and federal governments over the past few decades. The states and HCFA are encouraging managed care organizations to become involved with Medicaid in the hope that costs can be controlled. Currently three plans are available:

- Risk contracts—federally qualified or state-qualified HMOs contract with the state on a prepaid basis for providing covered services to eligible patients.
- Prepaid health plans (PHPs)—a PHP is an organization that contracts with the state to provide care for covered services on a risk and noncomprehensive basis.
- Primary care case management plans (PC-CMPs)—a PCCMP contracts with the state to provide services on a fee-for-service basis, with an additional fee for case management.

There is a wide variety of managed care plans available, and individual states will have to be surveyed to obtain information on the services provided.

CONCLUSION

Medicare and Medicaid are the two major federal third-party plans. Optometrists are intimately in-volved in both programs. An understanding of these programs is essential to a practitioner's financial and professional well-being. Because managed care is becoming more pervasive in these programs, optometrists need to remain vigilant about changes in eligibility and reimbursement.

BIBLIOGRAPHY

Allergan, Inc. Pathways in Optometry. Irvine, CA: Allergan, 1994.

American Optometric Association. An Optometrist's Guide to Managed Care. St. Louis: American Optometric Association, 1992.

American Optometric Association. Codes for Optometry. St. Louis: American Optometric Association, 1995.

American Optometric Association. Manual on Completion of Insurance Claim Forms (4th ed). St. Louis: American Optometric Association, 1994.

Boland P. Making Managed Health Care Work, A Practical Guide to Strategies and Solutions. Gaithersburg, MD: Aspen, 1993.

Kongstvedt PR. Essentials of Managed Health Care. Gaithersburg, MD: Aspen, 1995.

Newcomb RD, Marshall EC. Public Health and Community Optometry (2nd ed). Stoneham, MA: Butterworth, 1990.

Physician's Current Procedural Terminology (4th ed) (CPT-4). Chicago: American Medical Association, 1995.

Vision Service Plan. Vision Service Plan—Doctor's Procedure Manual. Rancho Cordova, CA: Vision Service Plan, 1995.

Chapter 27

Tax Reporting

John G. Classé

*Laws are like cobwebs, which may catch small flies
but let wasps and hornets break through.*
—Jonathan Swift
A Critical Essay Upon the Faculties of the Mind

One of the inviolable obligations of the practice of optometry is the payment of taxes to federal and state government. Taxes for income must be paid to the Social Security Administration and, in many states, to the unemployment compensation system. In some respects, this system is two-tiered, requiring payment to federal and state government, and the tax reporting itself is periodic, demanding quarterly and annual payments from the practitioner. This chapter clarifies these obligations and describes the applicable tax deadlines that must be met to satisfy reporting requirements.

This discussion considers the tax reporting obligations of self-employed practitioners in private practice. Optometrists who serve as independent contractors, however, are subject to these same requirements. Only employees do not have these obligations, since the withholding of taxes and the payment of these taxes are the responsibility of the employer. At the conclusion of the tax year, the employee receives a W-2 form describing the withholding of income for federal and state income taxes, Social Security taxes, and county or local taxes, if applicable.

The most important tax reporting requirements are for income, Social Security, and unemployment compensation. These obligations, which are summarized in Table 27.1, are described in terms of current reporting requirements. Tax counsel should always be consulted when preparing to report and pay taxes, for tax law is among the most ephemeral legislation, and changes are common.

BASIC REQUIREMENTS

Before a self-employed practitioner begins optometric practice, there are several important steps that must be taken. These depend, in part, on the type of business organization being used—individual proprietorship, partnership, limited liability company, or professional association/corporation—and on state requirements for the initiation of a new business. For the purpose of tax reporting, it is necessary for the practitioner to secure a federal tax identification number, which will be used for the payment of federal and state business income taxes. This number can be obtained by completing Form SS-4, Application for Employer Identification Number, and submitting it to the Internal Revenue Service (IRS). The employer identification number is used only for the reporting of business income. Any business tax return or reporting schedule should contain the employer identification number.

Table 27.1. Federal Income Tax Reporting

You may be liable for	If you are	Use form	Due on or before
Income tax	Sole proprietor	Schedule C (Form 1040)	Same day as Form 1040
Income tax	Individual who is a partner or S corporation shareholder	1040	15th day of 4th month after end of tax year
Income tax	Corporation	1120 or 1120-A	15th day of 3rd month after end of tax year
Income tax	S corporation	1120S	15th day of 3rd month after end of tax year
Self-employment tax	Sole proprietor, or individual who is a partner	Schedule SE (Form 1040)	Same day as Form 1040
Estimated tax	Sole proprietor or individual who is a partner or S corporation shareholder	1040-ES	15th day of 4th, 6th, and 9th months of tax year, and 15th day of 1st month after the end of tax year
Estimated tax	Corporation	1120-W	15th day of 4th, 6th, 9th, and 12th month of tax year
Annual return of income	Partnership	1065	15th day of 4th month after end of tax year
Social Security (FICA) tax and the withholding of income tax	Sole proprietor, corporation	941	4-30, 7-31, 10-31, and 1-31
	S corporation, or partnership	8109 (to make deposits)	—
Providing information on Social Security (FICA) tax and the withholding of income tax	Sole proprietor, corporation	W-2 (to employee)	1-31
	S corporation or partnership	W-2 and W-3 (to the Social Security Administration)	Last day of February
Federal unemployment (FUTA) tax	Sole proprietor, corporation	940	1-31, 4-30, 7-31, 10-31, and 1-31, but only if the liability for unpaid tax is more than $100
	S corporation, or partnership	8109 (to make deposits)	
Information returns	Sole proprietor, corporation, S corporation, or partnership transactions with other persons	1099 (to the recipient by 1-31)	For payments to nonemployees and to the IRS by 2-28

Source: Internal Revenue Service. Tax Guide for Small Businesses. Washington, DC: US Government Printing Office, 1995.

Sole Proprietorship

Tax reporting for an individual proprietor is the most straightforward for any type of business organization. IRS Form 1040 is used for reporting income and calculating taxes (Figure 27.1). If an optometrist is in practice as an individual proprietor, business income and allowable deductions are computed on a separate form (Schedule C). The business profit or loss calculated on this schedule is entered on Form 1040 and used for the determination of the optometrist's income tax.

Partnership

If an optometrist is in partnership, the partnership must report its income and the distributive share of profit or loss received by the partners on a separate tax return (Form 1065). The profit or loss received

Form **1040**   Department of the Treasury—Internal Revenue Service

U.S. Individual Income Tax Return 19**94** (5)   IRS Use Only—Do not write or staple in this space.

For the year Jan. 1–Dec. 31, 1994, or other tax year beginning _____, 1994, ending _____, 19___   OMB No. 1545-0074

Label
(See instructions on page 12.)

Use the IRS label. Otherwise, please print or type.

L A B E L   H E R E

Your first name and initial   Last name
John G   O'Dee

If a joint return, spouse's first name and initial   Last name
June B   O'Dee

Home address (number and street). If you have a P.O. box, see page 12.   Apt. no.
2020 Lazy Lane

City, town or post office, state, and ZIP code. If you have a foreign address, see page 12.
Anytown   AL   12345

Your social security number
123 : 45 : 6789

Spouse's social security number
987 : 65 : 4321

For Privacy Act and Paperwork Reduction Act Notice, see page 4.

Presidential Election Campaign (See page 12.)

	Yes	No	Note: *Checking "Yes" will not change your tax or reduce your refund.*
Do you want $3 to go to this fund?	✔		
If a joint return, does your spouse want $3 to go to this fund?	✔		

Filing Status
(See page 12.)

Check only one box.

1 ☐ Single
2 ✔ Married filing joint return (even if only one had income)
3 ☐ Married filing separate return. Enter spouse's social security no. above and full name here. ▶ _____
4 ☐ Head of household (with qualifying person). (See page 13.) If the qualifying person is a child but not your dependent, enter this child's name here. ▶ _____
5 ☐ Qualifying widow(er) with dependent child (year spouse died ▶ 19___). (See page 13.)

Exemptions
(See page 13.)

If more than six dependents, see page 14.

6a ✔ **Yourself.** If your parent (or someone else) can claim you as a dependent on his or her tax return, **do not** check box 6a. But be sure to check the box on line 33b on page 2.
b ✔ **Spouse**

c	**Dependents:** (1) Name (first, initial, and last name)	(2) Check if under age 1	(3) If age 1 or older, dependent's social security number	(4) Dependent's relationship to you	(5) No. of months lived in your home in 1994
	Brad W. O'Dee	✔		child	1

No. of boxes checked on 6a and 6b   **2**

No. of your children on 6c who:
• lived with you   **1**
• didn't live with you due to divorce or separation (see page 14)
Dependents on 6c not entered above

d If your child didn't live with you but is claimed as your dependent under a pre-1985 agreement, check here ▶ ☐
e Total number of exemptions claimed

Add numbers entered on lines above ▶   **3**

Income

Attach Copy B of your Forms W-2, W-2G, and 1099-R here.

If you did not get a W-2, see page 15.

Enclose, but do not attach, any payment with your return.

7	Wages, salaries, tips, etc. Attach Form(s) W-2	7	3,700
8a	**Taxable** interest income (see page 15). Attach Schedule B if over $400	8a	100
b	**Tax-exempt** interest (see page 16). DON'T include on line 8a	8b	
9	Dividend income. Attach Schedule B if over $400	9	
10	Taxable refunds, credits, or offsets of state and local income taxes (see page 16)	10	
11	Alimony received	11	
12	Business income or (loss). Attach Schedule C or C-EZ	12	41,020
13	Capital gain or (loss). If required, attach Schedule D (see page 16)	13	
14	Other gains or (losses). Attach Form 4797	14	
15a	Total IRA distributions. 15a ___ b Taxable amount (see page 17)	15b	
16a	Total pensions and annuities 16a ___ b Taxable amount (see page 17)	16b	
17	Rental real estate, royalties, partnerships, S corporations, trusts, etc. Attach Schedule E	17	
18	Farm income or (loss). Attach Schedule F	18	
19	Unemployment compensation (see page 18)	19	
20a	Social security benefits 20a ___ b Taxable amount (see page 18)	20b	
21	Other income. List type and amount—see page 18 ___	21	
22	Add the amounts in the far right column for lines 7 through 21. This is your **total income** ▶	22	44,820

Adjustments to Income

Caution: See instructions . . ▶

23a	Your IRA deduction (see page 19)	23a	2,000		
b	Spouse's IRA deduction (see page 19)	23b			
24	Moving expenses. Attach Form 3903 or 3903-F	24			
25	One-half of self-employment tax	25	2,898		
26	Self-employed health insurance deduction (see page 21)	26	300		
27	Keogh retirement plan and self-employed SEP deduction	27			
28	Penalty on early withdrawal of savings	28			
29	Alimony paid. Recipient's SSN ▶ ___	29			
30	Add lines 23a through 29. These are your **total adjustments** ▶			30	

Adjusted Gross Income

31	Subtract line 30 from line 22. This is your **adjusted gross income**. If less than $25,296 and a child lived with you (less than $9,000 if a child didn't live with you), see "Earned Income Credit" on page 27 ▶	31	39,622

Cat. No. 11320B   Form **1040** (1994)

Figure 27.1. Sample Form 1040.

Form 1040 (1994)   Page **2**

Tax Computation	32	Amount from line 31 (adjusted gross income)	**32** 39,622

33a Check if: ☐ **You** were 65 or older, ☐ Blind; ☐ **Spouse** was 65 or older, ☐ Blind. ☑
Add the number of boxes checked above and enter the total here . . . . ▶ **33a**

b If your parent (or someone else) can claim you as a dependent, check here . ▶ **33b** ☐

(See page 23.)

c If you are married filing separately and your spouse itemizes deductions or you are a dual-status alien, see page 23 and check here . . . . ▶ **33c** ☐

34 Enter the larger of your:
> **Itemized deductions** from Schedule A, line 29, **OR**
> **Standard deduction** shown below for your filing status. **But if you checked any box on line 33a or b,** go to page 23 to find your standard deduction. If you checked **box 33c,** your standard deduction is zero.
> • Single—$3,800   • Head of household—$5,600
> • Married filing jointly or Qualifying widow(er)—$6,350
> • Married filing separately—$3,175

34 6,350

35 Subtract line 34 from line 32 . . . . **35** 33,272

If you want the IRS to figure your tax, see page 24.

36 If line 32 is $83,850 or less, multiply $2,450 by the total number of exemptions claimed on line 6e. If line 32 is over $83,850, see the worksheet on page 24 for the amount to enter . **36** 7,350

37 **Taxable income.** Subtract line 36 from line 35. If line 36 is more than line 35, enter -0- **37** 25,922

38 Tax. Check if from **a** ☑ Tax Table, **b** ☐ Tax Rate Schedules, **c** ☐ Capital Gain Tax Worksheet, or **d** ☐ Form 8615 (see page 24). Amount from Form(s) 8814 ▶ **e** _____ **38** 3,889

39 Additional taxes. Check if from **a** ☐ Form 4970 **b** ☐ Form 4972 . . . . . **39**

40 Add lines 38 and 39 . . . . ▶ **40** 3,889

Credits

(See page 24.)

41 Credit for child and dependent care expenses. Attach Form 2441 | **41**
42 Credit for the elderly or the disabled. Attach Schedule R . | **42**
43 Foreign tax credit. Attach Form 1116 | **43**
44 Other credits (see page 25). Check if from **a** ☐ Form 3800
b ☐ Form 8396 **c** ☐ Form 8801 **d** ☐ Form (specify) _____ | **44**

45 Add lines 41 through 44 . . . . **45** ∅

46 Subtract line 45 from line 40. If line 45 is more than line 40, enter -0- . . . . . ▶ **46** 3,889

Other Taxes

(See page 25.)

47 Self-employment tax. Attach Schedule SE **47** 5,796
48 Alternative minimum tax. Attach Form 6251 . . . . **48**
49 Recapture taxes. Check if from **a** ☐ Form 4255 **b** ☐ Form 8611 **c** ☐ Form 8828 . **49**
50 Social security and Medicare tax on tip income not reported to employer. Attach Form 4137 **50**
51 Tax on qualified retirement plans, including IRAs. If required, attach Form 5329 . . **51**
52 Advance earned income credit payments from Form W-2 . . . . **52**
53 Add lines 46 through 52. This is your **total tax** . . . . ▶ **53** 9,685

Payments

Attach Forms W-2, W-2G, and 1099-R on the front.

54 Federal income tax withheld. If any is from Form(s) 1099, check ▶ ☐ | **54** 9,000
55 1994 estimated tax payments and amount applied from 1993 return . | **55**
56 **Earned income credit.** If required, attach Schedule EIC (see page 27). Nontaxable earned income: amount ▶ _____ and type ▶ .... | **56**
57 Amount paid with Form 4868 (extension request) . . . . | **57**
58 Excess social security and RRTA tax withheld (see page 32) | **58**
59 Other payments. Check if from **a** ☐ Form 2439 **b** ☐ Form 4136 | **59**

60 Add lines 54 through 59. These are your **total payments** . . . . ▶ **60** 9,000

Refund or Amount You Owe

61 If line 60 is more than line 53, subtract line 53 from line 60. This is the amount you **OVERPAID**. ▶ **61**
62 Amount of line 61 you want **REFUNDED TO YOU**. . . . . ▶ **62**
63 Amount of line 61 you want **APPLIED TO YOUR 1995 ESTIMATED TAX** ▶ **63**
64 If line 53 is more than line 60, subtract line 60 from line 53. This is the **AMOUNT YOU OWE**. For details on how to pay, including what to write on your payment, see page 32 . . **64** 685
65 Estimated tax penalty (see page 33). Also include on line 64 | **65**

Sign Here

Keep a copy of this return for your records.

Under penalties of perjury, I declare that I have examined this return and accompanying schedules and statements, and to the best of my knowledge and belief, they are true, correct, and complete. Declaration of preparer (other than taxpayer) is based on all information of which preparer has any knowledge.

Your signature ▶ _O'Dee_   Date _Apr 15, 1995_   Your occupation _Optometrist_

Spouse's signature. If a joint return, BOTH must sign. ▶ _June O'Dee_   Date _April 15, 1995_   Spouse's occupation

Paid Preparer's Use Only

Preparer's signature ▶ _____ Date _____ Check if self-employed ☐   Preparer's social security no. _____

Firm's name (or yours if self-employed) and address ▶ _____ E.I. No. _____ ZIP code _____

Figure 27.1. (continued)

by the partners from the partnership is reported on their individual Form 1040. Income tax is not paid by the partnership, only by the partners, who are taxed on the profit or loss they receive. Most limited liability companies are partnerships and thus file Form 1065.

Professional Association or Corporation

If an optometrist is a shareholder in a professional association or corporation (PA or PC), the association or corporation is regarded as a separate, tax-paying entity that must report all business income and claim all business deductions on its own tax form (Form 1120). The optometrist-shareholder is also the employee of the association or corporation, which withholds the optometrist's income tax and issues the optometrist a W-2 form at the conclusion of the tax year, just as with any other employee. The optometrist reports this income on Form 1040, claims allowable personal adjustments, exemptions, or deductions, and calculates the additional tax payment or refund. With a professional association or corporation, therefore, the association or corporation and the optometrist can pay income taxes to the federal government.

Because of the complexity of these various reporting requirements, and because the most common type of business organization used by optometrists is the individual proprietorship, the tax reporting described in this chapter emphasizes the obligations of an individual proprietor.

INCOME TAX REPORTING

Federal income tax reporting for an individual proprietor requires quarterly payments to the federal government. Payments must be made for the optometrist's income and for the income of employees. To determine the appropriate withholding of taxes, the optometrist must consult IRS publication 15, Circular E, Employer's Tax Guide. This publication provides guidelines and tables that can be used to determine the amount of withholding to be forwarded to an authorized federal bank. The deadlines for payment of these taxes are—for practitioners on a calendar year—April 15, June 15, September 15, and January 15 (see Table 27.1). At each quarterly payment, the optometrist must submit the proper amount of income taxes for employer and employees. A stiff penalty results if there is failure to make payment or submission of an improper payment. Thus, this system obligates the optometrist to forward income taxes to the federal government every few months, rather than sending the entire sum at the conclusion of the tax year.

The forms that are used for income tax reporting are Form 1040-ES, Estimated Tax for Individuals, which describes the estimated income tax for the self-employed optometrist, and Form 941, Employer's Quarterly Tax Return, which is used to describe the income tax withholding for employees (Figure 27.2).

These payments are estimates of the annual income tax. At the conclusion of the tax year, the optometrist is obligated to calculate the exact amount of income tax owed. The optometrist's business income and any necessary and ordinary business deductions are described on Schedule C (Figure 27.3), and the profit or loss determined is then entered on Form 1040 (see line 12, Figure 27.1). After adjustments, exemptions, and deductions are calculated and subtracted, the income tax is determined. The estimated income taxes that were paid quarterly are then subtracted from the income tax owed, and, if the result is less than the amount owed, an additional payment must be made to the IRS. If the taxes paid exceed the amount actually owed, the optometrist receives a refund.

State business income tax for individual proprietors is usually determined by the profit or loss calculated on Schedule C. The optometrist lists the profit or loss on the state income tax return, computes the allowable adjustments, exemptions, and deductions, and determines the tax due. From this amount, the optometrist can usually subtract the quarterly estimated taxes paid by the optometrist to the federal government. If payment is less than the income tax owed, additional payment must be made; if it is less, a refund can be collected.

The payment of income tax is intimately connected to the payment of Social Security taxes, which must be forwarded to the federal government in much the same manner as income taxes.

Form **941**		**Employer's Quarterly Federal Tax Return**		
(Rev. April 1994) Department of the Treasury Internal Revenue Service	4141	▶ See separate instructions for information on completing this return. Please type or print.		

Enter state code for state in which deposits made . ▶ ☐ (see page 2 of instructions).

Name (as distinguished from trade name): **John G O'Dee**

Trade name, if any

Address (number and street): **2020 Vision St**

Insight, AL 12345

Date quarter ended: **Dec 31, 1994**

Employer identification number: **098765432**

City, state, and ZIP code

OMB No. 1545-0029

T	
FF	
FD	
FP	
I	
T	

If address is different from prior return, check here ▶ ☐   IRS Use

1 1 1 1 1 1 1 1 1 1   2   3 3 3 3 3 3   4 4 4

5 5 5   6   7   8 8 8 8 8   9 9 9   10 10 10 10 10 10 10 10 10 10

If you do not have to file returns in the future, check here ▶ ☐   and enter date final wages paid ▶

If you are a seasonal employer, see **Seasonal employers** on page 2 and check here (see instructions) ▶ ☐

1	Number of employees (except household) employed in the pay period that includes March 12th ▶			*1*
2	Total wages and tips subject to withholding, plus other compensation		2	*8,000*
3	Total income tax withheld from wages, tips, and sick pay		3	*810*
4	Adjustment of withheld income tax for preceding quarters of calendar year		4	
5	Adjusted total of income tax withheld (line 3 as adjusted by line 4—see instructions) .		5	*810*
6a	Taxable social security wages	$ *8,000*	× 12.4% (.124) =	6a	*992*
b	Taxable social security tips	$	× 12.4% (.124) =	6b	
7	Taxable Medicare wages and tips	$ *8,000*	× 2.9% (.029) =	7	*232*
8	Total social security and Medicare taxes (add lines 6a, 6b, and 7). Check here if wages are not subject to social security and/or Medicare tax . . . . ▶ ☐		8	*1,224*
9	Adjustment of social security and Medicare taxes (see instructions for required explanation) Sick Pay $ _____ ± Fractions of Cents $ _____ ± Other $ _____ =		9	
10	Adjusted total of social security and Medicare taxes (line 8 as adjusted by line 9—see instructions)		10	*1,224*
11	**Total taxes** (add lines 5 and 10)		11	*2,034*
12	Advance earned income credit (EIC) payments made to employees, if any		12	
13	Net taxes (subtract line 12 from line 11). **This should equal line 17, column (d) below** (or line D of Schedule B (Form 941))		13	*2,034*
14	Total deposits for quarter, including overpayment applied from a prior quarter		14	*2,034*
15	**Balance due** (subtract line 14 from line 13). Pay to Internal Revenue Service . . .		15	
16	**Overpayment,** if line 14 is more than line 13, enter excess here ▶ $ _____			

and check if to be: ☐ Applied to next return   **OR**   ☐ Refunded.

- **All filers:** If line 13 is less than $500, you need not complete line 17 or Schedule B.
- **Semiweekly depositors:** Complete Schedule B and check here . . . . ▶ ☐
- **Monthly depositors:** Complete line 17, columns (a) through (d) and check here . . . . . . ▶ ☑

17	Monthly Summary of Federal Tax Liability.			
	(a) First month liability	**(b)** Second month liability	**(c)** Third month liability	**(d)** Total liability for quarter
	666.67	*666.67*	*666.68*	*2,000*

Sign Here   Under penalties of perjury, I declare that I have examined this return, including accompanying schedules and statements, and to the best of my knowledge and belief, it is true, correct, and complete.

Signature ▶ *JG O'Dee*   Print Your Name and Title ▶ *John G O'Dee*   Date ▶ *Jan 31, 1995*

For Paperwork Reduction Act Notice, see page 1 of separate instructions.   Cat. No. 17001Z   Form **941** (Rev. 4-94)

*U.S. Government Printing Office: 1994 — 301-628/00153

Figure 27.2. Sample Form 941.

SCHEDULE C
(Form 1040)

Department of the Treasury
Internal Revenue Service   (5)

Profit or Loss From Business
(Sole Proprietorship)
▶ Partnerships, joint ventures, etc., must file Form 1065.
▶ Attach to Form 1040 or Form 1041.   ▶ See Instructions for Schedule C (Form 1040).

OMB No. 1545-0074

1994

Attachment
Sequence No. **09**

Name of proprietor	Social security number (SSN)
John G O'Dee	*123 45 6789*

A	Principal business or profession, including product or service (see page C-1)	B Enter principal business code
	Optometry	(see page C-6) ▶ *9 2 9 0*

C	Business name. If no separate business name, leave blank.	D Employer ID number (EIN), if any
		0 9 8 7 6 5 4 3 2

E Business address (including suite or room no.) ▶ *2020 Vision St*
City, town or post office, state, and ZIP code   *Insight, AZ 12345*

F Accounting method: (1) ☑ Cash   (2) ☐ Accrual   (3) ☐ Other (specify) ▶ ....

G	Method(s) used to value closing inventory:	(1) ☑ Cost	(2) ☐ Lower of cost or market	(3) ☐ Other (attach explanation)	(4) ☐ Does not apply (if checked, skip line H)	Yes	No
H	Was there any change in determining quantities, costs, or valuations between opening and closing inventory? If "Yes," attach explanation						✓
I	Did you "materially participate" in the operation of this business during 1994? If "No," see page C-2 for limit on losses.					✓	
J	If you started or acquired this business during 1994, check here . . . . ▶ ☑						

Part I   Income

1	Gross receipts or sales. **Caution:** If this income was reported to you on Form W-2 and the "Statutory employee" box on that form was checked, see page C-2 and check here . . . . ▶ ☐	1	*100,000*
2	Returns and allowances	2	
3	Subtract line 2 from line 1	3	*100,000*
4	Cost of goods sold (from line 40 on page 2)	4	*32,000*
5	**Gross profit.** Subtract line 4 from line 3	5	*68,000*
6	Other income, including Federal and state gasoline or fuel tax credit or refund (see page C-2) . . .	6	*2,100*
7	**Gross income.** Add lines 5 and 6 . . . . ▶	7	*70,100*

Part II   Expenses. Enter expenses for business use of your home only on line 30.

8	Advertising	8	19 Pension and profit-sharing plans	19	
9	Bad debts from sales or services (see page C-3) . .	9 *0*	20 Rent or lease (see page C-4):		
			a Vehicles, machinery, and equipment .	20a	
10	Car and truck expenses (see page C-3)	10 *2,030*	b Other business property . .	20b	*6,000*
11	Commissions and fees. . .	11	21 Repairs and maintenance . .	21	
12	Depletion.	12	22 Supplies (not included in Part III) .	22	*600*
13	Depreciation and section 179 expense deduction (not included in Part III) (see page C-3) .	13 *4,150*	23 Taxes and licenses	23	*1,085*
			24 Travel, meals, and entertainment:		
			a Travel	24a	*385*
14	Employee benefit programs (other than on line 19) . . .	14	b Meals and entertainment .		
15	Insurance (other than health) .	15 *2,100*	c Enter 50% of line 24b subject to limitations (see page C-4) .		
16	Interest:		d Subtract line 24c from line 24b .	24d	
a	Mortgage (paid to banks, etc.) .	16a	25 Utilities	25	*1,800*
b	Other	16b *1,000*	26 Wages (less employment credits) .	26	*8,000*
17	Legal and professional services	17 *1,500*	27 Other expenses (from line 46 on page 2)	27	*250*
18	Office expense	18 *180*			

28	**Total expenses** before expenses for business use of home. Add lines 8 through 27 in columns. . ▶	28	*29,080*
29	Tentative profit (loss). Subtract line 28 from line 7	29	
30	Expenses for business use of your home. Attach **Form 8829**	30	
31	**Net profit or (loss).** Subtract line 30 from line 29.		
	• If a profit, enter on **Form 1040, line 12,** and ALSO on **Schedule SE, line 2** (statutory employees, see page C-5). Estates and trusts, enter on Form 1041, line 3.	31	*41,020*
	• If a loss, you MUST go on to line 32.		
32	If you have a loss, check the box that describes your investment in this activity (see page C-5).		
	• If you checked 32a, enter the loss on **Form 1040, line 12,** and ALSO on **Schedule SE, line 2** (statutory employees, see page C-5). Estates and trusts, enter on Form 1041, line 3.	32a ☐ All investment is at risk.
	• If you checked 32b, you MUST attach **Form 6198.**	32b ☐ Some investment is not at risk.

For Paperwork Reduction Act Notice, see Form 1040 instructions.   Cat. No. 11334P   Schedule C (Form 1040) 1994

Figure 27.3. Sample Schedule C.

SOCIAL SECURITY TAX REPORTING

The Federal Insurance Contributors Act (FICA) was established by the federal government to ensure that employers and employees would have at least some income at retirement, for disability, or as a survivor's benefit at the death of a working spouse. The Social Security system requires that payments be made by workers to the federal government, through the imposition of taxes established by the U.S. Congress. The collection and submission of these taxes to the government, for both employer and employees, is the responsibility of the employer. IRS Publication 15, Circular E, Employer's Tax Guide, must be consulted to determine the appropriate withholding of Social Security taxes.

Social Security tax is expressed as a percentage, which is imposed on the taxpayer's income, up to a stated ceiling amount. The tax has two components: a retirement tax and a Medicare tax.

Retirement Tax

In 1995, the percentage of retirement tax for employees was 6.2%, which could be imposed on wages up to $61,200. Therefore, for an employee earning $61,200, the withholding would be the maximum—$3,794. The Social Security law also requires the employer to contribute 6.2% of wages. This means that an optometrist with an employee who earns $61,200 would also have to pay $3,794 to the Social Security Administration on behalf of the employee. Therefore, the total amount that must be paid as Social Security retirement taxes for each employee was, as of 1995, 12.4% of the employee's wages—with the employee contributing 50% and the employer contributing 50%.

Medicare Tax

Since 1991, Social Security tax payments have also been required to support Medicare, which provides health care benefits to people 65 years old and older. Like its retirement tax counterpart, the Medicare portion is calculated as a percentage, but, unlike Social Security, there is no ceiling. The percentage imposed for Medicare payments is 2.9% of wages, regardless of the amount earned. Employer and employee contribute equally to the tax.

Therefore, the Social Security Administration requires a total payment of 15.3% of an employee's wages, with the employer contributing half, or 7.65%, to a specific ceiling amount for the Social Security tax and without a ceiling for the Medicare tax. Payment is made quarterly, at the same times and with the same form (Form 941) as for income tax (see Figure 27.2). This amount contributed on behalf of the employee can be listed on the employer's Schedule C and claimed as a business deduction.

The Social Security tax for employers is calculated in a slightly different manner.

Self-Employment Tax

The Social Security payments of an individual practitioner are based on the income or loss reported on Schedule C. If this amount does not exceed $400, no Social Security tax need be paid. If the amount is in excess of $400, the Social Security tax must be determined on Schedule SE (Figure 27.4). The calculation again depends on the use of a percentage, which is applied to a stated maximum of income. As of 1995, the percentage was 15.3%, to a maximum of $61,200. If income exceeds $61,200, a percentage of 2.9% is applied, without ceiling. Thus an individual practitioner pays to the Social Security Administration 15.3% of income, up to $61,200, and 2.9% thereafter.

The payment of Social Security taxes is made quarterly by the self-employed optometrist using Form 941, which includes the optometrist's estimated income tax payments. At the end of the tax year, when the optometrist completes Form 1040, Schedule SE is used to calculate the exact amount of Social Security tax owed, and that amount is entered on Form 1040 (see line 47, Figure 27.1). Quarterly payments made to Social Security are deducted from the total tax owed; if less tax has been paid than is owed, the balance must be remitted to the IRS. If an excess has been paid, a refund can be collected.

Social Security taxes do not have to be paid to state government. Failure to pay Social Security taxes on time or payment made in improper amounts is punishable by sizable fines—both for

SCHEDULE SE	Self-Employment Tax	OMB No. 1545-0074

SCHEDULE SE
(Form 1040)

Department of the Treasury
Internal Revenue Service

Self-Employment Tax

▶ **See Instructions for Schedule SE (Form 1040).**

▶ **Attach to Form 1040.**

OMB No. 1545-0074

19 94

Attachment
Sequence No. **17**

Name of person with **self-employment** income (as shown on Form 1040)
John G O'Dee

Social security number of person
with **self-employment** income ▶   *123 45 6789*

Who Must File Schedule SE

You must file Schedule SE if:

• You had net earnings from self-employment from other than church employee income (line 4 of Short Schedule SE or line 4c of Long Schedule SE) of $400 or more, **OR**

• You had church employee income of $108.28 or more. Income from services you performed as a minister or a member of a religious order **is not** church employee income. See page SE-1.

Note: *Even if you have a loss or a small amount of income from self-employment, it may be to your benefit to file Schedule SE and use either "optional method" in Part II of Long Schedule SE. See page SE-2.*

Exception. If your only self-employment income was from earnings as a minister, member of a religious order, or Christian Science practitioner, **and** you filed Form 4361 and received IRS approval not to be taxed on those earnings, **do not** file Schedule SE. Instead, write "Exempt–Form 4361" on Form 1040, line 47.

May I Use Short Schedule SE or MUST I Use Long Schedule SE?

Did you receive wages or tips in 1994?

No

Are you a minister, member of a religious order, or Christian Science practitioner who received IRS approval **not** to be taxed on earnings from these sources, **but** you owe self-employment tax on other earnings? **Yes** ▶

No

Are you using one of the optional methods to figure your net earnings (see page SE-2)? **Yes** ▶

No

Did you receive church employee income reported on Form W-2 of $108.28 or more? **Yes** ▶

No

Yes

Was the total of your wages and tips subject to social security or railroad retirement tax **plus** your net earnings from self-employment more than $60,600? **Yes** ▶

No

Did you receive tips subject to social security or Medicare tax that you **did not** report to your employer? **Yes** ▶

No ◀

YOU MAY USE SHORT SCHEDULE SE BELOW	YOU MUST USE LONG SCHEDULE SE ON THE BACK

Section A—Short Schedule SE. Caution: *Read above to see if you can use Short Schedule SE.*

1	Net farm profit or (loss) from Schedule F, line 36, and farm partnerships, Schedule K-1 (Form 1065), line 15a	**1**	
2	Net profit or (loss) from Schedule C, line 31; Schedule C-EZ, line 3; and Schedule K-1 (Form 1065), line 15a (other than farming). Ministers and members of religious orders see page SE-1 for amounts to report on this line. See page SE-2 for other income to report	**2**	*41,020*
3	Combine lines 1 and 2	**3**	*41,020*
4	**Net earnings from self-employment.** Multiply line 3 by 92.35% (.9235). If less than $400, **do not** file this schedule; you do not owe self-employment tax . . . . ▶	**4**	*37,881*
5	**Self-employment tax.** If the amount on line 4 is:		
	• $60,600 or less, multiply line 4 by 15.3% (.153). Enter the result here and on **Form 1040, line 47.**		
	• More than $60,600, multiply line 4 by 2.9% (.029). Then, add $7,514.40 to the result. Enter the total here and on **Form 1040, line 47.**	**5**	*5,796*
6	**Deduction for one-half of self-employment tax.** Multiply line 5 by 50% (.5). Enter the result here and on **Form 1040, line 25**	**6**	*2,898*

For Paperwork Reduction Act Notice, see Form 1040 instructions.   Cat. No. 11358Z   Schedule SE (Form 1040) 1994

Figure 27.4. Sample Schedule SE.

the employer's payments and for those made on behalf of employees.

UNEMPLOYMENT TAX REPORTING

The federal government, in concert with the states, has devised a system of unemployment compensation under the Federal Unemployment Tax Act (FUTA). The system is funded exclusively by employers, most of whom must pay taxes to federal and state government. Some states do not require unemployment tax, and payment must be made exclusively to the federal government.

The tax is paid for each employee, with the amount being a percentage of the employee's wages, to a stated ceiling. In 1995, the federal unemployment tax became 6.2% of wages, to a maximum of $7,000. Thus, if an employee earns $7,000 or more, the employer must contribute $434. This tax is not taken from the wages of the employee; rather, it is paid exclusively from the earnings of the employer. The federal government allows a credit for unemployment taxes paid by an employer to the state, up to 5.4% of wages. In such a state, the employer must pay only the balance to the federal government. If the employer pays the maximum—5.4% of wages—to the state, only 0.8% of wages must be paid to the federal government.

Reporting of federal unemployment taxes is performed on Form 940, Employer's Annual Federal Unemployment Tax Return (Figure 27.5). Payment must be made quarterly, unless the tax owed is less than $100, in which case the quarterly deposit does not have to be submitted until the amount owed exceeds $100. Form 940 is submitted with the final payment, which must be sent to the IRS within 1 month of the end of the tax year (January 31 if the tax year is a calendar year).

State unemployment tax deposits usually must be made on a quarterly basis, and a form must be submitted annually by April 15 if the employer's tax year is a calendar year.

The employer receives a business tax deduction for the unemployment tax paid to state or federal government. This deduction is claimed on Schedule C if the employer is an individual proprietor.

FEDERAL TAX PENALTIES

Because an individual practitioner must file Schedules C and SE along with Form 1040, and because most individual practitioners will use a calendar year as the tax year, the deadline for submission of annual tax returns is April 15. An automatic 2-month extension will be granted if Form 4868 is filed on or before this date. Payment of the estimated tax must accompany the request for an extension. Application for further extensions will be granted only if there is hardship. There are penalties for failure to pay by the due date and for substantially underpaying the tax due, and these penalties will be applied if the unpaid amount is more than 10% of the final tax owed or more than $5,000. These penalties are also applicable if quarterly income tax and Social Security tax payments are not filed by the due date or are substantially underpaid. The employer is responsible for the collection and payment of these taxes and will be held liable for any amounts due.

Form **940**	**Employer's Annual Federal Unemployment (FUTA) Tax Return**	OMB No. 1545-0028
Department of the Treasury Internal Revenue Service (O)	▶ For Paperwork Reduction Act Notice, see separate instructions.	**1994**

Name (as distinguished from trade name)	Calendar year		T
John G O'Dee	1994		FF
Trade name, if any			FD
2020 Vision St.			FP
Address and ZIP code	Employer identification number		I
Insight, AL 12345	09: 8765432		T

A Are you required to pay unemployment contributions to only one state? (If no, skip questions B and C.) . . ☑ Yes ☐ No

B Did you pay all state unemployment contributions by January 31, 1995? (If a 0% experience rate is granted, check "Yes.") (If no, skip question C.) . . . . ☑ Yes ☐ No

C Were all wages that were taxable for FUTA tax also taxable for your state's unemployment tax? . . . . . ☐ Yes ☑ No

If you answered "No" to any of these questions, you must file Form 940. If you answered "Yes" to all the questions, you may file Form 940-EZ, which is a simplified version of Form 940. You can get Form 940-EZ by calling 1-800-TAX-FORM (1-800-829-3676).

If you will not have to file returns in the future, check here, complete, and sign the return . . . . ▶ ☐
If this is an Amended Return, check here . . . . ▶ ☐

Part I   Computation of Taxable Wages

1	Total payments (including exempt payments) during the calendar year for services of employees .	**1**	8,000	
2	Exempt payments. (Explain each exemption shown, attach additional sheets if necessary.) ▶ -----------------------------	Amount paid		
	-----------------------------	**2**		
3	Payments of more than $7,000 for services. Enter only amounts over the first $7,000 paid to each employee. Do not include payments from line 2. The $7,000 amount is the Federal wage base. Your state wage base may be different. Do not use the state wage limitation	**3**	1,000	
4	Total exempt payments (add lines 2 and 3)		**4**	1,000
5	Total taxable wages (subtract line 4 from line 1) . . . . ▶		**5**	7,000

Be sure to complete both sides of this return and sign in the space provided on the back.   Cat. No. 11234O   Form **940** (1994)

DO NOT DETACH

Form **940-V**	**Form 940 Payment Voucher**	**1994**
Department of the Treasury Internal Revenue Service		

Complete boxes 1, 2, 6, and 7. Do not send cash and do not staple your payment to this voucher. Make your check or money order payable to the Internal Revenue Service. If tax due is over $100, make the deposit with Form 8109.

1 Your employer identification number	2 Enter the first four letters of your business name	3 MFT	4 Tax year	5 Transaction code
09 : 8765432	O D E E	1 0	9 4 1 2	6 1 0
	6 Your business name and address		7 Amount of payment	
Do not staple your payment to this voucher.			$ 108 . 50 Do not send cash.	

Figure 27.5. Sample Form 940.

Form 940 (1994)   Page 2

Part II   Tax Due or Refund

1   Gross FUTA tax. Multiply the wages in Part I, line 5, by .062 . . . . | 1 | 434
2   Maximum credit. Multiply the wages in Part I, line 5, by .054 . . . | 2 | 432 |
3   Computation of tentative credit (Note: *All taxpayers must complete the applicable columns.*)

(a) Name of state	(b) State reporting number(s) as shown on employer's state contribution returns	(c) Taxable payroll (as defined in state act)	(d) State experience rate period		(e) State experience rate	(f) Contributions if rate had been 5.4% (col. (c) x .054)	(g) Contributions payable at experience rate (col. (c) x col. (e))	(h) Additional credit (col. (f) minus col.(g)). If 0 or less, enter -0-.	(i) Contributions actually paid to state
			From	To					

3a Totals . . . ▶
3b Total tentative credit (add line 3a, columns (h) and (i) only—see instructions for limitations on late payments) ▶ | | 0

4
5
6   Credit: Enter the smaller of the amount in Part II, line 2, or line 3b . . . . | 6 | 0
7   **Total FUTA tax** (subtract line 6 from line 1) . . . . | 7 | 434
8   Total FUTA tax deposited for the year, including any overpayment applied from a prior year . . | 8 | 325 | 50
9   **Balance due** (subtract line 8 from line 7). This should be $100 or less. Pay to the Internal Revenue Service. See page 3 of the Instructions for Form 940 for details . . . . ▶ | 9 | 108 | 50
10 **Overpayment** (subtract line 7 from line 8). Check if it is to be: ☐ **Applied to next return,** or ☐ **Refunded** . . . . ▶ | 10 |

Part III   Record of Quarterly Federal Unemployment Tax Liability *(Do not include state liability)*

Quarter	First	Second	Third	Fourth	Total for year
Liability for quarter	108.50	108.50	108.50	108.50	434

Under penalties of perjury, I declare that I have examined this return, including accompanying schedules and statements, and to the best of my knowledge and belief, it is true, correct, and complete, and that no part of any payment made to a state unemployment fund claimed as a credit was or is to be deducted from the payments to employees.

Signature ▶ *JE O Dee*   Title (Owner, etc.) ▶ *Owner*   Date ▶ *Jan 31, 1995*

Figure 27.5. (continued)

BIBLIOGRAPHY

IRS publication 15, Employer's Tax Guide (Circular E).
IRS publication 15-A, Employer's Supplemental Tax Guide.
IRS publication 17, Your Federal Income Tax (For Individuals).
IRS publication 334, Tax Guide for Small Businesses.
IRS publication 463, Travel, Entertainment, and Gift Expenses.
IRS publication 505, Tax Withholding and Estimated Tax.
IRS publication 533, Self-Employment Tax.
IRS publication 535, Business Expenses.
IRS publication 538, Accounting Periods and Methods.
IRS publication 541, Tax Information on Partnerships.
IRS publication 542, Tax Information on Corporations.
IRS publication 583, Starting a Business and Keeping Records.
IRS publication 589, Tax Information on S Corporations.
IRS publication 917, Business Use of a Car.
IRS publication 946, How to Depreciate Property.

Chapter 28

Analysis of Practice Economics and Growth

John Rumpakis and Craig Hisaka

Living well is the best revenge.

—George Herbert
Jacula Prudentum

The ability to develop a systematic, universal method for determining the economic status of a professional practice is essential for survival in today's competitive atmosphere. Optometric practice economics involves data gathering, formulation, and analysis of all financial information to determine the economic status of a business. Without the ability to formulate and analyze financial data, the practicing optometrist would not be able to survive in the business world.

It is important to understand the specialized vocabulary used in financial transactions. Just as the language of clinical care is learned, so must the language of business be learned in order to communicate better with business professionals, colleagues, and other individuals. Table 28.1 provides a list of basic business financial terms used in the day-to-day operations of a professional practice.

The day-to-day recordkeeping of financial transactions in a professional practice can be a nightmare for the poorly organized optometrist. If an accurate means of tracking income and expenses is not used, a practitioner cannot manage the practice profitably. Optometrists have developed sophisticated methods for maintaining patient records to ensure that proper care is rendered and to provide protection from potential liability, yet all too often the average optometrist does not maintain an accurate, efficient method of financial recordkeeping. This deficiency obviously leads to poor financial management and increases the risk of incurring financial liability. Documentation of financial records is an essential component of a successful practice. Greater profitability, enhanced financial security, and reduced risk of financial liability are all benefits of proper financial management.

BASIC FINANCIAL STATEMENT CONSTRUCTION

In organizing the financial records of a practice, the optometrist should prepare a balance sheet and an income statement.

Balance Sheet

The balance sheet is a financial document that summarily depicts a company's or an individual's financial status at a specific point in time. It balances the amount of assets a business has against its liabilities and the owner's equity. In simplest terms, it shows how much a company owns versus how much a company owes. The difference between the two is the net worth of the company.

The balance sheet is composed of four basic areas: title, assets, liabilities, and net worth (Figure 28.1).

Table 28.1. Common Business Terms

Business: A series of activities coordinated and integrated toward the production of goods or services, the end purpose being the generation of profit.

Assets: Items of value owned by a business, including cash and bank accounts, material inventory, equipment, buildings, and land. Fixed assets are items of value that have a lifetime of greater than 1 year. Current assets are items of value that have a lifetime of less than 1 year.

Liabilities: Claims of creditors against the assets of a business. Fixed liabilities are claims of creditors that will last for longer than 1 year. Current liabilities are claims of creditors that will last for less than 1 year.

Owner's equity: Items of value, or money contributed that the owner or owners have invested in the business.

Balance sheet: A financial statement that shows a business's assets, liabilities, and the owner's equity at a particular point in time. A balance sheet provides a snapshot of the company's asset-to-debt status.

Income statement: A financial statement that summarizes all the revenue and expense transactions that will result in a profit or loss over a specific period of time. The income statement provides an assessment of the company's financial profitability over time.

Profit and loss statement: A financial analysis related to the income statement that shows total received income compared against total actual expenditures for a given period of time. The profit and loss statement does not take into consideration non-cash expenditures that are included in an income statement.

Accounts receivable: Money owed to the business by patients or customers for goods and services they have already received.

Accounts payable: Money owed by the business to some other business or individual for goods and services already received by the business.

Principal: When borrowing or loaning money, the principal is the amount of money either borrowed or loaned.

Loan term: The time period that is allowed for repayment of the principal. This is not always the time period used to calculate the allocation of interest and principal per payment.

Interest rate: The percentage rate fee that is charged by a lender for the funds that are borrowed. Legal requirements obligate lenders to express the interest rate as an annual percentage rate (APR).

Amortization schedule: A financial statement that summarizes a loan by showing the principal borrowed, the interest rate charged, the payment frequency, and the payment-by-payment allocation of principal and interest throughout the term of the loan.

Credit terms: The terms by which money is either owed to or by a business. Terms include principal amount, interest rate, and the time period in which the money is due.

Credit risk: The rating factor used by lenders to judge a borrower for the purpose of determining credit terms for that borrower. If an individual or business is a high risk, the loan terms will be less favorable; the lower the risk, the more favorable the loan terms will be.

Points: A service fee charged by the lender to process a loan that is usually expressed in the form of a percentage based on the principal amount of the loan.

Effective interest rate: The actual interest rate calculated by incorporating the associated service fees into the total cost of borrowing the principal amount. Ths effective service rate generally differs from the stated interest rate of a loan.

Cosigner: An individual who assumes liability for a debt in the event of a default by the primary borrower.

Cash basis of accounting: A form of accounting that is strictly determined by the amount of cash received and cash paid out.

Accrual basis of accounting: A form of accounting that incorporates accounts receivable, accounts payable, depreciation, and inventory.

Cash flow: A term that refers to the flow of funds within a company, reflecting actual funds received and actual funds expended for a specific time period. Cash flow is usually calculated on a daily or monthly basis.

Title

The title area of the balance sheet contains the name of the business, the title of the financial document, and the specific date that the information was valid.

Assets

The asset area is usually on the left side of the document or on the top. The asset section is defined by subsections that itemize "fixed" and "current" assets. These two subsections list the specific items

Acme Vision Clinic, P.C.
30–Jun-97
Balance Sheet

ASSETS		**LIABILITIES**	
Current Assets		**Current Liabilities**	
Bank Accounts	$ 12,000.00	Accounts Payable	$ 27,500.00
Cash On Hand	2,000.00	Contracts Payable	4,000.00
Merchandise Inventory	35,000.00	Short Term Note Payable	5,000.00
Accounts Receivable	30,000.00		
Total Current Assets	$ 79,000.00	**Total Current Liabilities**	$36,500.00
Fixed Assets		**Fixed Liabilities**	
Store fixtures	$ 47,500.00	Personal notes payable	$ 56,000.00
Office furniture	25,000.00	Equipment notes payable	25,000.00
Optometric equipment	87,000.00	Line of credit payable	5,000.00
Computer equipment	15,000.00		
		Total Fixed Liabilities	$86,000.00
Total Fixed Assets	$ 174,500.00		
		Total Liabilities	$122,500.00
Total Assets	$ 253,500.00		
		Net Worth	
		Owners Equity	$131,000.00
		Total Liabilities & Net Worth	$253,500.00

Figure 28.1. Balance sheet—assets and liabilities.

within each category. At the bottom of the asset section is the sum total of all fixed and current assets for the business.

Liabilities

The liabilities area is located either on the right side of the balance sheet or under the asset section. Like the asset section, the liability section is broken into two subsections, which consist of "fixed" and "current" liabilities. These subsections are further subdivided by individual components that constitute the total. The subtotals for fixed and current liabilities are added together at the bottom of this section to provide a sum for total liabilities.

Net Worth

The net worth area is also referred to as the owner's equity. The net worth figure represents the financial contribution the owner or owners have made to the business. It is determined by calculating the mathematical difference between the total assets and the total liabilities. If a business owns more than it owes, it has a positive net worth. If a business has incurred more debt than it owns in assets, it has a negative net worth. Therefore, the sum of the total liabilities and the net worth must equal the total assets of the business. This relationship is the reason the document is called a balance sheet.

Income Statement

The income statement is one of the most informative of all financial statements. It provides a summary of all revenues and expenses that will ultimately result in a profit or loss. The construction of this statement is significantly more complex than the balance sheet but, when properly constructed,

Acme Vision Clinic, P.C.
1997 Income Statement
1 January - 31 March 1997
Quarterly Report

GROSS SALES REVENUE:

Practice Revenue	January	February	March	Quarterly Grand Total	Percentage of Gross Income
Services:	$22,000.00	$23,500.00	$24,750.00	$70,250.00	56.09%
Materials:	$15,000.00	$18,000.00	$22,000.00	$55,000.00	43.91%
Subtotal	$37,000.00	$41,500.00	$46,750.00	$125,250.00	100.00%
Less credit/adjust	$2,405.00	$2,697.50	$3,038.75	$8,141.25	6.50%
Net Sales Revenue	$34,595.00	$38,802.50	$43,711.25	$117,108.75	93.50%
Cost of Goods Sold	$12,210.00	$13,695.00	$15,427.50	$41,332.50	33.00%
Gross Margin on Sales	$22,385.00	$25,107.50	$28,283.75	$75,776.25	60.50%

OPERATING EXPENSES:
Fixed Expenses:

	January	February	March	Quarterly Grand Total	Percentage of Gross Income
Advertising Yellow Pages	$500.00	$500.00	$500.00	$1,500.00	1.20%
Depreciation	$1,200.00	$1,200.00	$1,200.00	$3,600.00	2.87%
Dues AOA	$100.00	$100.00	$100.00	$300.00	0.24%
Dues Employees	$0.00	$0.00	$0.00	$0.00	0.00%
Dues Business Club	$75.00	$75.00	$75.00	$225.00	0.18%
Dues Athletic Club	$75.00	$75.00	$75.00	$225.00	0.18%
Insurance Basic Overhead	$100.00	$100.00	$100.00	$300.00	0.24%
Insurance Disability	$50.00	$50.00	$50.00	$150.00	0.12%
Insurance Major Medical	$250.00	$250.00	$250.00	$750.00	0.60%
Insurance Property/Liability	$100.00	$100.00	$100.00	$300.00	0.24%
Insurance Worker's Compensation	$50.00	$50.00	$50.00	$150.00	0.12%
Lease Professional Equipment	$548.00	$548.00	$548.00	$1,644.00	1.31%
Lease Office Equipment	$200.00	$200.00	$200.00	$600.00	0.48%
Licenses	$6.67	$6.67	$6.67	$20.00	0.02%
Plant Service	$65.00	$65.00	$65.00	$195.00	0.16%
Rent (including utilities)	$3,000.00	$3,000.00	$3,000.00	$9,000.00	7.19%
Salary Dr. Acme	$5,000.00	$5,000.00	$5,000.00	$15,000.00	11.98%
Salary Staff #1	$1,239.58	$1,239.58	$1,239.58	$3,718.75	2.97%
Salary Staff #2	$1,097.92	$1,097.92	$1,097.92	$3,293.75	2.63%
Taxes Federal Income	$900.00	$900.00	$900.00	$2,700.00	2.16%
Taxes State Income	$400.00	$400.00	$400.00	$1,200.00	0.96%
Taxes Personal Property	$395.00	$395.00	$395.00	$1,185.00	0.95%
Taxes Payroll Federal	$3,283.75	$3,283.75	$3,283.75	$9,851.25	7.87%
Taxes Payroll State	$798.75	$798.75	$798.75	$2,396.25	1.91%
Telephone Basic Service	$65.00	$65.00	$65.00	$195.00	0.16%
Telephone Cellular	$50.00	$50.00	$50.00	$150.00	0.12%
Telephone Long Distance	$35.00	$35.00	$35.00	$105.00	0.08%
Telephone Maintenance	$29.00	$29.00	$29.00	$87.00	0.07%
Total Fixed Expenses:	$19,613.67	$19,613.67	$19,613.67	$58,841.00	46.98%

Figure 28.2. Income statement—quarterly report.

can offer a wealth of information at a glance. The income statement is divided into four major sections: income, operating expenses, profit and loss statement, and break-even analysis.

Income

In the practice of optometry, income is derived from the services provided and the materials sold. It is important to specify which income is generated by services and which is generated by materials. Services revenue and materials revenue are both subsections of the category termed "gross sales revenue" (Figure 28.2). When services and materials revenues for a given month are added together, the total gross income for the specified time period is obtained. The credits and adjustments are then subtracted from this figure to obtain the "net sales revenue." This figure represents the actual amount of income that was earned after all credits and adjustments to gross income were made.

The next item incorporated into the income statement is the "cost of goods sold," which represents the actual costs of all items purchased for retail sales in the practice. In a typical practice, these expenditures would represent optical laboratory bills, purchases of contact lenses, frame inventory purchases, purchases of ophthalmic

Figure 28.2 (continued)

Variable Expenses:					
Accounting	$100.00	$100.00	$100.00	$300.00	0.24%
Advertising General	$0.00	$0.00	$0.00	$0.00	0.00%
Attorney/Legal	$0.00	$0.00	$0.00	$0.00	0.00%
Automotive	$80.00	$80.00	$80.00	$240.00	0.19%
Bank Card Discount	$130.00	$130.00	$130.00	$390.00	0.31%
Bank Charges	$40.00	$40.00	$40.00	$120.00	0.10%
Continuing Education Staff	$20.00	$20.00	$20.00	$60.00	0.05%
Continuing Education O.D.'s	$50.00	$50.00	$50.00	$150.00	0.12%
Entertainment	$150.00	$0.00	$0.00	$150.00	0.12%
Equipment Purchase Dispensary	$0.00	$0.00	$0.00	$0.00	0.00%
Equipment Purchase Front Office	$0.00	$0.00	$0.00	$0.00	0.00%
Equipment Purchase Professional	$0.00	$0.00	$0.00	$0.00	0.00%
Equipment Purchase Lab	$0.00	$0.00	$0.00	$0.00	0.00%
Equipment Repairs	$0.00	$0.00	$0.00	$0.00	0.00%
Furnishings	$0.00	$0.00	$0.00	$0.00	0.00%
Miscellaneous	$60.00	$60.00	$60.00	$180.00	0.14%
Office Supplies	$75.00	$75.00	$75.00	$225.00	0.18%
Optometric Supplies	$50.00	$50.00	$50.00	$150.00	0.12%
Postage	$250.00	$250.00	$250.00	$750.00	0.60%
Postage Meter Reset Fees	$7.50	$7.50	$7.50	$22.50	0.02%
Printing	$0.00	$0.00	$0.00	$0.00	0.00%
Publication	$0.00	$0.00	$0.00	$0.00	0.00%
Refunds	$150.00	$150.00	$150.00	$450.00	0.36%
Shipping	$30.00	$30.00	$30.00	$90.00	0.07%
Subscriptions Front Office	$8.33	$8.33	$8.33	$25.00	0.02%
Subscriptions Professional	$4.17	$4.17	$4.17	$12.50	0.01%
Temporary Services	$0.00	$0.00	$0.00	$0.00	0.00%
Tenant Improvements	$0.00	$0.00	$0.00	$0.00	0.00%
Travel	$200.00	$150.00	$175.00	$525.00	0.42%
Tuition	$0.00	$0.00	$0.00	$0.00	0.00%
Uncollectable Debt	$185.00	$207.50	$233.75	$626.25	0.50%
Total Variable Expense:	$1,590.00	$1,412.50	$1,463.75	$4,466.25	3.57%
Total Expenses	$21,203.67	$21,026.17	$21,077.42	$63,307.25	50.54%
Net Income On Operations	$1,181.33	$4,081.33	$7,206.33	$12,469.00	9.96%
DEBT SERVICE					
Line of Credit Interest	$50.00	$50.00	$50.00	$150.00	0.12%
Line of Credit Principal	$43.00	$43.00	$43.00	$129.00	0.10%
Term Note Interest	$200.00	$200.00	$200.00	$600.00	0.48%
Term Note Principal	$195.00	$195.00	$195.00	$585.00	0.47%
Total Debt Service:	$488.00	$488.00	$488.00	$1,464.00	1.17%
Net Cash Available:	$693.33	$3,593.33	$6,718.33	$11,005.00	8.79%

solutions, and any accessory items. This figure is particularly important. The difference between net sales revenue and the cost of goods sold is called the "gross margin on sales." This figure represents the amount of income that remains after payments for material costs have been made. The gross margin on sales is the last figure in the income section of the income statement.

Operating Expenses

The operating expenses area of the financial statement is broken down into two subsets, called fixed and variable expenses (see Figure 28.2). "Fixed expenses" are independent of the number of patients seen or the amount of business done. "Variable expenses" depend on the number of patients seen or the volume of business done. Typical examples of fixed expenses are rent, salaries, and insurance premiums. Typical examples of variable expenses are laboratory bills, supplies, and commissions. Fixed and variable expenses are listed and a total (called "total expenses") for the two categories is obtained. The mathematical difference between the gross margin on sales and the total operating expenses yields the "net income on operations."

In a practice without debt this figure is the bottom-line net income (see Figure 28.2). However, most practices have incurred some debts, described in a different section termed "debt service." This section breaks down the principal and interest portion of each payment according to the amortization schedule that is created for the loan. It is important for the interest portion to be itemized separately because it is tax deductible. The sum of the principal and interest should equal the "total debt service."

The difference between the net income on operations and the total debt service will result in the true net income of the business.

Profit and Loss Statement

The profit and loss statement is a condensation of the income statement and shares most of the same information as the income statement (Figure 28.3). The profit and loss statement, however, provides a more timely and dollar-relevant picture of the financial status of the company. Definitively, the profit and loss statement reveals the cash flow status of the company, recording only the amount of actual payments received by the company and the actual paid expenses of the company. It specifically does not include non-cash expenditures such as depreciation, credits and adjustments, or uncollectable debts. Thus, it reveals a true cash picture of the profitability of a business and aids management in determining if adjustments are needed in collections policies or spending habits.

The profit and loss statement strictly compares cash in and cash out. There is no differentiation between fixed and variable expenses. The cost of goods sold and the debt service are considered ordinary expenses. It does not make any difference if the amount varies with the amount of business done or if it is fixed, because only the actual income received and actual dollars spent for a particular time period need to be measured to derive the profitability (or loss) for the business.

A profit and loss statement is generally produced every month for most businesses. However, how often this information is needed is highly individualized for each particular practice and is often based on the degree of management that is needed or desired.

Break-Even Analysis

Having the ability to perform a break-even analysis for day-to-day situations is highly desirable in the private practice of optometry. Whether a practice is started cold or purchased from a practitioner, costs are incurred to purchase assets, finance inventory, and fund operating expenses. For effective financial management and prudent fiscal planning, it is es-

sential to see how quickly the revenues generated can satisfy the overhead costs and cause the practice to become profitable. Optometrists, like other health care providers, also face the financial burden of having to keep offices technologically current. This cost of new equipment and supporting technology is significant. Thus, it is very important to be able to show that the cost of this equipment is justified by the revenue it can generate. These simple concepts show the necessity of being able to quickly calculate or graphically produce a break-even analysis. It is important to remember that the definition of the break-even point is "total revenues equal to total expenses;" this means that no profit or loss has been incurred. In fact, the entire purpose of performing a break-even analysis is to determine the point at which—or the number of procedures performed after which—the first dollar of profit will be generated.

The essential elements for constructing a break-even analysis are the total revenues, total expenses, total fixed expenses, and total variable expenses. These values are derived from the income statement. Non-cash expenditures, such as depreciation, should not be included in the total fixed expenses or the total expenses, because such expenditures will artificially raise or increase the break-even point. By eliminating these items from the break-even analysis, only the actual income generated and the actual expenses incurred or paid out are considered.

When constructing the break-even graph, it is important to establish some standards for comparison (Figure 28.4). The Y axis will always represent the income values generated. The X axis will represent either the amount of time passed or the number of procedures performed until break-even is reached. Total revenues are placed on the graph, with the starting point at the origin. Thus, if time is zero, or if the number of procedures performed is zero, the total revenue is zero. Total fixed costs will start at some income level on the Y axis, but will be at zero on the X axis. These costs will be the same regardless of time or number of procedures performed. Total expenses (the total fixed costs added to the total variable costs) will use the intersection of the fixed cost line and the Y axis as its starting point. The slope of the total expense line will represent the variable costs incurred. The area between the total expense line and the fixed ex-

Figure 28.3. Profit and loss statement—quarterly report.

Acme Vision Clinic, P.C.
1997 Profit & Loss Statement
1 January - 31 March 1997
Quarterly Report

GROSS SALES REVENUE:	January	February	March	Quarterly Grand Total	Percentage of Gross Income
Practice Revenue					
Net Sales Revenue	$34,595.00	$38,802.50	$43,711.25	$117,108.75	100.00%
OPERATING EXPENSES:					
Accounting	$100.00	$100.00	$100.00	$300.00	0.26%
Advertising General	0.00	0.00	0.00	0.00	0.00%
Advertising Yellow Pages	500.00	500.00	500.00	1,500.00	1.28%
Attorney/Legal	0.00	0.00	0.00	0.00	0.00%
Automotive	80.00	80.00	80.00	240.00	0.20%
Bank Card Discount	130.00	130.00	130.00	390.00	0.33%
Bank Charges	40.00	40.00	40.00	120.00	0.10%
Continuing Education O.D.'s	50.00	50.00	50.00	150.00	0.13%
Continuing Education Staff	20.00	20.00	20.00	60.00	0.05%
Cost of Goods Sold	12,210.00	13,695.00	15,427.50	41,332.50	35.29%
Dues AOA	100.00	100.00	100.00	300.00	0.26%
Dues Athletic Club	75.00	75.00	75.00	225.00	0.19%
Dues Business Club	75.00	75.00	75.00	225.00	0.19%
Dues Employees	0.00	0.00	0.00	0.00	0.00%
Entertainment	150.00	0.00	0.00	150.00	0.13%
Equipment Purchase Dispensary	0.00	0.00	0.00	0.00	0.00%
Equipment Purchase Front Office	0.00	0.00	0.00	0.00	0.00%
Equipment Purchase Lab	0.00	0.00	0.00	0.00	0.00%
Equipment Purchase Professional	0.00	0.00	0.00	0.00	0.00%
Equipment Repairs	0.00	0.00	0.00	0.00	0.00%
Furnishings	0.00	0.00	0.00	0.00	0.00%
Insurance Basic Overhead	100.00	100.00	100.00	300.00	0.26%
Insurance Disability	50.00	50.00	50.00	150.00	0.13%
Insurance Major Medical	250.00	250.00	250.00	750.00	0.64%
Insurance Property/Liability	100.00	100.00	100.00	300.00	0.26%
Insurance Worker's Compensation	50.00	50.00	50.00	150.00	0.13%
Lease Office Equipment	200.00	200.00	200.00	600.00	0.51%
Lease Professional Equipment	548.00	548.00	548.00	1,644.00	1.40%
Licenses	6.67	6.67	6.67	20.01	0.02%
Line of Credit Principal	43.00	43.00	43.00	129.00	0.11%
Line of Credit Interest	50.00	50.00	50.00	150.00	0.13%
Miscellaneous	60.00	60.00	60.00	180.00	0.15%
Office Supplies	75.00	75.00	75.00	225.00	0.19%
Optometric Supplies	50.00	50.00	50.00	150.00	0.13%
Plant Service	65.00	65.00	65.00	195.00	0.17%
Postage	250.00	250.00	250.00	750.00	0.64%
Postage Meter Reset Fees	7.50	7.50	7.50	22.50	0.02%
Printing	0.00	0.00	0.00	0.00	0.00%
Publication	0.00	0.00	0.00	0.00	0.00%
Refunds	150.00	150.00	150.00	450.00	0.38%
Rent (including utilities)	3,000.00	3,000.00	3,000.00	9,000.00	7.69%
Salary Dr. Acme	5,000.00	5,000.00	5,000.00	15,000.00	12.81%
Salary Staff #1	1,239.58	1,239.58	1,239.58	3,718.75	3.18%
Salary Staff #2	1,097.92	1,097.92	1,097.92	3,293.75	2.81%
Shipping	30.00	30.00	30.00	90.00	0.08%
Subscriptions Front Office	8.33	8.33	8.33	24.99	0.02%
Subscriptions Professional	4.17	4.17	4.17	12.51	0.01%
Taxes Federal Income	900.00	900.00	900.00	2,700.00	2.31%
Taxes Payroll Federal	3,283.75	3,283.75	3,283.75	9,851.25	8.41%
Taxes Payroll State	798.75	798.75	798.75	2,396.25	2.05%
Taxes Personal Property	395.00	395.00	395.00	1,185.00	1.01%
Taxes State Income	400.00	400.00	400.00	1,200.00	1.02%
Telephone Basic Service	65.00	65.00	65.00	195.00	0.17%
Telephone Cellular	50.00	50.00	50.00	150.00	0.13%
Telephone Long Distance	35.00	35.00	35.00	105.00	0.09%
Telephone Maintenance	29.00	29.00	29.00	87.00	0.07%
Temporary Services	0.00	0.00	0.00	0.00	0.00%
Tenant Improvements	0.00	0.00	0.00	0.00	0.00%
Term Note Interest	200.00	200.00	200.00	600.00	0.51%
Term Note Principal	195.00	195.00	195.00	585.00	0.50%
Travel	200.00	200.00	200.00	600.00	0.51%
Tuition	0.00	0.00	0.00	0.00	0.00%
Uncollectable Debt	185.00	207.50	233.75	626.25	0.53%
Total Expenses	$32,701.67	$34,059.17	$35,817.92	$102,578.76	87.59%
Net Income From Operations	$1,893.33	$4,743.33	$7,893.33	$14,529.99	12.41%

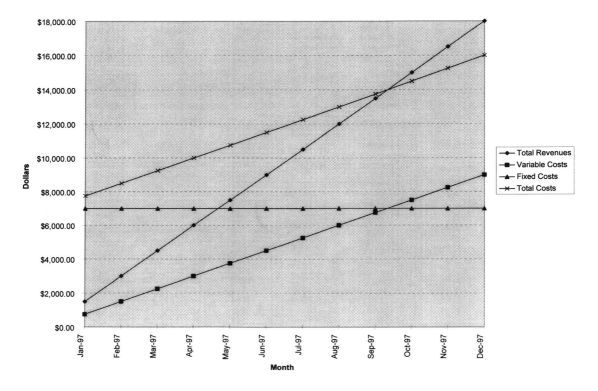

Figure 28.4. Graph illustrating a break-even analysis.

pense line represents the total variable costs. The point at which the total expense line and the total revenue line intersect is the break-even point. The area between the total expense line and the total revenue line, before the break-even point, represents the loss incurred. The area between the total expense line and the total revenue line, after the break-even point, represents the profit gained. A bar graph can also be used to perform a break-even analysis (Figure 28.5).

An optometrist can use this type of analysis to gain insightful financial information that is crucial to the necessary planning that makes a practice successful.

FINANCIAL STATEMENT ANALYSIS

Analysis of these financial statements is critical to assess a practice's financial status. It is not only important to assess the performance of the

practice for the time period in question but also to analyze the financial history of the practice. This analysis enables the optometrist to predict and plan the practice's financial future. Determining the financial status or health of a practice can be approached by using methodology that is similar to the approach taken for patient care. A practitioner takes a case history, gathers data, performs some form of data analysis, determines a diagnosis, and prescribes a plan for treatment. In financial terms, when a practitioner takes a case history of a business, information that is relevant to the business is gathered from various sources. How many patients did the practice see? What was the gross income of the practice? What was the inventory turnover? What was the recall percentage? These are but a few of the many questions a business owner needs to ask. Gathering the data is fairly simple once it is determined what one needs to know. Obtaining the financial statements in the proper format is es-

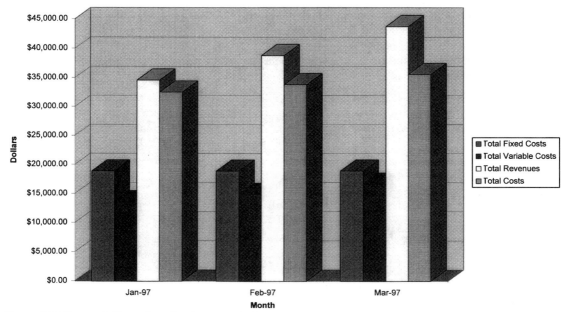

Figure 28.5. Bar graph illustrating a break-even analysis.

sential if a practitioner is to glean necessary information about the practice. Standardization of financial statements and the information they contain is somewhat lacking in optometric practices; thus analysis can be more difficult until the information is placed into a format where industry standards can be compared. Unless the practitioner is comparing "apples to apples," the analysis performed and the conclusions reached will not be valid.

Ratio Analysis

To determine if a business is healthy, there are different ratios that can be applied to a balance sheet to analyze the relationships between different variables of assets, liabilities, and net worth or owner's equity. When the ratios are applied, it is important to use them as a means of answering questions about a business. This goal can be accomplished by comparing the business's current data to past performance, as well as to industry standards. Standard ratios used for analysis include balance sheet ratios and various income statement ratios.

Balance Sheet Ratios

Standard balance sheet ratios that are considered useful include the current ratio, the quick ratio, and the estimate of working capital.

Current Ratio. The current ratio shows the relationship between current assets and current liabilities. Current assets are those presumed to be convertible into cash within 90 days. Current liabilities are those debts due within 1 year. The current ratio measures the business's liquidity or cash position. It is used to measure the business's ability to satisfy short-term debt. Standard accounting norms indicate that a sound current ratio would be 2:1. Interpreting this ratio means that a business has twice as many current or liquid assets as it has current debts.

Quick Ratio. The quick ratio compares the business's available cash, plus receivables, to current liabilities. The quick ratio is commonly known as the "acid test" of liquidity. It compares only the most liquid assets with current liabilities. Only available cash and accounts receivable are used as assets in this case. A desirable quick ratio is 1:1.

An optometrist purchases a corneal topography unit for $18,000. What utilization is needed in terms of additional gross income to cover the unit's cost?

The contibution margin is the amount by which the revenue derived from the use of the unit exceeds the cost of its use.

If the contribution margin is .55 or 55%, the $\dfrac{\$18,000}{.55}$ = $32,727 of additional gross income.

If the contribution margin is .40 or 40%, then $\dfrac{\$18,000}{.40}$ = $45,000 of addtional gross income.

Figure 28.6. Use of contribution margin.

Working Capital. Working capital is the mathematical difference—expressed in dollars—between current assets and current liabilities. In everyday business operations, the net working capital enables the business to meet all obligations as they become due.

Income Statement Ratios

There are various income statement figures that can be analyzed. Among the most important are the gross margin percentage, inventory turnover, and income as a percentage of gross sales.

Gross Margin Percentage. The gross margin percentage is the difference between the cost of products sold and their sales price. This important figure is used to determine if the difference between the purchase cost and the selling price is adequate.

Inventory Turnover. The inventory turnover ratio is determined by dividing the cost of goods sold by the average inventory. To calculate the average inventory, the beginning and ending inventory for the period in question are added and this sum is divided by two. Inventory turnover allows the practitioner to compare the turnover of the practice with that of industry standards.

Income as a Percentage of Gross Sales. Income as a percentage of gross sales is probably the most important ratio that can be obtained from an income statement. It is calculated by subtracting total expenses from total sales and dividing this figure by total sales. It shows, on a percentage basis, the portion of every dollar of sales that results in profit. It also allows the practitioner to derive, on a line item basis, what percentage of every sales dollar goes to operational expenses. This figure is very helpful, for it enables the practitioner to see how and where practice dollars are spent.

Contribution Margin. The contribution margin is the amount by which revenue exceeds the variable cost of producing revenue. It indicates the marginal income after variable cost is covered. It is calculated by subtracting variable costs from total sales and dividing by total sales. This ratio can be quite helpful in determining the income necessary to cover the purchase price for equipment or the cost of additional employees (Figure 28.6).

These ratios are a few of many figures that financial analysts work with when analyzing a practice. These relationships are not inclusive, and there are many others that can be applied to analyze different financial relationships within a business.

Analysis of Chair Cost

Although most optometrists have heard about or seen calculations on chair cost, many do not realize that this type of analysis is the most effective method of establishing professional fees. This con-

Figure 28.7. Example: calculation of chair cost.

There are several assumptions made in this example:

• Sole practitioner

• Yearly gross income	$400,000.00
• Monthly gross income	$33,333.33
• Cost of goods sold	$9,999.99 @ 30% of gross income
• Gross margin on sales	$23,333.33 @ 70% of Gross Income
• Operating costs	$11,666.66 @ 35% of Gross Income
• Pre-tax net income	$9,999.99 @ 30% of Gross Income

• Comprehensive examination fee $55.00
• Monthly prorated operating expenses
　　　70% professional = $8,166.66
　　　30% dispensary   = $3,499.99

• Professional overhead/hours
　　　Doctor hours per month = 160 hours
　　　5 days per week
　　　250 days per year
　　　20 days per month
　　　160 hours per month

Chair Cost Calculation

Chair Cost = $\dfrac{\text{Professional overhead per month}}{\text{Practitioner hours per month}}$

Chair Cost = $\dfrac{\$8166.66}{160}$ = $51.04 per hour

Profit Margin on the Services Provided

$55.00 - $51.04 = $3.96 per examination or a 7.75% profit margin on services alone.

　　　If the doctor needs to have a higher profit margin, then it should be calculated appropriately. For example, if a 20% margin is desired then the appropriate examination fee would be $61.25.

cept is used in many industries, but it is seldom used by optometrists due to lack of understanding, misinterpretation of results, and reluctance to change existing financial methods.

　　　Chair cost is a formula that is based on analyzing a practice's overhead as it relates to professional services and the number of practitioner production hours. This concept is hard for many practitioners to understand because the optometric profession has, historically, relied much too heavily on the retail sale of frames, lenses, and contact lenses as the major source of practice revenue. In these changing times, practitioners must be able to determine what it actually costs to produce service revenues only, without the sale of retail items. True profitability in the service portion of a practice can then be accurately analyzed, and prices for services can be accurately determined. An example can be used to illustrate how chair cost is analyzed (Figure 28.7).

　　　From this example, it can be seen that chair cost is one financial tool that a practitioner simply cannot do without. With increasing third-party involvement in optometry, it also becomes the best analytical tool to evaluate professional service fees for profitability and to determine whether an optometrist can afford to participate in a vision service plan offered by a third-party carrier.

Productivity Statistics

One important application of economic analysis is the generation of productivity statistics. The purpose of these statistics can be to provide a financial goal for the practice or to analyze the financial performance of the practice. In the former case, a goal worksheet can be prepared. This worksheet should describe the productivity desired for a specific period of time. For example, the practice productivity goal for 1 month can be described in terms of the daily, weekly, and monthly revenues needed to meet the goal (Figure 28.8), or the financial performance of the practice can be ana-

October Productivity				
1997				
Work Days In Month	Goal for Month			
23	$ 63,000.00			
Week Ending	10/6/97	10/13/97	10/20/97	10/31/97
# of Days Past:	5	10	15	23
Gross Charges	$21,039.69	$43,038.09	$56,555.00	$66,537.29
Total Receipts	$23,057.83	$43,208.55	$55,428.66	$61,484.06
Net Charges	$19,121.83	$39,283.37	$42,879.61	$63,448.93
Gross Charges/Day	$4,207.94	$4,303.81	$3,770.33	$2,892.93
Total Receipts/Day	$4,611.57	$4,320.86	$3,695.24	$2,673.22
Net Charges/Day	$3,824.37	$3,928.34	$2,858.64	$2,758.65
Monthly Projections				
Gross Charges	$96,782.57	$98,987.61	$86,717.67	$66,537.29
Total Receipts	$106,066.02	$99,379.67	$84,990.61	$61,484.06
Net Charges	$87,960.42	$90,351.75	$65,748.74	$63,448.93
Daily Billing Requirement				
To Reach Goal	$2,437.68	$1,824.36	$2,515.05	($448.93)

Figure 28.8. Productivity goals.

Acme Vision Clinic, P.C.					
Productivity Statistics					
Calendar Year 1997					ANNUAL
	Q1	Q2	Q3	Q4	TOTAL RECEIPTS
Gross Receipts per Quarter	$129,583.49	$134,338.00	$168,492.00	$177,762.00	$610,175.49
Total Variable Costs per Quarter	$48,384.00	$45,260.00	$61,528.00	$62,420.00	$217,592.00
Operating Costs per Quarter	$60,385.00	$57,544.00	$66,093.00	$80,985.00	$265,007.00
Professional Costs per Quarter	$ 42,269.50	$ 40,280.80	$ 46,265.10	$ 56,689.50	$185,504.90
Dispensing Costs per Quarter	$ 18,115.50	$ 17,263.20	$ 19,827.90	$ 24,295.50	$79,502.10
	Q1	Q2	Q3	Q4	ANNUAL TOTALS
Doctor Hours per Quarter	571.56	571.56	571.56	571.56	2286.24
Full Time Staff per Quarter	3	3	3	3	
Part Time Staff per Quarter	0.5	0.5	0.5	0.5	
					ADJUSTED
1997 Examination Fee = $89.00	Quarter 1	Quarter 2	Quarter 3	Quarter 4	YEARLY AVERAGE
Chair Cost per Quarter	$73.95	$70.48	$80.95	$99.18	$81.14
Contribution per Quarter	$81,199.49	$89,078.00	$106,964.00	$115,342.00	$98,145.87
Contribution Margin per Quarter	62.66%	66.31%	63.48%	64.89%	64.33%
Staff Productivity/Hour per Quarter	$79.74	$82.67	$103.69	$109.39	$93.87

Figure 28.9. Productivity statistics.

lyzed over a period of time to evaluate the productivity of the practitioner and staff and the costs of operation, and to calculate the chair cost, contribution margin, and other economic issues of significance (Figure 28.9). Practitioners should use this information to assess the practice's financial performance and to identify where change or improvement is needed.

CONCLUSION

Providing a practice with the proper financial documentation and observing sound financial practices will allow the optometrist to manage and properly assess the practice's financial condition at any time. It will also allow comparisons to industry-wide financial norms. If a practitioner is to be an effective manager, he or she must have the proper reporting methods and financial information available and must use that information to the best effect. U.S. health care has become a highly competitive environment, and, if survival is the rule and numbers are the playing field, then optometrists must be able to grasp basic business concepts and apply them to the eye care industry.

BIBLIOGRAPHY

Classé JG. Legal Aspects of Optometry. Stoneham, MA: Butterworth, 1989.

Dun & Bradstreet Information Services. Industry Norms and Key Business Ratios. Murray Hill, NJ: Dun & Bradstreet Information Services, 1996.

Steinhoff D. Small Business Management Fundamentals (6th ed). New York: McGraw-Hill, 1993.

Part V
Maintaining a Practice

Chapter 29

Marketing

Lawrence S. Thal and Craig Hisaka

You can tell the ideals of a nation by its advertisements.

—Norman Douglas
South Wind

Like a nation, the ideals of an optometric practice can probably be determined by its advertisements. However, advertising should not be confused with marketing. Comparing the definition of these two terms illustrates their differences. As applied to optometry, marketing can be defined as "the total of activities by which the provision of services and transfer of materials from optometrist to patient are effected." In comparison, advertising would be defined as "the art or practice of calling public attention to one's product, service, needs, or related matters—especially by paid announcements in newspapers and magazines or over radio, television, or other media."

As these definitions indicate, an advertisement is a message—printed in a newspaper or magazine, broadcast on radio or television, sent to individuals through the mail, or disseminated in some other fashion—that attempts to convince readers or listeners to favor a particular optometrist or buy a particular product. Surveys of optometrists have revealed that more than 25% of patients choose their optometrist or ophthalmologist on the recommendation of friends and, for an established practice, about 65% of patient flow is derived from previous patients. In many practices, therefore, advertising could be used only to compete for the remaining 10% of patients. This might explain why many practitioners have concluded that advertisements, in the long run, do not really increase earnings.

It is because of marketing, not advertising, that the majority of patients continue to return to optometrists year after year for care. The goal of marketing is to acquire, satisfy, and retain patients. It is clear that optometrists who understand the needs of their patients and seek to satisfy them tend to be more successful than optometrists who do not. While marketing has evolved into a potentially complex and diverse field, which includes a wide variety of special functions—such as advertising, public relations, market research, and so forth—the basic needs of most patients are not usually complex. Their needs are best satisfied by listening, providing education, and being able to convey a caring attitude. It is unfortunate that patients are usually not qualified to determine how much a practitioner knows. It is easy, however, for a patient to gain a sense of how much a practitioner cares.

EXTERNAL MARKETING

The most commonly used external marketing technique is advertising.

Advertising

The aim of advertising is to influence consumer choice. A magazine, television program, or any

297

other advertising medium is judged by an advertiser according to "exposure opportunity"—the number of people who might see the advertisement—and "message opportunity"—the way an advertisement communicates via a particular medium.

In considering "exposure," advertisers speak of "reach," which signifies the number of people who see the advertisement at least once, and of "frequency," which is the average number of times each person is "reached." An advertisement's total impact is indicated by its number of "gross impressions"—reach times frequency. A further aspect of exposure is cost, which is usually stated as "cost per thousand gross impressions" (CPM). Another aspect is "target reach," which is the number of people within a specific audience who have seen the advertisement. Often, advertisers want to reach only one segment of an audience—for example, women, teenagers, presbyopic individuals, or new residents of a particular community. Exposure, reach, and frequency are factors that influence the selection of advertising media, including television, radio, newspapers, magazines, or direct mail.

Television provides high exposure and low CPM. It is not efficient for specific targets. Because it supplies sound, pictures, and movement, it offers the most complete message opportunity. Unlike printed media, however, its messages are ephemeral, disappearing after being broadcast. Television earns approximately 21% of total advertising expenditures in the United States.

Television is the most striking communications medium in the world today, and radio is listened to as never before. Exposure through broadcast media reaches an extensive audience. Television and radio stations often allot time for public service programming, including interviews and listener call-in shows. These formats are excellent opportunities for participation as an eye care expert.

Radio is good for targeting various geographic, age, or interest groups. Its CPM is very low. Like television, its messages are conveyed only when being broadcast. Because radio offers nothing but sound, it is the most limited medium. Radio earns approximately 7% of the total advertising expenditures in the United States.

Broadcast promotion is expensive and requires considerable expertise in writing, production, and media selection. To be effective, broadcast promotions must air for a sustained length of time. Intermittent announcements are costly and often ineffective. With the exception of those practitioners who have practices in extremely competitive environments, most optometrists find the paid use of broadcast media to be expensive and unnecessary.

Newspapers have much lower exposure than television or radio but reach a higher percentage of the areas they cover. They are excellent for geographic targeting. Newspapers earn the highest proportion of total advertising expenditures (approximately 30%). Many optometrists have instituted media relations programs, which consist of sending short news releases to local newspapers on a regular, year-round basis. The news release usually offers helpful eye care advice or provides information on optometric public service activities. By sending out releases on a regular basis, the optometrists establish visibility and credibility among editors, increasing the probability that they will be written about in the newspapers or consulted on eye-related articles.

Other optometrists have received positive media exposure by supplying an eye care column for the local newspaper. The American Optometric Association (AOA) offers a series of columns with accompanying art work for this purpose.

Paid announcements in large newspapers and magazines are usually not necessary for most optometric practices. When used, announcements must be published over a substantial period of time to attract attention, gain acceptance, and foster recall. Many optometrists find that other, more targetable communications are more effective.

Magazines provide less exposure than television, radio, or newspapers but are highly selective with respect to audience interests. Magazines reproduce more attractively than newspapers, but newspapers are printed more frequently. Magazines earn approximately 9% of total advertising expenditures in the United States.

Direct mail is not inexpensive, but it is the most selective of all media. The advertiser typically uses mailing lists containing only the names of people within the selected audience. Listings are chosen for particular features, such as age, geography, sex, income, or other characteristics. Direct mail can offer lengthy messages, but it has the disadvantage of being easily discarded by the recipient before being examined. Direct mail earns approximately 14% of total advertising expenditures in the United States.

A variety of printed materials can be used effectively to keep the optometrist's name before current patients and to raise his or her profile in the community. Some proven strategies include the use of brochures and pamphlets, literature published by the AOA, letters and mailings, news releases, practice newsletters, personal letters, and telephone listings.

Brochures and Pamphlets

Distributing educational brochures is an excellent way to increase patient and community awareness of professional services, to build an identity with civic and community organizations, and to educate and inform individual consumers. Sending brochures not only gets eye care information into patients' homes but at the same time reminds them that the practitioner is a concerned professional. Patients might pass the brochure on to neighbors or friends—all potential patients.

Regardless of where or when literature is distributed, it is important for it to contain the practitioner's identity. Literature should be tastefully printed with the optometrist's name, office address, and telephone number, making it easy for a recipient to obtain more information or make an appointment.

AOA Literature

An excellent source of educational literature is the American Optometric Association. Member optometrists can obtain professionally written and designed materials covering nearly every aspect of eye care.

Letters and Mailings

Another effective technique for keeping a continuous flow of information to patients is to create special mailings. Birthdays, holidays, and other special occasions offer opportunities for optometrists to personalize their relationship with patients.

News Releases

Many optometrists have found that sending news releases to local newspapers is an effective public relations strategy. A news release might focus on a new staff member or associate, a new service, a screening that the optometrist is sponsoring, or a human interest story about the optometrist or one of the optometrist's patients.

Practice Newsletter

Newsletters are versatile, economical, and well-received marketing tools. They help the optometrist keep in touch with patients between office visits and provide information about the office staff, patients, new products and services, and advances in eye care.

Personal Letters

Personal letters or announcements, sent to patients and referral sources, are good vehicles for announcing a new location, additional services, a new partner or associate, or a change in office hours. Direct mail adds importance to an announcement that otherwise might be hidden in a newsletter.

In general, printed media—newspapers, magazines, or direct mail—offer a significant advantage: They can be saved for future reference.

Telephone Listing

Another form of printed media is the telephone book. The Yellow Pages is the one form of advertising that all optometrists use. There are two types of Yellow Pages listings—trademark listings and display advertising. The trademark listing is a 1-inch by 1-column advertisement that can include a name line, a certain number of words, and the logo of a society, with a listing of local members beneath it. A display advertisement can be up to half a page in size and can refer readers to the trademark listing. Regardless of whether an optometrist chooses to use a display advertisement, a trademark listing for the local optometric society is considered a necessity.

While advertising is a very effective method for reaching a large audience quickly, it is an extremely expensive option for most health care professionals. By effectively using less aggressive and less costly communication techniques, many op-

Table 29.1. Sample Marketing Plan for an Optometric Practice

Mission statement

To provide high-quality, reasonably priced primary eye care with special emphasis on services for children, and to educate patients and the community about the importance of ongoing, routine eye care.

Goal #1

Attract 50 patients (under age 12) during the next 6 months by improving communications with parents of school-aged children.

    Strategy: Write articles for practice newsletter on eye conditions that affect children. Emphasize the practice's special expertise in diagnosing and treating these problems.

    Strategy: Write a news release for the local newspaper discussing children's eye problems and treatments.

    Strategy: Volunteer to speak at a meeting of a parent-teacher organization or other community group whose members are parents of school-aged children.

    Strategy: Organize a children's eye screening at a local shopping center, or participate in community-wide health-screening or "Save Your Vision Week" event.

Goal #2:

In the next 12 months, make children's frames account for 20% of dispensary business.

    Strategy: Increase by 20% the number of children's frames in the dispensary.

    Strategy: Create a children's corner in the dispensary with special decor and display area.

    Strategy: Write an article for practice newsletter on children's frames—e.g., special features, how to select children's frames. Create an attractive "fact sheet" using this same information, and display it prominently in the office or use as a handout to parents of school-aged children.

Source: Adapted from Allergan, Inc. Pathways in Optometry. Irvine, CA: Allergan, 1994.

tometrists find that a telephone directory listing is the only form of paid promotion they need to market their practices. If a practitioner decides to use some form of advertising, however, it will be necessary to devise a marketing plan.

COMPONENTS OF A MARKETING PLAN

There are four parts to a marketing plan: mission statement, goals, strategies, and tactical plan. A sample marketing plan is illustrated in Table 29.1.

Mission Statement

The mission statement describes the basic purpose of the practice and what the optometrist seeks to accomplish through it. The marketing goals break down the mission statement into the five or six major tasks that the practitioner will have to accomplish to achieve or come close to achieving the mission. Once the practitioner has set these goals, the ways in which they will be met can be established. These methods constitute the practitioner's marketing strategies. After strategies have been set,

the practitioner can develop a tactical plan to implement each strategy.

Marketing Goals

Before a practitioner decides on marketing goals, the current marketing situation must be analyzed. For example, the practitioner might want to work with young children and increase the number of patients seen so that more than 50% of the practice is devoted to pediatric care. If the school population is decreasing, however, and if there are several other optometrists in the community who specialize in pediatric care, this goal might not be realistic. Therefore, goals must reflect reality. That reality includes the opportunities and problems that impact on the practice.

Suppose, for example, that a department store chain is going to offer eye care at a shopping mall near a practitioner's office. The optometrist might see this as a real threat—patients could be lost to the store. In response, the practitioner might set a goal to minimize the risk that the store represents to the practice. On the other hand, the optometrist might see department store eye care as an opportunity. It could be a chance for the practitioner to highlight and contrast the services being offered by his or her practice compared to those offered by the store. By having this store nearby, the practitioner can capitalize on the differences. Either way, the practitioner has identified the effect that this external factor has on the practice and can plan to respond to it.

Marketing Strategies

Strategies are the way that a practitioner meets the goals that have been set. Strategies are based on target markets, competitive position, and the marketing mix.

Before selecting a strategy, two things must be decided about the current market. First: Is the practitioner going to provide services to all segments of the market, or will the practitioner concentrate marketing efforts on one particular target segment? Second: Should the practitioner choose to target one or more market segments, and which would they be? The major benefit of target marketing is that it allows the practitioner to concentrate marketing efforts and resources.

Another factor that affects the selection of strategies is the marketing mix. There are four basic considerations. An optometrist's "service" is eye care, "place" is the setting in which that care is delivered, "price" is the fee charged for services, and "promotion" refers to the way the practitioner communicates with current and potential patients. The practitioner analyzes each of the four areas and looks for ways to enhance them when formulating marketing strategies.

Only after a practitioner has analyzed the market and formulated goals is that practitioner ready to begin marketing activities. Participating in marketing activities without a clear set of goals is a scatter-shot approach, one that can keep the practitioner busy without producing significant results.

ADVERTISING EFFECTIVENESS

A 1991 study of the amount spent on advertising by 3,432 California optometrists in solo practice found several characteristics to be statistically significant. Practices that spent the most on advertising had:

- More patients seen per week
- More total time spent fitting contact lenses
- Less time spent with individual patients receiving contact lenses
- Higher gross income
- More technicians employed
- Lower fees
- Less time spent per patient examination
- Less time spent on health portions of examinations
- Patients on a more frequent recall schedule

Practices that spent the least on advertising had:

- More time spent per patient examination
- Higher net-to-gross income ratio
- Larger patient backlog

Because many studies of advertising effectiveness have been performed, with highly variable results reported, it is left to each practitioner to determine how to use advertising within a specific community. Since an advertisement conveys the ideals of a practice, a practitioner must be very careful not to damage an otherwise good public impression. Advertising can actually be destructive if it is aimed at a target audience but is considered inappropriate by that audience. Most Americans have seen advertising that they find to be offensive. While it can be assumed that an advertisement in poor taste will alienate consumers from the product, the advertiser who uses it has apparently been convinced that this method of advertising is, in fact, effective.

An example of advertising with a poor effect is "price advertising." Lower prices are thought to be synonymous with lower quality. As some ophthalmic chains have found, the power of advertising—when based strictly on cost—does not serve the advertiser in the long run. Although price advertising is known to be effective in building a short-term response, it can also destroy the consumer's perception of the advertiser's professional abilities, hindering the advertiser's capacity to develop a loyal customer base for the long term. As a result, the traditional means of attracting patients to chains—advertising low prices, convenience, and variety of products—has not met with long-term success.

Some of the commercial chains have, in fact, chosen to abandon the discount market—a small

Table 29.2. Example State Restrictions on Advertising

- Optometrists must be able to substantiate all claims made in advertisements and any claims must be accurate. It is unlawful to disseminate any form of public communication containing a false, fraudulent, misleading, or deceptive statement.
- Guarantees, if stated, must be adhered to and spelled out.
- Reference to price in an advertisement should be exact. Terms such as "from $19.99," "as little as," or "as low as," should not be used since these are potentially misleading.
- Advertising professional superiority or advertising that an optometrist performs professional services in a superior manner is prohibited.
- It is illegal to employ or use solicitors (cappers or steerers).
- It is illegal to advertise professional services as being free or without cost.
- If costs of services are mentioned, they should be clearly identifiable. All variables and other material factors should be specifically disclosed.
- The price advertised for products should include charges for any related professional services, including dispensing and fitting services, unless the advertisement specifically and clearly indicates otherwise.

Source: Authors' review of state optometry laws, 1995.

and low-profit segment of the industry—in favor of advertising campaigns aimed toward the value market, which is made up of patients who desire quality care. This market belongs largely to independent optometrists, who in the 1990s are estimated to provide 52% of all eye examinations and 43% of all eyewear.

State laws and board rules can include specific regulations about advertising. They should be consulted before an advertising program is initiated as part of a marketing effort.

LEGAL AND ETHICAL ASPECTS OF ADVERTISING

Optometry boards have a long history of opposition to advertising. Despite the advent of precedent-setting decisions by the United States Supreme Court recognizing the right of professionals to advertise, boards may continue to initiate actions to prevent unfair or deceptive advertising of ophthalmic goods or services.

The ban on advertising by professionals began in the 1930s. In the 1950s the U.S. Supreme Court stated that it could "see no constitutional reason why a state may not treat all who deal with the human eye as members of a profession who should use no merchandising methods for obtaining customers." In the majority of states, the high court's opinion resulted in laws or board rulings that prohibited or restricted advertising by optometrists.

Deceptive tactics that led to these restrictive state statutes and regulations included "bait and switch" advertising. Cut-rate prices would be advertised by the business, but the low-priced items would be either "unavailable" or "unsuitable" for the potential purchaser, who would end up buying an expensive item instead. Another reprehensible tactic was "capping and steering," in which advertising was used to lure people seeking ophthalmic materials to an unscrupulous practitioner. After the practitioner had "capped" the individual by determining the spectacle prescription, the individual was "steered" to the business for the sale of expensive eyewear. Underlying these and other despicable practices was the power of advertising, which, although undeniably abused, achieved its single purpose—to attract business. Advertising is not profitable unless a volume business is sought, and it is this fundamental purpose of advertising that is at odds with the concept of professionalism.

Since the 1970s the Supreme Court has recognized that certain commercial advertising by professionals should be afforded constitutional protection. However, states are still allowed to set reasonable restrictions to ensure that consumers receive truthful and nondeceptive advertising (Table 29.2).

Advertising by optometrists might be required to include certain information. Examples of these requirements are provided in Table 29.3. Exact provisions vary from state to state, and state laws and board regulations must be consulted to determine the specific restrictions in any particular jurisdiction.

COMMUNITY OUTREACH

A community outreach program involves offering eye care and education. Among the most common and proven methods for community outreach are participation in eye care events and health fairs, and the use of public speaking.

Eye Care Events

A well-organized special event can focus much attention on eye care within a short period, and it offers many opportunities to inform consumers about optometry.

There are also several national eye care events that provide optometrists with an ideal opportunity to build public exposure while offering a much-needed public service. The AOA-sponsored "Save Your Vision Week" is announced by Presidential proclamation each year and takes place during the first full week of March. A major focal point of this event is "Give One Day," which promotes volunteer services for working individuals who are in need of eye care but not covered by insurance.

The AOA offers several tools to help practitioners participate in such events. Planning guides for national events, such as "Save Your Vision Week" and "Older Americans Month," are included in the *AOA News* periodically.

Especially effective are screenings for vision problems, cataracts, and glaucoma. Screenings attract positive attention from the media, as well as from potential patients. Target populations, such as high school athletes, children, or older adults, are excellent choices for screening programs. Good locations for vision screenings include schools, senior centers, banks, and shopping malls.

Different opportunities for exposure also arise at other times of the year. For example, an optometrist can volunteer to screen local high school football and basketball players. In many states, high school athletes must be given a physical examination before the start of the season. The optometrist might be able to work with local physicians and other health care providers while providing this service.

Health Fairs

Health fairs present excellent marketing opportunities for the optometrist. Most health fairs are sponsored by at least one health-oriented group, such as a hospital or health organization. National Health Fair Week, which takes place in the spring, is sup-

Table 29.3. Example Requirements for Optometric Advertising

- Statement of the practioner's name or the corporate name.
- Statement of the office's addresses and telephone numbers.
- Statement of regular office hours.
- Statement of languages, other than English, fluently spoken by the practitioner or a person in the practitioner's office.
- Statement that the practitioner limits the practice to specific fields.
- Statement that the practitioner provides services under a specified private or public insurance plan or health care plan.
- Statement of schools and postgraduate clinical training programs from which the practitioner has graduated, with the degrees received.
- Statement of publications authored by the practitioner.
- Statement of teaching positions currently or formerly held by the practitioner, with pertinent dates.
- Statement of affiliations with hospitals or clinics.
- Statement of charges or fees for services or commodities offered by the practitioner.
- Statement that the practitioner regularly accepts installment payments.
- Picture of a practitioner, office, or ophthalmic materials, but not of a person with an eye disease or injury.
- Picture of a person wearing eyeglasses or contact lenses.
- Statement of the manufacturer, designer, style, make, trade name, brand name, color, size, or type of commodities advertised.
- Statement, or statements, providing public health information encouraging preventative or corrective care.
- Statement of all optometrists' names practicing at the designated location when an optometrist or an optometric corporation uses a fictitious name.

Source: Authors' review of state optometry laws, 1995.

ported by thousands of national, regional, and local groups that represent all levels of government; media; business and industry; and health, academic, and civic organizations.

Speaking Engagements

As a doctor of optometry, a practitioner is considered an expert in eye care in the community. As part of a public relations program, optometrists should endeavor to speak to as many groups as possible. To obtain speaking opportunities, practitioners can volunteer to be part of the speakers bureau of a state or local optometric association.

Speaking engagements offer the advantage of a meeting with a large audience. The practitioner can promote optometry in an informal yet educational way that can provide new patients, while raising the level of consciousness about the need for eye care in the community. To help optometrists become effective speakers, the AOA has developed the *Optometric Speaker's Guidebook* (St. Louis: American Optometric Association, 1978), which contains helpful statistics and guidelines for speech preparation.

In addition to public education, an aim of community outreach is to positively influence the way practitioners and the services provided by practitioners are perceived. This means enhancing the image of optometrists as providers of quality eye care.

INTERNAL MARKETING

Internal marketing involves the dissemination of information to an existing patient population to educate them about services, ophthalmic materials, new developments, and related matters that will motivate patients to return for further care.

Patient Perceptions

Patients can perceive changes. The most common and obvious change is when the practitioner decreases the time spent with patients. When this "quality time" begins to diminish, patients often remark, "When the doctor started the practice, he spent time with me. The doctor cared for his patients, but now the doctor is just too busy." The underlying message is that the practitioner is too busy to care anymore and, perhaps, is "chasing the dollar." Today, it is very common to hear patients openly complain about "greed among doctors" and how they miss their old doctor, their old optometrist, or their old dentist. They feel that these practitioners cared about their patients, always had time, and showed compassion for them. What a sad commentary about our generation of health care providers—technically more skillful, but lacking in care and compassion for their patients.

The key to successful internal marketing is to adopt a philosophy that is committed to furthering the best interests of patients, to treating patients in the same manner as we would all wish to be treated, and to maintaining that philosophy.

Public opinion surveys regarding doctor-patient relationships come to the same conclusion over and over. Patients are most infuriated when practitioners convey an impression that they don't care. Such an attitude is indicated when patients comment that a practitioner:

- "Doesn't care about the patients' feelings or personal comfort"
- "Is impressed with his or her own importance"
- "Is cold, distant, and patronizing"
- "Acts as though he or she knows everything"
- "Is a terrible listener"
- "Causes undue waiting, with no respect for the patient's time"
- "Is abrupt, rude, and rushed"
- "Turns patients over to a technician"
- "Has bad personal habits and mannerisms"
- "Gave the impression that I was just another patient and didn't remember my name"
- "Had an overcrowded waiting room"
- "Used too many technical terms"
- "Has inconvenient hours, parking, and location"
- "Speaks too fast or too slow; has pauses that go unnoticed; repeatedly clears the throat; speaks in a monotone; has a high-pitched voice; uses sloppy speech patterns; drops consonants; and slurs pronunciation"
- "Makes it seem like an assembly line—interest in money, not in patients"
- "Is disrespectful to patients and staff"
- "Didn't listen or give me enough time"
- "Belittled me and treated me like a child"

How to Obtain Patient Referrals

It has been said that a satisfied patient is one who gets what was bargained for—competent and skilled services—and that an enthusiastic patient is one who gets more than was expected—something "extra." Whenever a patient receives more in return than was given, that patient not only feels that something is owed in return but also feels motivated to reward the practitioner. An enthusiastic patient does this by providing the best form of "advertising"—recommending the practitioner to family and friends—which results in patient referrals.

Extras can make a big difference in the way people feel and respond. Common examples of this difference include the courteous waiter who supplies water, coffee, and other service without being asked and the hotel staff member who performs all the extras that make a stay or vacation a pleasant experience. Many success stories in business have been built on this concept of providing more than was expected. To provide extras, a practitioner should be creative. Being creative does not require genius. It means thinking of those little things that make a difference. For top-quality hotels, it means leaving a newspaper each morning outside the guest's door and allowing easy access to coffee service. For practitioners, it can include keeping a good supply of current magazines in the reception area, allowing patients to take the magazine if they have not finished it, putting coins in the reception room with a sign reading "For the parking meter," having the receptionist call patients to let them know that appointments are running late, and similar courtesies intended to provide that something extra.

A patient fully expects a professional examination. Even if a practitioner has the best technical skills, however, a patient is not competent to judge them. It is also difficult to impress a patient with professional skills because the patient is inevitably more aware of the results than the techniques. If all that is provided is a professional examination, the patient will not complain, but the patient will probably not become an active source of referrals. Taking that extra step makes for an enthusiastic patient. Because of this often subtle distinction, the line is very thin that separates a successful practice from a mediocre practice.

To increase patient referrals, a practitioner must learn to reinforce services by adding psychological value. For example, if appreciation is shown to a patient for having made a referral, it will increase the likelihood that the patient will recommend the practitioner again. The more unique, personal, and individual a practitioner can make each "thank you," the more the patient will feel appreciated. One reason a "thank you" provides powerful reinforcement is that gratitude itself is an "extra," a bonus. Also, if a patient is a frequent source of referrals, something extra is truly required—such as flowers, a plant, or some other small gift that shows appreciation for the patient's support. It is important to send "thank you" notes to professional colleagues who provide referrals. In such cases, the practitioner should endeavor to turn the referred patient into an "enthusiastic" patient—the referring professional's reputation is also at stake.

Another way to increase referrals is by hiring friendly, outgoing assistants. This can help build referrals in two ways. First, the assistant is the first one to provide a greeting when the patient enters the office and the last one to say goodbye. Having a cheerful assistant can leave a good, lasting impression on patients. The cheerful assistant also helps others in the office become more cheerful and friendly. The second way the assistant helps is outside the office. When the assistant talks about the practice to family, neighbors, and friends, a positive message will be conveyed about the practitioner and optometry.

Internal marketing involves sharing information with patients. Various means can be used to provide this information. The most common have already been identified—brochures, newsletters, personal letters, and the like. But more personalized means of marketing involve the sharing of information and time with patients, often while the patient is in the office. Examples include:

- Showing deep consideration for a patient's time
- Providing a sympathetic and caring demeanor in direct ratio to the concerns and fears of each patient
- Being available to come to the phone
- Giving what is free to give (pharmaceutical samples will be much more appreciated by patients than by family members or personal friends)
- Giving what is not free to give (e.g., a magazine that the patient did not get to finish reading)
- Charting a patient's personal interests and family situation
- Being effusive in acknowledging gifts from patients
- Having a duplicate set of patient education materials in each examination room and in the patient consultation room
- Keeping a suggestion box in the office for both patient and staff use
- Being on time

- Learning all that can be learned about the patient
- Impressing the patient with a cohesive team
- Taking the time to teach the patient habits for better health, even if not eye related
- Having a good physical appearance and dressing professionally
- Offering something more in the waiting room than old magazines (do not overlook a professional journal that is less technical)
- Avoiding patient surprises by explaining what is going to be done before it is attempted
- Communicating clearly and honestly
- Treating patients as equals
- Having the receptionist convey an attitude of appreciation (the last thing a patient needs to hear after paying the bill is a sincere "thank you")
- Touching patients (practitioners should make it a point to greet patients with a handshake or pat at the first and last encounter in the office)

Having a good bedside manner will result in a direct positive financial impact on the practice. Patients will be retained longer, and a higher rate of patient referrals will be generated.

Other suggestions for that something extra to increase patient enthusiasm include:

- Before performing any procedure, explain in advance what is going to be done, why it is going to be done, and what the patient can expect to happen. Always explain the benefits of a procedure to the patient.
- Provide an extra service. If it is late and if it is appropriate, ask where the patient is parked and offer to provide an escort. If there is an emergency and the patient needs new glasses, lives near the office, but cannot come in, offer to deliver the glasses to the patient.
- The finishing touch of any eye examination or office visit is a "thank you!"

Today, most patients want information from their optometrists. They desire to take an active role and participate in their own well-being. They want a sense of control, which includes the use of options and alternatives. Many polls and surveys indicate that consumers feel that the "best doctors are those who explain in a manner that the consumer understands." It is also true that most patients who are dissatisfied will not return to complain.

In contemporary health care, decreases in reimbursement rates, decreases in "market share" due to competition, rising costs of operating a practice, costs of expensive technological instrumentation, economic recession, and other economic factors have forced many practitioners to decrease the time spent with patients. This can "dehumanize" the practice. In such practices, the practitioner allocates time to solve the patients' optometric, medical, or dental problems, but the time to "bond" with patients is significantly reduced or eliminated. The result is that the patient perceives the practitioner to have a "quantity" practice rather than a "quality" practice.

The major difference between a quality practice and a quantity practice is that in a quality practice, the range of services is emphasized to a limited number of patients while in a quantity practice the emphasis is on patient volume, with limited services and procedures being provided. In a quality practice, growth results in an upward curve that accelerates at an increasingly faster rate until the demands on the practitioner reach a point of diminishing returns, resulting in a slowing and eventual flattening of growth. As the quality of services begins to deteriorate, there will inevitably be a decline in the number of referrals, and patients will begin to seek services from other practitioners. The reason will be the "dehumanization" of the practice, brought on by the demands of quantity and resulting in decreased time and attention for each patient.

CONCLUSION

Marketing is a useful tool to help build and maintain a patient base. Through the use of marketing techniques, the practitioner can communicate with patients, prospective and established, while conveying a positive image of the practice and the profession. The use of marketing plans is an accepted part of professional practice, and practitioners should make use of external and internal marketing techniques as appropriate for their setting and circumstances. It should never be forgotten, however, that the most successful practices are built on the basis of service and that such practices provide something extra that sets them apart from their competitors. There are no marketing techniques that can satisfy patients and motivate them to return for future care if this highly personal element, inherent in the doctor-patient relationship, is not provided.

BIBLIOGRAPHY

Allergan, Inc. Pathways in Optometry. Irvine, CA: Allergan, 1994.

Bagdasar S, Chew I, Smith C, et al. The Relationship Between Practice Characteristics of Solo Practices and Amount Spent on Advertising: An Analysis of the California Survey of 1988. An unpublished thesis submitted in partial fulfillment of the requirements for the degree, Doctor of Optometry, University of California at Berkeley, School of Optometry, 1991.

Classé J. Legal Aspects of Optometry. Stoneham, MA: Butterworth, 1989.

Elmstrom G. Advanced Management for Optometrists. Chicago: Professional Press, 1974.

Levoy RP. The $100,000 Practice and How to Build It. Englewood Cliffs, NJ: Prentice-Hall, 1966.

Pinto JB, Shepard DD. Marketing Your Ophthalmic Practice. Thorofare, NJ: Slack, 1987.

Chapter 30

Quality Assurance

Craig Hisaka

There is nothing that any man can make
that another man cannot make cheaper.

—John Ruskin
Unto This Last

The assurance of quality in health care would seem to be guaranteed by the various regulatory mechanisms established by the government and the professions. Unfortunately, over the past few decades government has increasingly looked at health care as an expenditure that must be reduced—often without fully considering the effect on quality. The health care professions have been reluctant to institute aggressive quality assurance programs and have consistently resisted government regulatory efforts. The result has been a lack of attention to the problems posed by quality assurance in the private practice setting.

Because of these evolving changes in the U.S. health care system, the question must be asked: "Can private practitioners survive the next decade in a highly competitive marketplace, with increased commercialization of health care services and in the face of rising costs and decreasing revenues?" These are formidable obstacles. Therefore, to survive the next decade and to thrive despite the competitiveness of the environment, optometrists must rely and refocus on traditional values—cultivating the doctor-patient relationship, making decisions that best serve the interests of patients, and providing high-quality care. This chapter discusses some of the problems that confound the delivery of care in today's competitive environment and describes a record review process

that can be used by private practitioners to provide quality assurance.

ADOPTION OF A PHILOSOPHY OF CARE

Each practitioner should develop a philosophy about patient care (Table 30.1). These feelings should be put into words and transformed into a concept of care for a practice. Doctors' philosophies of care are rarely analyzed, tested, or defined.

Moreover, there appear to be few mechanisms of accountability for health care services while almost all other products and services provided in society are constantly scrutinized by consumer groups, government agencies, and media. A business that provides substandard services or products is usually exposed for its shortcomings. In contrast, health care has been one of the few segments of society in which providers offering services have enjoyed considerable autonomy from this type of exposure. In addition, health care providers have, in many cases, failed to practice self-policing. To provide "quality care" is always a goal of practice, but it is not always achieved. Practitioners must devise workable means of ensuring that quality is provided, even in the face of economic pressures that tend to exert an opposing effect.

Table 30.1. Sample Philosophy of Care

- Provide thorough visual analysis with the most modern technology and instrumentation.
- Provide health education models, photographs, and slides.
- Allow for 1-hour examinations: an extensive case history and consultation are taken in an office before every examination, which is performed in a separate and adjacent room (to personalize the care).
- Make followup telephone calls to determine whether the treatment solved the problem (by the doctor).
- Write letters to school nurses, physicians, and other health care providers regarding findings that are significant and relevant to the care, treatment, and best interest of patients.
- Organize office so that patients are seen punctually. If a patient is more than 15 minutes late, the appointment is rescheduled, making tardiness rare.
- Commit to continuing education for maintenance and update of knowledge and skills.

IDENTIFYING CHALLENGES TO QUALITY CARE

There are several areas of practice in which the challenge to provide quality care is most evident—clinical problem solving, adhering to the standard of care, providing appropriate ophthalmic materials, and billing properly for services.

Clinical Problem Solving

The examination is a problem-solving exercise. Every patient schedules an examination for a specific reason. It might be because of a refractive problem or because of ocular pathology, or because the patient just feels it is time for an evaluation. This chief complaint voiced by the patient must be addressed during the examination. The practitioner attempts to determine the cause of the chief complaint and devises a means of addressing it. Therefore the diagnosis and treatment plan, and how well they relate to the chief complaint, are essential components of any effort to ensure quality. The patient record must reflect that the problem solving was directed at the chief complaint, and there must be a clear treatment regimen for the problem found.

The reimbursement of practitioners by third parties for eye care services also depends on this rela-

tionship. Where patient records do not indicate the link between complaint and findings or even the appropriate level of examination, payment will be withheld or denied.

Adhering to the Standard of Care

During the ocular health examination, the practitioner must adhere to the standard of care. This standard is often described as "doing what a reasonable practitioner would do under the same or similar circumstances." Whether the patient is receiving an annual examination, a follow-up assessment for the treatment of glaucoma, or a contact lens progress check, the practitioner must adhere to reasonable standards for examination and management.

During an eye health assessment a practitioner usually screens for existing pathology and establishes a baseline against which to measure future changes. Both of these functions need to be accomplished in accordance with professional standards. To do so requires that the practitioner keep up with the changing elements of optometric care. Keeping up with these changes requires a commitment to learning on the part of the optometrist, and this leads to several assumptions.

First, the equipment used for pathology detection must be current. Advances in stereo viewing, in visual field analysis, in viewing the interior of the eye, and in recording and documentation of ocular pathology have significantly improved the ability to detect and measure eye disease. Repeatability is important if change is to be measured, monitored, and interpreted by the treating optometrist. Current technology provides for more accurate and cost-effective examinations. A practice must be prepared to invest in technology for pathology detection (e.g., binocular indirect ophthalmoscope, automated perimetry, retinal cameras), and this technology must be incorporated into routine visual analysis.

A second assumption is that the proper techniques will be used during examination. Quite often, proper examination requires that pharmaceutical agents be used. Tonometry, dilation of the pupil, and gonioscopy are common procedures that require the use of pharmaceutical agents. To survive and thrive in the next decade, a practice needs to incorporate into its concept of care the use of these agents. Informing and educating patients about the relationship between these agents and the quality of examination should be a goal of every practitioner.

Third, to provide quality care, there is an inevitable effect on patient scheduling. Adequate time must be allocated for examinations, and patient flow must be planned to make efficient use of patient time in the office.

Providing Ophthalmic Materials

Refractive services are the cornerstone of optometric care, and the usual end result of these services is the prescribing of ophthalmic materials. To provide quality care, these materials—spectacles, contact lenses, low vision devices—must be accurate and appropriate for the patient's needs. Every practice is required to verify lens orders to ensure that they meet appropriate standards for accuracy before dispensing. Well-run practices will also determine the percentage of lens orders that result in remakes because of errors by the practitioner or adaptation problems by patients.

Quality assurance concerns go beyond these matters to consider more fundamental issues. Do the clinical findings justify the prescribing of eyewear? Were the appropriate lens material and frame type prescribed? Was the proper use of the eyewear explained and documented? Does the patient record reflect that the materials were verified before dispensing? Practitioners must determine the answers to these questions by a record review.

Payment for Services

Proper billing for payment for services is a necessary component of quality care. The traditional method of payment, fee for service, is rapidly being replaced by third-party payment. Payment for eye care services by third parties has had a significant impact on examinations by private practitioners. For example, a third-party payer will set the fees for an examination and will establish a reimbursable recall schedule. The practitioner is obligated to do what the plan requires to be reimbursed for services, but the plan should not dictate the exact scope of the examination or when the patient is to be recalled for periodic followup. Otherwise, a conflict is created, and the following question

arises: Is the clinical decision-making process based on reimbursement and economics, or is the clinical decision-making process based on what is in the best interest of the patient?

Through a record review process, the practitioner can identify whether examination decisions are based on concerns about reimbursement or on quality of care. If patients whose examinations are paid for by third parties receive a lower quality of care than patients who pay for examinations themselves, quality care is not being ensured. The practitioner must change the care for patients on the third-party program (or quit the program). Legally, the quality of care does not depend on the amount being paid for services, and a practitioner cannot provide unequal services to patients based on the amount of reimbursement for services.

Systematic Record Review

Before beginning the record review process, it should be recognized that the purpose is to determine if quality care is being provided. The exercise should be planned and carried out periodically, depending on the needs of the practice—a reasonable goal is at least once annually.

The review can easily be carried out in half a day and can be performed solely by the practitioner or by practitioner and staff or exclusively by staff members.

To begin the review, a reasonable number of records of patients seen over the preceding year should be randomly selected. The number of records pulled should probably constitute 5% of the patients seen. For example, if 2,000 full examinations were performed, about 100 records should be obtained.

The practitioner needs to make a checklist for examiners to follow (Figure 30.1). This checklist enables the examiners to look for specific items during the review and to mark findings on a relative scale. Examiners must be instructed in what to look for and how to mark the checklist. Usually, all that is needed is to go through the review of a few records with the examiners for them to learn how to use the checklist. Then, each examiner is assigned a certain number of records and marks the checklist for each one reviewed. At the conclusion of the exercise, the completed checklists are given to the practitioner.

Optometry Record Audit Form

Reviewer: Laura Leah

Review Date: 4/24/96

Scoring
0 = not met; 1 = partially met; 2 = fully met
No score if item was not necessary

Chart	Doctor (first init & last name)	Patient (both initials & last four)	Patient history (& reason for visit)	Neuro screening (pupils, EOM, VF)	Best corrected visual acuity	External exam, or Slit lamp exam	Tonometry	Internal exam, or (DFE)	Additional tests (as needed)	Diagnosis	Management (treatment)	Pt/Fam health ed (as needed)	Average
1	M. Harris	T. Patterson	1	2	2	2	2	2		2	2	2	
2	M. Harris	C. Roberts	2	2	2	2	2	2		2	2	2	
3	M. Harris	J. Wallace	2	2	2	2	2	2	1	2	2	1	
4	M. Harris	E. Langford	2	2	2	2	2	2		2	2	2	
5	M. Harris	E. Ferrell	2	2	2	2	2	2		2	2	0	
6	M. Harris	O. Cochran	2	2	2	2	2	2	2	2	2	0	
7	M. Harris	J. Renfroe	1	2	2	2	2	2		2	2	2	
8													
9													
10													
	Average												

Comment as needed on reverse side

Figure 30.1. Sample quality assurance audit form. (Courtesy of Lyman Norden, OD.)

Examination of the checklist should allow the practitioner to determine if:

- The chief complaint was addressed by the diagnosis and treatment
- Examination findings were fully and accurately described
- The diagnosis and treatment were supported by examination findings
- Prescriptions for ophthalmic materials were justified by examination findings
- Billing for services was correct and justified by the procedures performed
- Referrals or recalls were properly managed

The review might reveal that deficiencies or omissions rarely occur or that certain types of errors recur with surprising frequency. The information can be used to correct any clinical or documentary problems that are discovered. In so doing, the quality of care rendered by the practice will be improved.

CONCLUSION

Patients entrust practitioners with their care and rely on practitioners always to do what is best. Despite practitioners' best intentions, the highest quality care might not always be provided. Quality assurance assesses and modifies care to ensure that it meets patient expectations. Perhaps the most difficult aspect of the quality assurance process is taking the time to review records to ascertain if quality care is being provided. Given the growing influence of third-party providers, and the increasing likelihood that they will implement quality assurance measures of their own, it is prudent for private practice optometrists to adopt a record review process. Although time will be required to perform the review and changes might need to be implemented in office procedures, practitioners should not forget that there is one important clinical benefit to be realized by this effort—improvement in the quality of care rendered to patients.

BIBLIOGRAPHY

Bailey RN. The doctor-patient relationship: communication, informed consent and the optometric patient. J Am Optom Assoc 1994;€5(6):418–22.

Drew R. Solving complaints professionally. Optom Econ 1993;3(3):38–40.

Gabel WK. National practitioner data bank. J Am Optom Assoc 1993;64(2):133–5.

Harris MG, Thal LS. Retention of patient records. J Am Optom Assoc 1992;63(6):430–5.

Hubler RS. Confident, competent referrals. Optom Econ 1992;2(8):15–17.

Keller JT. What is the standard of care? J Am Optom Assoc 1991;62(2):88–9.

Lebow KA. Is your planning on target? Optom Econ 1993;3(60):30–4.

Lookabaugh RE. How to double your patient-pleasing power. Optom Manage 1992;27(3):16–20.

Marshall EC. Assurance of quality vision care in alternative health care delivery systems. J Am Optom Assoc 1989;60(11):827–31.

Muellerleile JM. Forms follow function. Optom Econ 1991;1(6):22–6.

Newcomb RD. Total quality improvement (TQI) for optometric practice in the Department of Veterans Affairs (VA). J Am Optom Assoc 1993;64(8):538–42.

Pollard A. QA, UR, and you. Optom Econ 1994; 4(10): 10–14.

Ruskiewicz J. How to keep more powerful patient records. Optom Manage 1993;28(1):47–52.

Schwartz CA. Total quality optometry. Optom Econ 1992;2(9):13–16.

Sherburne SO. Communications breakdown. Optom Econ 1993; 3(3): 24–6.

Shuman B. Quality assurance: the evolution of practice guidelines. N Engl J Optom 1992;44(4):15–17.

Shuman B. Quality assurance: outcome criteria. N Engl J Optom 1993; 45(2):37–40.

Shuman B. Quality assurance: process criteria. N Engl J Optom 1993;45(1):11–14.

Shuman B. Quality assurance: structure criteria. N Engl J Optom 1992;44(5):17–21.

Williams B, Bowen T, Nolan W. Make no-shows a non-issue. Optom Manage 1993;28(8):36–7.

Wingert TA, McAlister WH, Bachman JA. State board requirements for CPR certification for licensure in independent health professions. J Am Optom Assoc 1993;64(2):117–9.

Winslow C. Do you disappear after office hours? Rev Optom 1994;131(4):43–5.

Winslow C. Follow a new road to quality management. Rev Optom 1993;130(11):33–6.

Winslow C. Sensitize your staff, satisfy your patients. Rev Optom 1992;129(10):32–4.

Winslow C. Your staff is the key to practice excellence. Rev Optom 1993;130(12):21–3.

Chapter 31

Risk Management

John G. Classé and Lawrence S. Thal

The die is cast.

—Jean-Paul Sartre
Les Jeux Sont Faits

The need to manage risk is an integral part of health care and is as important to the practitioner in private practice as to the clinician within an institutional setting. Through the use of appropriate communication, testing, and treatment, the risk of injury to patients can be minimized. By providing adequate documentation of care, the details of management can be preserved. Only by attending to both aspects of care—appropriate testing and adequate documentation—can it be said that risk is truly managed.

Risk management, when properly applied, results in optimum patient care. One beneficial effect of proper care is a reduced likelihood of malpractice litigation. Professional liability has become a serious concern for medicine, and this is reflected in the sizable malpractice insurance premiums that physicians must pay. Premiums are a reflection of liability risk and can be used to determine the frequency of claims. In 1989, the average physician in the United States paid $10,950 annually for $1 million of professional liability insurance coverage. Because the litigation risk in ophthalmology is about average for all medical specialties, the cost of professional liability insurance for ophthalmologists is currently about this amount. In comparison, the malpractice risk in optometry is much less, resulting in significantly lower expenditures for premiums.

In 1986, $1 million of professional liability insurance coverage for optometrists cost about $450 per year. A decade later, this premium cost had not substantially changed. Although laws defining the scope of practice for optometrists vary from state to state, there is no differentiation in premium costs based on whether optometrists are permitted to use therapeutic drugs or are limited to diagnostic drugs. The reason can be found in the types of liability claims brought against optometrists (Table 31.1). Most claims for substantial damages allege failure to diagnose disease rather than treatment errors. The most important claims involve failure to diagnose open-angle glaucoma, retinal detachment, and tumors affecting the visual system. Because of the pre-eminence of these diseases, about three-fourths of the claims alleging misdiagnosis of disease involve the posterior segment of the eye. For the anterior segment, injuries to the cornea are the most important. Contact lenses are a significant contributor to corneal injury; in fact, 40–50% of all malpractice claims involve contact lens practice. The majority of these claims are for minor damages, however, with a minority of claims involving bacterial or herpetic injury to the cornea. Ocular injury from shattered spectacle lenses is another cause of malpractice claims. The usual allegation is that polycarbonate plastic should have been prescribed rather than a less impact-resistant lens material. Injury from the adverse effects of ophthalmic drugs is a rare cause of litigation involving optometrists.

Table 31.1. Optometric Malpractice Claims

Misdiagnosis of intraocular disease (56% of claims)
Leading types of claims (in order of significance):
    Glaucoma
        Primary open-angle glaucoma
        Pigmentary glaucoma
        Angle closure glaucoma
    Retinal detachment
    Tumors
        Intraocular tumors
        Brain tumors
    Diabetic retinopathy
    Toxoplasmosis
    Histoplasmosis
Ophthalmic materials (21% of claims)
    Contact lenses
        Complications of lens-related corneal abrasions
        Misdiagnosis of corneal disease
        Misdiagnosis of intraocular disease
        Failure to comply with informed consent (mono-
            vision)
    Spectacles
        Failure to prescribe polycarbonate plastic
        Defective frame design (sports frames)
Misdiagnosis of anterior segment disease (13% of claims)
    Corneal disease
        Herpes simplex
        Fungal infection
    Ocular foreign bodies
    Tumors of the anterior adnexa
Binocular vision practice (8% of claims)
    Failure to treat amblyopia
    Failure to diagnose brain tumors causing strabismus
        or decreased acuity
    Failure to diagnose retinoblastoma causing strabis-
        mus or decreased acuity
Ophthalmic drugs (2% of claims)
    Adverse effects of diagnostic agents

Source: Author's 1996 review of claims. Types of claims are listed in order of decreasing frequency.

Legislative changes in optometry's scope of practice, which have conferred greater clinical and legal responsibilities on optometrists, have caused remarkably little alteration in the profession's liability posture. Before the 1970s, when state legislatures began to amend optometry practice acts to permit the use of drugs, the cost of malpractice insurance coverage represented less than 1% of an optometrist's net income. Current premium costs remain at the same level—less than 1% of net income. Risk management seeks to maintain this favorable liability posture for the profession.

ELEMENTS OF PROFESSIONAL LIABILITY

To apply risk management to the practice of optometry, the legal elements of malpractice must be understood. Malpractice is more properly termed "medical negligence." It is a civil action brought by an injured party seeking monetary compensation. If negligence is alleged in a professional liability claim, the injured party (the plaintiff) must establish that:

- The doctor-patient relationship existed.
- The defendant practitioner did not act reasonably (conduct is measured against the "standard of care," which is the conduct that is deemed to be reasonable under the circumstances by members of the profession).
- There was actual physical injury to the patient (e.g., loss of visual acuity, visual field, or ocular motility).
- There was a legal link between the practitioner's act (or failure to act) and the patient's injury (termed "proximate cause").

All four elements must be supported by the preponderance of the evidence, which is provided through expert testimony. Expert witnesses explain technical information and offer opinions concerning the standard of care. If misdiagnosis or improper treatment of ocular disease is at issue, an ophthalmologist can be deemed competent to offer expert testimony. Thus, an optometrist can be held to a medical standard of care with respect to the diagnosis and treatment of eye disease.

STANDARDS OF CARE IN CLINICAL PRACTICE

Risk management is based on understanding clinical standards of care and the stringent observance of them. Because proper diagnosis is a key consideration, the procedural aspects of care receive the greatest emphasis—what to ask during the history, which tests to perform, when to periodically re-evaluate the patient, and when to refer to another practitioner. Because adherence to standards of care must be established to avoid liability, proper documentation of communications, test results, and recall and referral appointments is essential. Examples of standards of care and of documentation are provided below for those areas of practice most likely to produce a negligence claim—misdiagnosis of ocular disease, use of ophthalmic drugs, and the prescribing of contact lenses and spectacles.

Diagnosis of Ocular Disease

The three ocular diseases most likely to result in allegations of misdiagnosis are open-angle glaucoma, retinal detachment, and tumors affecting the visual system. The most common reason for diagnostic errors is failure to dilate the pupil. Clearly, the most important step in limiting the risk of misdiagnosis is to develop a protocol for the use of pupillary dilation. Examination of the fundus should include both the retinal periphery and the posterior pole and should entail the use of the appropriate instrumentation (e.g., 78 or 90 D fundus lenses, direct and binocular indirect ophthalmoscopes). Communication of findings and planned follow-up are also significant aspects of care and should not be neglected.

Open-Angle Glaucoma

Failure to diagnose open-angle glaucoma has often been linked with failure to perform tonometry; however, a significant number of glaucoma suspects will have applanation intraocular pressures (IOPs) that are normotensive, and patients with low-tension glaucoma will possess IOPs in the mid- to low teens. Although tonometry is a test that should be performed liberally, without regard to the age of the patient, it will not detect glaucoma suspects who are normotensive. Although open-angle glaucoma diminishes the field of vision, few practitioners perform a sensitive test of the visual field (e.g., automated perimetry) unless there is clinical justification for it. A screening test, such as confrontation fields, is often used as part of the general examination, but this test will not reveal diminution of visual field until the disease has reached an advanced stage. For these rea-

sons, examination of the optic nerve is often the most crucial aspect of diagnosis. Assessment through a dilated pupil, with the advantage of stereopsis offered by fundus biomicroscopy, can offer the best opportunity to detect disease, for often one eye will precede the other in degree of involvement. Distinct or subtle differences in the cupping of the neuroretinal rim can provide the clue that leads to further testing and to differential diagnosis.

If a patient is a glaucoma suspect, testing of the visual field with automated perimetry must be performed. This obligation extends to ocular hypertensive patients, who have about a 10% risk of contracting the disease. Periodic reassessment of intraocular pressures and visual fields must be performed, and this creates a long-term obligation for management. The risk of disease and the rationale for testing must be explained to the patient and documented in the record of care.

Retinal Detachment

There is a timeliness to the diagnosis of retinal detachment that, if not observed, can lead to significant loss of vision. Therefore, patients who are symptomatic for retinal detachment—having blurred vision, seeing sparks or lights, experiencing reduced visual field—must receive a timely dilated fundus examination and a thorough assessment of the retina. Both the periphery and the posterior pole must be examined. Failure to perform a dilated fundus examination will inevitably be construed as negligence. Prompt referral is necessary if a detachment is found.

Patients who are at risk for retinal detachment should also receive a dilated fundus examination. These patients include individuals with:

- Significant myopia
- Aphakia or pseudophakia
- YAG laser capsulotomy
- Open-angle glaucoma and significant myopia that is treated with miotic drugs
- Lattice degeneration
- Proliferative retinopathy (e.g., proliferative diabetic retinopathy, sickle cell hemoglobinopathy, branch retinal vein occlusion)
- Nonpenetrating trauma to the eye
- Retinal detachment in the fellow eye

Patients with acute onset, symptomatic posterior vitreous detachment (PVD) must also receive a timely, thorough evaluation of the ocular fundus. Between 8–15% of patients with symptomatic PVD will have suffered a retinal tear, and approximately one-third of these tears will progress to retinal detachment. The retinal break might not be present at the time of examination; a partial PVD can produce a retinal tear afterward, when there is complete separation of the vitreous. Even if the initial assessment is negative, the patient must be reexamined 2–4 weeks later, because the risk of retinal detachment remains significant, especially during the 2 months following the onset of symptoms. The patient must be warned of the symptoms of detachment and instructed to return for assessment immediately if they occur. These communications should be carefully documented in the patient's record.

Tumors

Intraocular tumor is an exceedingly rare disease, but if a tumor produces symptoms, misdiagnosis caused by failure to perform a dilated fundus examination can result in litigation. Even tumors as rare as intraocular malignant melanoma, retinoblastoma, and von Hippel-Lindau have been the source of malpractice claims. Failure to examine the peripheral retina in symptomatic cases is considered to be a breach of the standard of care.

Silent intraocular tumors pose a genuine diagnostic challenge to practitioners. The most troublesome situation is an asymptomatic first presenting patient. Does the standard of care require a dilated fundus examination and evaluation of the peripheral retina of these patients? The growing medical orientation of the standard of care is moving inexorably in that direction, as indicated by recent litigation. Therefore, it is wise to include a dilated fundus examination as part of the general assessment of "routine" first presenting patients.

Misdiagnosis of external tumors such as basal cell and squamous cell carcinoma can also be construed as negligence. Questionable lesions of the adnexa should be referred for biopsy and, when appropriate, for surgical removal. Patients with visual field loss indicative of intracranial neoplasms must likewise receive referral for definitive diagnosis. For patients with a suspicious history (e.g., headaches, neurologic symptoms) or findings (e.g., decreased acuity, acute strabismus, papilledema), perimetry is indicated. Tumors can threaten life as well as vision, and optometrists must remain vigilant for these rare but potentially devastating diseases.

Use of Ophthalmic Drugs

Although the adverse effects of drug use are a liability issue for ophthalmologists, they are rarely a source of litigation for optometrists. In fact, considering the importance of the diagnosis of intraocular disease, failure to use a mydriatic drug (to obtain pupillary dilation) is a much more likely source of litigation than an adverse effect of drug use (e.g., acute angle closure). All drugs have side effects, however, and ophthalmic drugs are no exception. For convenience of this discussion, drugs will be categorized as diagnostic or therapeutic.

Diagnostic Drugs

The most frequently used drugs are anesthetics and mydriatics. Anesthetics should not be applied copiously to a cornea with a compromised epithelium—a permanent corneal opacity can result. Mydriatics should not be administered without first assessing the anterior chamber angle. If the angle is anatomically narrow and has the potential to precipitate an angle closure during pupillary dilation, the patient must be warned of this risk, and an informed consent to proceed must be obtained (Figure 31.1). Provisions must also be made for management of the angle closure, should it occur. Alternatively, patients may be referred for laser peripheral iridotomy. Patients who have received pupillary dilation during general examination should be advised that blurred vision and photophobia will persist for several hours and that caution is needed while operating a motor vehicle or performing other potentially hazardous tasks. The same warning must be given to patients who have received cycloplegia. In some instances (e.g., uncorrected hyperopes with significant refractive error) it is prudent to have a third party

Figure 31.1. Informed consent agreement for dilation of the pupil when the anterior chamber angle is narrow enough to close.

EXAMPLE INFORMED CONSENT DOCUMENT FOR DILATION OF THE PUPIL WHEN A PATIENT HAS A NARROW ANTERIOR CHAMBER ANGLE

Dilation of the pupil is a common diagnostic procedure used by optometrists to better examine the interior of the eye. It allows a more thorough examination by making the field of view wider and by permitting the doctor to see more of the inside of the eye. Being able to examine the inside of the eye is essential to determining that your eye is healthy.

To dilate the pupil, eye drops must be administered. They require roughly half an hour to take effect. Once your pupils are dilated, it is common to be sensitive to light, a symptom that is usually alleviated by sunglasses. If you do not have any sunglasses, a disposable pair will be provided for you. Another common symptom is blurred vision, especially at near. It will require about 4-6 hours for your vision to return to normal. During this time you must exercise caution when walking down steps, driving a vehicle, operating dangerous machinery, or performing other tasks that may present a risk of injury. If you have any special transportation needs, please let us know so that they can be arranged prior to dilation.

In about 2% of people there is a possible complication of dilation of the pupil; it has been determined that you fall into this category. You must understand this complication before you give your consent to have this procedure performed.

The doctor's examination has revealed that there is a possibility of elevating the pressure inside your eye when dilation is performed. The medical term for this eventuality is "angle closure glaucoma". Because of this possibility, once your eye is dilated and the interior of the eye has been examined, the pressure will be checked again. Should it become elevated, it will be necessary to lower the pressure by administering eyedrops and oral medication. Afterwards, it may be necessary to refer you to an eye surgeon for treatment with a laser to prevent further occurrences of this kind.

Because of the structure of your eyes, it is possible for an angle closure to occur at some other time, when the symptoms may not be recognized and treatment may not be immediately provided. Such an eventuality could seriously affect your vision. Therefore, there is a benefit to you in having dilation perfomed today and in allowing this complication, if it occurs, to be diagnosed and treated immediately.

The decision to undergo dilation is yours. You may choose not to have dilation performed, but because of your history, symptoms, or examination findings, the doctor recommends that dilation of the pupil be used today to examine your eye for disease. If you have any questions concerning the procedure, please ask them so that we may answer them. Then please sign your name in the appropriate place below to signify your decision.

[]   I understand the risks and benefits of pupillary dilation and I consent to have the procedure performed.

[]   The risks and benefits of pupillary dilation have been adequately explained to me and I understand them, but I do not wish to undergo the procedure.

_____   _____
Date   Signature of Patient

---

transport the patient during the period that acuity is reduced.

Therapeutic Drugs

Litigation from therapeutic drug use most often involves topical steroids. Adverse side effects of long-term use include cataracts and open-angle glaucoma. Patients who must undergo a long-term regimen of use must be warned of side effects and monitored with sufficient frequency to detect these effects if they occur. Prescriptions should specify the number of permissible refills. If no refills are permitted, the prescription should contain language to this effect.

A second source of litigation is the use of systemic steroids, which often have significant side effects. These drugs should not be used unless it can be ascertained that a topical route of administration would not be adequate. Warnings of expected side effects should be given and documented.

Drugs used for the treatment of open-angle glaucoma can also produce undesirable side effects. Beta blockers can significantly affect individuals with heart block or chronic obstructive pulmonary disease, miotics can precipitate a retinal detachment in patients who are significantly myopic, and systemic carbonic anhydrase inhibitors can cause adverse effects ranging from kidney stones to aplastic anemia. Patients must receive adequate warnings of drug side effects and must be examined periodically to ensure that injurious effects have not occurred. In all cases, oph-

Figure 31.2. Fitting/informed consent agreement for extended wear lenses.

University Optometric Group
908 19th Street South
Birmingham, AL 35294
(205) 934-5161

Fitting Agreement for Extended Wear (Overnight) Contact Lenses

Extended wear (overnight) contact lenses present both patient and doctor with special obligations and requirements. To ensure successful lens wear, a specially designed program of fitting, lens care, and followup evaluation has been designed for you. To receive the benefits of this program, however, you must adhere to recommended lens care and wear procedures and must return as required for periodic progress evaluations. The details of our program are explained in the paragraphs that follow.

Eligibility

Extended wear contact lenses are available only to patients who have received an eye health examination at University Optometric Group during the past 12 months and who have no obvious contraindications to wear. The use of overnight lenses is not for everyone, and your doctor will advise you concerning the suitability of extended wear lenses for you. Because it is not always possible to determine in advance of lens wear whether you will enjoy a successful response to overnight use of lenses, frequent examination is necessary at the beginning of wear. Various personal, physiological and environmental factors may necessitate a change in the recommended wearing schedule or even termination of extended wear. These factors include, but are not limited to:

- inability or unwillingness to return for followup care
- inability or unwillingness to follow instructions for lens care and maintenance
- poor lens hygiene
- manual dexterity problems that prevent periodic lens removal and cleaning
- severe emotional stress
- use of certain medications
- dryness of the eye
- ocular allergic response

If you suspect that these or other factors may affect your ability to wear overnight lenses successfully, please discuss your concerns with the doctor before initiating the lens fitting process.

All patients must have a pair of spectacles which can be worn in place of contact lenses as needed.

Contact Lens Fitting

Your doctor will perform a careful fitting and lens evaluation which will include the following:

- assessment of any contraindications to lens wear
- examination of external eye and tear film
- measurements for the fit of lenses
- placement of trial lenses in the eye
- determination of appropriate lens power and design
- evaluation of ocular response to trial lens wear

You will have an opportunity to wear trial lenses and to assess the sharpness of your vision through them. If after this evaluation it is determined that you do not wish to wear overnight lenses, you will be charged a fee of $35 for the fitting and examination.

If you decide to wear overnight lenses, you will be charged an additional fee for lenses, solutions needed for cleaning and disinfection, training in lens insertion and removal, education in lens cleaning and maintenance procedures, and for progress evaluations that are part of the fitting period. The total cost is dependent upon the type of lenses selected for you, the solutions needed for maintenance, and the number of progress evaluations. We will be happy to review these costs with you at the time of payment.

Progress Evaluations

Evaluation of lens wear is a necessary aspect of the proper care of patients using overnight lenses. Complications can occur rapidly, and periodic examination is needed to safeguard eye health and prevent injury. For these reasons, progress evaluations will be scheduled for:

- 24 hours after beginning overnight wear
- 3 days after beginning overnight wear
- 10 days after beginning overnight wear
- 4 weeks after beginning overnight wear

The initial schedule for your progress evaluations is as follows:

Examination	Date/Time
24 hour	_____
3 days	_____
10 days	_____
4 weeks	_____

© 1992 John G. Classé

---

thalmic drug use must be adequately documented in the patient's record of care.

Contact Lenses

Risk management in contact lens practice is most easily described by type of lens modality—daily wear or extended wear. Although the risk of significant complication is greater for patients fitted with extended wear lenses, the much larger number of individuals wearing daily wear lenses causes more legal claims to be brought by members of this population. Because of the greater likelihood of complications found in extended wear, estimated to be 4–15 times that for daily wear, patients must be informed of the risks, and a structured program of care should be devised. Fitting agreements are used to satisfy informed consent requirements and to describe management,

Figure 31.2 (continued)

Additional examinations may be necessary, depending upon your response to overnight wear.

It is important for the health of your eyes that you return as required for examination, follow the recommended wearing schedule, and clean and disinfect your lenses as directed. Failure to fulfill these obligations may result in termination of lens wear.

Wear of Lenses

You have been fitted with the following type and brand of extended wear contact lenses:

Type	Manufacturer/Brand
gas permeable	_____
soft	_____
disposable	_____

As with any other medical device, the use of extended wear contact lenses is not without risk. This risk is higher than for daily wear lenses (lenses that are not worn overnight). A small but significant percentage of individuals wearing extended wear lenses develop potentially serious complications that can lead to permanent eye injury and vision loss.

Therefore, it is important that you recognize the symptoms of potentially serious complications of wear, which include the following:

- **decreased (blurry) vision**
- **eye pain or irritation**
- **redness of the eye**
- **watering or discharge**
- **sensitivity to light**

If you experience any of these symptoms, you should immediately remove your lenses, call the clinic, and schedule an appointment. Do not delay in calling for an appointment and do not resume lens wear until advised to do so by your doctor.

A proper wearing schedule is essential to reducing the risk of complications. Although extended wear lenses are intended to be worn overnight, the US Food and Drug Administration has issued an advisory letter recommending that lenses be worn continuously for no more than 6 nights. After wear for the period recommended by your doctor, lenses are to be left off one night and cleaned and disinfected before wear is resumed.

You are advised to wear your lenses no more than _____ nights continously. After removal, the lens must be properly cleaned, disinfected, and stored overnight.

Lens Care

Proper care of lenses is necessary for successful wear, proper vision, good eye health and normal lens life. You will be instructed in the proper methods of lens care and handling and provided with the proper solutions and materials for the cleaning, disinfection and storage of extended wear (overnight) lenses.

You should not hesitate to ask your doctor or a staff assistant about lens care and maintenance, and you should become familiar with the lens care products listed below, for they have been prescribed specifically for your eyes and lenses. **You should never change or substitute brands without first checking with your doctor.** The use of improper solutions may result in eye irritation or lens damage.

The following products have been selected for use with your lenses:

Lens cleaner _____

Lens disinfectant _____

Soaking solution _____

Rinsing solution _____

Wetting solution _____

Eyedrops _____

If a lens accumulates deposits which cannot be removed, it must be replaced. Lens life is unpredictable, and frequent replacements may be necessary. The cost of replacing damaged lenses is $_____ per lens during the period this agreement is in effect. Lost lenses may be replaced for this same fee.

A successful lens fit cannot be guaranteed, despite the best efforts of your doctor and full compliance on your part with all requirements for lens wear and care. If a change of lens type is required, a fee of $_____ per lens will be charged. If the decision is made to terminate extended lens wear, you will be eligible for a refund of $_____ per lens if the lenses are returned within _____ days of beginning wear.

Disposable Lenses

Disposable lenses are a type of extended wear (overnight) lens used to reduce the likelihood of certain ocular complications of contact lens wear. If disposable lenses are prescribed for you, they must be removed and discarded in accordance with the schedule that has been advised. As with other types of extended

---

and these agreements should obligate patients to return at stated periods for follow-up (Figure 31.2). Agreements can be tailored to meet the specific patient needs—daily wear, extended wear, disposable wear, or monovision for presbyopia. An important component of any fitting agreement is the contact lens prescription. The practitioner's policy for release of the prescription, which must be in accordance with state law, should be made clear to the patient before the fitting. When a prescription is released to the patient, it should contain all the information necessary to allow the patient to obtain the lenses. Liability issues vary somewhat, based on the type of lens prescribed.

Daily Wear Lenses

There are six major areas of litigation involving daily wear lenses, requiring the application of risk management:

Figure 31.2 (continued)

wear lenses, continuous wear is limited to no more than 6 nights. After a night without wear, a new set of lenses is placed in the eye. Disposable lenses should not be used after being taken out of the eye, but if a lens is accidentally or deliberately removed, it should not be reused without first being cleaned and disinfected.

Your wearing schedule is listed below:

Remove lenses after _____ days of wear.

Do not wear lenses for 24 hours.

Replacement lenses can be worn for _____ days.

If no problems are encountered, repeat the above schedule for _____ weeks, after which time you will be scheduled to return for a progress evaluation and a new supply of lenses.

Because disposable lenses cannot be inspected by the doctor prior to dispensing, you should examine each lens prior to insertion in the eye. Defective lenses should be discarded or brought to the clinic for inspection. Lenses should be removed immediately if significant symptoms occur, such as blurred vision, pain, redness, ocular discharge, or sensitivity to light, and an appointment should be scheduled with your doctor.

Contact Lens Prescriptions

Until your doctor has had an opportunity to fit you with lenses and evaluate the response of your eyes to lens wear, the prescription for your contact lenses cannot be determined. For that reason, a contact lens prescription cannot be provided until the conclusion of the fitting period, which is generally about a month after lens wear has begun.

The contact lens prescription provided by your doctor will describe the exact lens parameters needed to ensure that, if it becomes necessary, you can obtain these same lenses from another practitioner. The prescription will be valid for a period of time which may range from 3 months to one year, depending upon the type of lenses you received. Patients who are fitted with disposable or planned replacement lenses usually require the shorter periods of time, because lenses may be modified at progress evaluations. There is no fee for providing you with a copy of your prescription.

Patient Responsibility

Please read carefully the five paragraphs that follow, for they constitute your obligations as a contact lens patient of University Optometric Group.

I understand that my cooperation and compliance is vital to my success with extended wear (overnight) contact lenses.

I have been instructed in the proper methods of lens care and handling. I understand the importance of adhering to proper lens care procedures and the need for periodic progress evaluations. I agree to follow the recommended wearing schedule and to keep scheduled appointments. I agree to follow my doctor's advice for the safe wear of lenses as indicated on this form and in my record of care. I will notify my doctor or University Optometric Group immediately if any eye or vision problems occur.

I understand that extended wear (overnight) contact lenses have many benefits but, as with any other drug or device, they are not without risks. I have been told that the risk of complications with extended wear (overnight) lenses is greater than for daily wear lenses. I have also been told that a small percentage of wearers develop serious complications, including conditions that can cause permanent eye injury and vision loss. For this reason, I agree to follow the advice and instructions provided by my doctor. I will remove my lenses and seek care immediately if I experience eye pain, redness, discharge, sensitivity to light, or decreased vision.

I have been told the nature, purpose, and benefits of extended wear (overnight) contact lenses. I know that there are feasible alternatives, including daily wear contact lenses and spectacles, available to me. I understand that I may not be able to wear extended wear (overnight) lenses successfully and that lens wear may have to be terminated. I know that I may ask any questions I wish concerning my lenses or the policies of University Optometric Group prior to the ordering of lenses.

By my signature I acknowledge that I have read, understood and received a copy of this fitting agreement. I agree to adhere to the policies, fees, and clinical requirements of University Optometric Group's **Fitting Agreement for Extended Wear (Overnight) Contact Lenses.**

Signature of Patient

Signature of Parent or Guardian

Date   Witness (initials)

• Fitting patients with nonapproved lenses or solutions, or using approved lenses or solutions in a nonapproved manner
• Inadequate disclosure of the limitations of monovision wear
• Failure to verify lens parameters before dispensing lenses to patients
• Negligence by a contact lens technician
• Misdiagnosis or inadequate management of contact lens–related corneal abrasions or infections
• Failure to periodically evaluate the ocular health (external and internal) of contact lens patients

The most important considerations are the management of contact lens–related abrasions and the periodic evaluation of the ocular health of contact lens wearers. If neglected, they create the biggest opportunity for significant injury and large damages.

Extended Wear Lenses

In addition to the problems enumerated above, there are special considerations that apply to patients fitted with extended wear lenses:

• Improper selection of patients for extended wear (e.g., patients with dry eye)

- Inadequate patient instruction (e.g., failure to inform patients of proper methods of lens disinfection and maintenance)
- Improper wearing schedule (e.g., recommending, without clinical justification, continuous wear beyond six nights)
- Improper management of contact lens–related complications (e.g., corneal abrasions that evolve into ulcerative keratitis)
- Inadequate monitoring of ocular health

A special concern is found in disposable lens wear. Because several months' supply of lenses are dispensed to patients at one time, a customary obligation—inspection and verification of lenses before dispensing—cannot be fulfilled. The patient must be informed of this deviation from usual practice and instructed to return immediately for re-evaluation if acute problems arise after insertion of lenses (e.g., pain, redness, decreased acuity, discharge). This information should be included in the informed consent agreement (see Figure 31.2).

Spectacle Lenses and Frames

Legal claims involving spectacles are brought because a lens or frame breaks and causes ocular injury. Spectacles are prescribed based on the primary purpose for which they will be used—dress wear, occupational or industrial use, or athletic competition or sporting activities. Protection from injury is always a consideration regardless of the type of use, but whenever protection becomes a key clinical concern, the lens material of choice must be polycarbonate plastic. Patients for whom ocular protection is of importance constitute a sizable group of individuals:

- Monocular persons
- Athletes
- Individuals whose occupation might place them at special risk for ocular injury (e.g., police officers)
- Children
- Persons with corneas that have been compromised by surgery (e.g., pseudophakia, penetrating keratoplasty, radial keratotomy)

Dress eyewear can be inadequate to protect patients from injury—industrial strength frames or athletic frames with polycarbonate lenses might be necessary. If secondary use (such as occasional participation in athletic events) poses a significant risk of injury, patients must be advised of the need for protective eyewear, and the proper lenses and frames must be prescribed for athletic use.

All lenses and frames prescribed for occupational or industrial use ("safety glasses") must meet specific federal standards for impact resistance. Eyewear must be inspected before dispensing to ensure that it meets these standards, which include a minimum lens thickness requirement (3 mm, regardless of lens material) and a "Z-87" logo for the frame.

Frames prescribed for athletic use, particularly for the racquet sports, should meet the requirements of American Society for Testing and Materials (ASTM) standard F803. Polycarbonate frames and lenses are mandatory.

RECORDKEEPING AND DOCUMENTATION

Even though care is provided in accordance with recognized standards, the defense of a legal claim can be impaired if the practitioner's record does not adequately describe the care rendered. The two key aspects of proper risk management are: use of an appropriate method of recordkeeping and diligent documentation of test results, important communications, and treatment plans.

Recordkeeping

To obtain efficient, clear, and thorough recordkeeping, a problem-oriented system should be used. Problem-oriented recordkeeping, as used in private practice, consists of three components:

- Data base
- Progress notes
- Documents for ophthalmic materials

Each of these components serves a specific purpose.

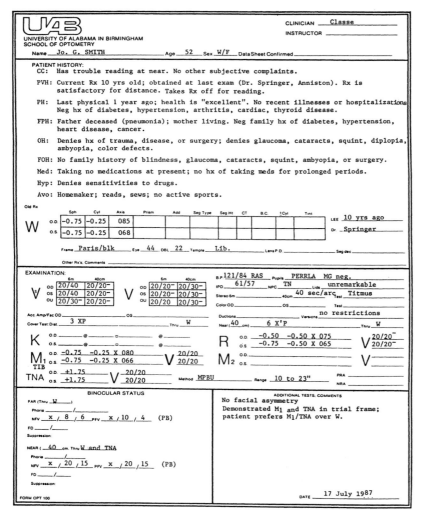

Figure 31.3. Sample form used as a data base. (Reprinted with permission from JG Classé. Legal Aspects of Optometry. Stoneham, MA: Butterworth, 1989.)

Data Base

The data base includes the history and all test results collected at each examination. Forms are often used for recording this information, for they provide completeness and uniformity (Figure 31.3). At the initial examination, and at subsequent general examinations, the form is completed or updated. There are three important aspects of the data base: the history, the examination findings, and the diagnosis and treatment plan. If short-term recall is required following examination, progress notes are used.

Progress Notes

Whenever a patient must return for further testing, for the assessment of therapy, or to evaluate treatment provided by another practitioner, progress notes are used (Figure 31.4). Recordkeeping is efficiently organized into four steps, commonly identified by the acronym SOAP:

- *S*ubjective complaint (the reason for the patient's return)
- *O*bjective findings (results of testing)
- *A*ssessment (diagnosis)

Figure 31.3 (continued)

BIOMICROSCOPY   Angle OD _1:½_ (T) _1:1_ (N)   OS _1:½_ (T) _1:½_ (N) Method: _SL_

    OD: Conjunctiva, cornea, media, iris unremarkable. 1⁺ posterior yellowing of lens.
          Neg. staining w/fluorescein. Anterior adnexa unremarkable.

    OS: as noted for OD.

T OD __14__ mm Hg   ANESTH. _Fluress_ ___%
    OS __15__ mm Hg   APPREHENSION Ⓛ M H
    (TAP) NCT MM   TIME: _2:00_ a.m./p.m.

OPHTHALMOSCOPY   (Dilation ĉ _1 gt Myd 1% and Neo 2½%_)

BIO _X_   OD: disc oval, no pallor, C/D=.2/.2, 1 D deep, margins distinct, NRR intact
DO _X_   A/V= 2:3, no crossing changes
MIO___   macular reflex present
         GRA unremarkable by BIO

       OS: as noted for OD except for 4 DD size nevus at 12:00 and 3 DD from disk

VISUAL FIELDS _full central fields OD/OS_ Method _TS_ Stimulus _2W_ Dist. _1000_
               Performed at 7 fc; good responses

ADDITIONAL TESTS/SKETCHES ATTACHED: _____

Dx / IMPRESSIONS:

Diag Code (COIT)*.   Diagnoses

1. _CMA OD and OS_
2. _Presbyopia_
3. _Choroidal nevus OS_
4. _____
5. _____
6. _____

*See Clinic Manual for listing

Comments:
Warned the patient of the risks of driving
while pupils dilated. Supplied mydriatic
glasses.

Tx / Px
1. Prescribe M₁ for full-time wear
2. Prescribe +1.75 add
3. Monitor at next exam
4.
5.
6.

RTC: _1 yr_
Comments: Photodocument nevus OS

SIGNATURES

Examiner _____
Staff _____ JF Classé O.D.
                     (10/82)

• *Plan* (future management, based on the diagnosis)

Progress notes are excellent means of recording episodic care, such as that found in contact lens practice, binocular vision therapy, or the treatment of ocular disease. These notes are used to supplement and expand the data base.

Documents for Ophthalmic Materials

Optometrists dispense spectacle lenses and frames, contact lens solutions and materials, and various types of binocular and low vision aids. An orderly account must be maintained of orders, verifications, and dispensings. In addition, prescriptions for spectacles must be provided for patients. Copies of all prescriptions should always be retained, and special attention should always be given to expiration dates and any pertinent limitations (e.g., "polycarbonate plastic only").

Problem-oriented recordkeeping is well accepted by both the legal and medical professions. Because it emphasizes an orderly and efficient approach to care, it achieves effective risk management and is the preferred method of recordkeeping for optometrists.

DOCUMENTATION

When documenting examination findings, descriptive terms should be used. Rather than empty

Patient   W.C. Jones   **Date**   June 15, 1996

S   Complains of gritty, sandy eyes; particularly crusty at awakening. Onset 3 weeks ago. Takes artificial tears for relief, which is temporary. No other complaints. History otherwise unchanged since last eye exam 3 months ago.

O   OD 20/60^{+1} OD -4.50 -1.00 x 095
        VA   @ 6m w/W   W
             OS 20/50^{-1} OS -4.00 -0.50 x 085

                                                        add + 2.50

        R   OD -4.75 -1.00 x 090   20/50^{-1}
             OS -5.00 -0.75 x 090   20/40^{-2}

        MVA OD -4.75 -1.00 x 095   20/50^{-1}
             OS -4.50 -0.50 x 085   20/40^{-1}

        Trial frame   Patient appreciates improved VA but does not want to change W

        SLE   OD 2$^+$ conjunctival injection; marginal blepharitis; anterior chamber clear; corneal SPK w/fluorescein; 1$^+$ papillae in bulbar conjunctiva; 2$^+$ NS cataract

             OS as noted for OD

        Ophthal   OD disc oval, no pallor, margins distinct, C/D=.1/1., NRRI
        1 gt T $_{1\%}$ A/V=2/3, no crossing changes
                        drusen in macula; no hemorrhages or exudates
        MDO/BIO   GRA unremarkable; no holes, breaks or lattice

             OS as noted for OD except C/D=.2/.2

A   1. 2$^+$ NS cataract OD/OS
        2. age-related maculopathy
        3. bacterial keratoconjunctivitis OD/OS

P   1. Discussed surgical consult with patient; he does not wish to see a surgeon at present. Warned patient of reduced acuity; advised patient to minimize driving, esp at night. RTC in 6 months.

        2. Discussed prognosis of ARM with patient; he was advised to RTC immediately if sudden change in VA occurs.

        3. Rx gentamycin 1 gt q 4 hours; hot compresses qid; RTC 3 days.

Figure 31.4. Example of a progress note. (Reprinted with permission from JG Classé. Legal Aspects of Optometry. Stoneham, MA: Butterworth, 1989.)

terms such as "normal," "unremarkable," and "WNL" ("within normal limits"), language describing the practitioner's observations should be employed. For example, the optic nerve might be recorded as "C/D .3/.4, margins distinct, no pallor, NRRI" ("neuroretinal rim intact"). Of particular importance are the findings of ophthalmoscopy and the slit lamp examination. In addition, the details of testing should also be recorded (e.g., instruments used, drugs administered). All aspects of the eye health assessment should be accorded this descriptive documentation, which constitutes a most important part of the defense if there is a malpractice claim.

Informed consent requirements arise in many aspects of practice. Examples include contact lens fittings, dilation of a narrow anterior chamber angle, and prescribing drugs for treatment. Printed forms are often used to ensure that the appropriate information is conveyed and to preserve a written record of the patient's consent. These forms expedite the process of adhering to informed consent requirements, and they provide excellent evidence if a legal dispute arises. These documents should be an integral part of clinical practice.

If patients require follow-up, a definite recall appointment should be scheduled, even if the date is remote (e.g., 3–6 months in the future). The patient should be contacted by mail or telephone (or both) just before the appointment date and reminded of the examination. If referral is necessary, a practitioner should be chosen and contacted and a definite appointment scheduled. The date of the appointment should be noted in the patient's record.

If practical, a letter describing the reason for the referral and requesting a description of the diagnosis and treatment plan should be sent to the practitioner to whom the patient is being referred.

Maintaining well-organized records is one of the most important steps that clinicians can take to manage risk. The importance of proper recordkeeping and documentation as a necessary component of risk management cannot be overemphasized.

PROFESSIONAL LIABILITY INSURANCE

All optometrists should purchase adequate professional liability insurance. No plan of risk management can be considered complete without it. The cost is reasonable and the protection is needed. Professional liability policies can provide insurance coverage for a host of legal woes (Table 31.2), but the main purpose is to provide insurance coverage, up to the policy's limits for negligence claims. There are two basic types of policies to choose from when obtaining this coverage: claims made and occurrence.

Claims-Made Policies

Claims-made policies provide insurance protection as long as the practitioner is paying premiums. After premium payments end, insurance coverage ends. To obtain protection after premium payments have ended but before statutes of limitation have expired, a reporting endorsement must be purchased. The purchase of this coverage adds to the claims-made policy cost, which is usually less expensive than an occurrence policy.

Occurrence Policies

Under occurrence policies, insurance protection is provided as long as the act that gave rise to the claim occurred during the period when insurance premiums were being paid. Therefore, a claim can be brought after premium payments have ended, and coverage will not be denied as long as the act that caused the claim occurred while the policyholder was paying premiums. Occurrence policies tend to be less flexible than

Table 31.2. Coverage Provided by Professional Liability Insurance

Personal liability coverage
    Malpractice
    Defamation
    Product liability
    Premises liability
    Vicarious liability (liability for the acts or omissions of employees)
    Injuries to employees
Fire insurance coverage
    Building
    Contents
Other property coverage
    Transit
    Theft and burglary
    Reproduction of records
    Embezzlement
    Accounts receivable
    Office overhead

claims-made policies in terms of coverage added to the basic policy.

Professional liability insurance pays for the costs of defending a claim (including attorney's fees) and for a judgment or settlement up to the policy limits. Coverage is usually expressed in amounts "per individual" and "per occurrence." For example, a policy limit of $1 million/$3 million would provide coverage of $1 million for each individual injured up to $3 million. Insurance coverage in this amount is recommended in an "umbrella" policy, which provides coverage for acts that are part of the practice of optometry even if they occur outside the practitioner's office. Optional coverage might be needed to obtain insurance protection for optometrist-employees, or for other liability risks that an individual practitioner can face.

There is a standard procedure followed for the management of claims. The insurer will investigate the claim, determine if liability exists, and decide whether to reach a settlement with the claimant. The right to settle a claim typically rests with the insurer; policies do not usually allow an optometrist to demand vindication in court. If a case goes to court and a judgment is rendered against the optometrist, the insurer will pay the judgment up to the limits of the policy. If the policy is insufficient to satisfy the judgment, the assets of the optometrist might be at risk. In the majority of cases, the claim is settled without benefit of trial. The insurance company pays damages to the plaintiff, or the claim is dropped for various reasons.

Professional liability policies cover only acts that are within the scope of optometry. If, for example, an optometrist negligently uses a therapeutic drug for treatment without being legally entitled to do so, the insurer could decline to defend the claim or refuse to pay any settlement or judgment. The optometrist would be required to use personal assets to hire an attorney, go to court, or pay a settlement. It is prudent, therefore, to perform only those acts that constitute the authorized practice of optometry.

CONCLUSION

The preceding discussion of risk management has emphasized the need to conform to prevailing standards of care when providing professional services and has described the importance of adequate recordkeeping and documentation. Because of the time, expense, and personal anguish of defending a malpractice claim, procedures that minimize the likelihood of such a claim should be given careful consideration and due implementation. To ensure that adequate resources are available to defend a claim, appropriate professional liability insurance should be obtained. With accepted standards of care, proper recordkeeping, and adequate insurance, a practitioner will perform the steps necessary to manage risk.

BIBLIOGRAPHY

Alexander LJ. Primary Care of the Posterior Segment (2nd ed). East Norwalk, CT: Appleton & Lange, 1994.

Alexander LJ, Scholles JR. Clinical and legal aspects of pupillary dilation. J Am Optom Assoc 1987;58: 432–7.

American Optometric Association. Scope of Practice: Patient Care and Management Manual. St. Louis: American Optometric Association, 1986.

Bettman JW. A review of 412 claims in ophthalmology. Int Ophthalmol Clin 1980;20(4):131–42.

Bettman JW. Seven hundred medicolegal cases in ophthalmology. Ophthalmology 1990; 97:1379–84.

Classé JG. Contractual considerations in contact lens practice. J Am Optom Assoc 1986;57:220–6.

Classé JG. The eye-opening case of *Keir v United States*. J Am Optom Assoc 1989;60:471–6.

Classé JG. Legal Aspects of Optometry. Stoneham, MA: Butterworth, 1989.

Classé JG. Legal aspects of sports vision. Optom Clin 1993;3(1):27–32.

Classé JG. Liability and ophthalmic drug use. Optom Clin 1992;2(3):121–34.

Classé JG. Liability and the primary care optometrist. J Am Optom Assoc 1986;57:926–9.

Classé JG. Liability for the treatment of anterior segment eye disease. Optom Clin 1991;1(4):1–23.

Classé JG. Pupillary dilation: an eye-opening problem. J Am Optom Assoc 1992; 63:733–41.

Classé JG. A review of 50 malpractice claims. J Am Optom Assoc 1989;60:694–706.

Classé JG, Harris MG. Medicolegal Complications of Contact Lens Wear. In J Silbert (ed), Anterior Segment Complications of Contact Lens Wear. New York: Churchill Livingstone, 1992;487–509.

Classé JG, Scholles JR. Liability for ophthalmic materials. J Am Optom Assoc 1986;57:470–7.

Classé JG, Snyder C, Benjamin WJ. Documenting informed consent for patients wearing disposable lenses. J Am Optom Assoc 1989;60:215–20.

Davis MD. Natural history of retinal breaks without detachment. Arch Ophthalmol 1974;92:183–94.

Harris MG, Classé JG. Clinicolegal considerations in monovision. J Am Optom Assoc 1988;59:491–5.

Harris MG, Classé JG. Contact lens prescriptions: a clinicolegal view. J Am Optom Assoc 1988;59:732–6.

Harris MG, Dister RE. Informed consent for extended wear patients. Optom Clin 1991;1(4):33–50.

Irvine AR. The pathogenesis of aphakic retinal detachment. Ophthalmic Surg 1985;16:101–7.

Lindner B. Acute posterior vitreous detachment and its retinal complications. Acta Ophthalmol 1977;87(Supp 1):1–108.

National Association of Insurance Commissioners. Malpractice Claims. Madison, WI: National Association of Insurance Commissioners, 1980; vol 2, no 2.

Poggio EC, Glynn RJ, Schein OD, et al. The incidence of ulcerative keratitis among users of daily wear and extended wear contact lenses. N Engl J Med 1989;321:779–83.

Schein OD, Glynn RJ, Poggio EC, et al. The relative risk of ulcerative keratitis among users of daily wear and extended wear soft contact lenses: a case study. N Engl J Med 1989;321:773–8.

Scholles JR. Malpractice: watch your step. Rev Optom 1986;123(4):26.

Sherr AE. Industrial safety glasses—an update. J Am Optom Assoc 1980;51:129–37.

Tasman W. Posterior vitreous detachment and peripheral retinal breaks. Trans Am Acad Ophthalmol Otolaryngol 1968;72:217–24.

Thal LS. *Gates v Jensen*: another precedent for glaucoma testing. J Am Optom Assoc 1981;52:349–53.

Wechsler S, Classé JG. *Helling v Carey*: caveat medicus (let the doctor beware). J Am Optom Assoc 1977;48:1526–9.

Weed L. Medical Records, Medical Education, and Patient Care. Cleveland: Press of Case Western Reserve, 1970.

Chapter 32

Estate Planning

John G. Classé and Gary Moss

Annual income twenty pounds, annual expenditure nineteen six, result happiness. Annual income twenty pounds, annual expenditure twenty pounds ought and six, result misery.

—Charles Dickens
David Copperfield

Although happiness might require more gain than sixpence, misery can quite properly be equated with greater expenditure than income. Indeed, a practitioner's professional life is driven by the need to earn more than is spent. Because there is also life after practice, practitioners face the perplexing problem of determining how to use earnings to maximum advantage for retirement. As with most difficult problems, there are no simple solutions and no easy answers to be followed dogmatically without exception throughout life. Furthermore, the problem is compounded by the lack of experience in financial planning, economics, and money management that is the lot of the average health profession graduate. This lack of experience is probably one of the reasons that young couples argue (and divorce) over money matters more often than for any other cause.

There are two ways to overcome this lack of knowledge: education and experience. Neither way is without cost and neither is, of itself, a sufficient foundation. Education and experience are both necessary for one to be truly knowledgeable. For the beginning practitioner, education offers an obvious starting point, and there are many sources that can be consulted to acquire a working knowledge of financial matters. Because financial planning is complex, opinions differ, even among experts, and it is important to obtain a broad perspective before investing money in a plan. Even so, there are certain fundamental concepts that are generally considered the bedrock of any plan. They, in fact, can be used to develop a philosophy of estate planning.

A PHILOSOPHY OF ESTATE PLANNING

For an optometry school graduate entering practice, retirement and estate planning are remote and easily relegated to future consideration. In fact, planning for the future can be viewed as being in conflict with more immediate, tangible goals that are related to practice, family life, and financial demands. Such a view is shortsighted and reflects a lack of understanding of the key role that estate planning—preparing for the future—plays in the life of a practitioner. One key aspect of such planning is to ensure that there is financial security not only for retirement but also for the education of children, in the event of disability, and to protect a spouse left alone by unexpected death. Estate planning provides for both the expected and the unexpected events of life by securing adequate fi-

Table 32.1. Net Mean Income by Year in Practice

First year: $61,636
Second year: $62,145
Third year: $63,646
Fourth year: $71,377
Fifth year: $77,158
Tenth year: $88,690

Source: 1995 American Optometric Association. Caring for the Eyes of America—A Profile of the Optometric Profession. St. Louis: American Optometric Association, 1996.

nancial resources to manage these events when or if they occur.

Estate planning begins with four fundamental steps: adequate income, a home, a cash reserve sufficient to meet emergencies, and affordable, comprehensive insurance coverage. Once these four fundamental requirements have been met, a fifth step can be considered—investment. Each of these steps will be briefly described, in the usual order of acquisition.

Income

Although optometry is one of the half dozen highest paying professions in America, statistics show that individuals in high income brackets overextend themselves with a regularity that is not remarkably different from that of individuals with more modest incomes. Therefore, the relative affluence offered by a career in optometry does not insulate a practitioner from the financial tribulations of life. Nor does this affluence, of itself, ensure that a practitioner will be able to attain financial security. It probably does establish great expectations, but these expectations must be tempered by reality.

Studies conducted by the American Optometric Association (AOA) over the past 50 years have created a relatively clear picture of the income levels of optometrists (see Chapter 1). For all optometrists, income growth was quite sluggish until the late 1950s. At that time technological achievements such as the contact lens and the tonometer expanded the scope of practice and caused a concurrent increase in earnings. Economic growth was quite vigorous during the 1960s and 1970s, and although the eroding effects of inflation during the

late 1970s and early 1980s prevented real increases in income from being realized, the effect of changes in the scope of practice and in the Medicare law resulted in steady growth during the late 1980s and early 1990s. Of course, the majority of optometrists are in private practice, which still represents the most affluent career option in the profession. The net income earned by a private practitioner, however, is related to the number of years that practitioner has been in practice. Therefore, to obtain an accurate picture of the income a practitioner should expect to earn, the number of years in practice must be known. The AOA surveys are most useful in this regard (Table 32.1).

An optometrist's income is subject to diminution by inflation and taxes no matter what the stage of practice, but the income of a beginning practitioner is further diminished by the economics of entry into private practice. The AOA economic surveys have shown that 5–7 years are required to establish a practice that is started "cold" and to pay off educational debts. In addition, the usual period that is required to rise from associate to full partner in a practice is generally the same. Payment for the purchase of an existing practice usually takes 5–10 years. Surveys have also revealed that, on the average, a private practitioner reaches the national net mean income for optometrists after 10 years. A young practitioner must consider these 5–10 years for building a practice when organizing an estate plan and must take care not to formulate unrealistic goals or expectations.

After this initial period is passed, however, net income continues to rise until after 20 years of practice. The relative affluence of this second phase in private practice is challenged by the financial responsibilities of raising a family. After 20 years, net earnings tend to drop slowly until retirement.

These statistics suggest that during the first years of practice a young practitioner should ignore any thoughts of estate planning and instead should concentrate on the demanding task of establishing a financial base. Such a suggestion would, however, be false. In fact, estate planning is vital during the initial period of building a practice, when discipline and a calculated approach toward achieving financial goals are essential. Budgeting will be necessary and will have much to do with the practitioner's ability to obtain adequate housing and savings, two prerequisites of estate planning.

A budget is a necessity, both in professional and private life. Effort must be made to stay within its guidelines; this means that income and expenditures must be carefully monitored to ascertain whether that extra "sixpence" is being earned or a deficit is being generated. Good financial recordkeeping will permit adjustments to be made for the cost of living, inflation, and changes in tax laws. It is essential to maintain adequate recordkeeping so that realistic budgeting can be achieved.

There are two simple but important rules of personal budgeting:

- Limit the cost of renting or purchasing a home to no more than 28% of net income
- Put 10% of net income into a liquid fund that can be used for emergencies

This approach allows 62% of net income to be used for other needs—such as subsistence, servicing of automobiles and appliances, entertainment and vacations, and insurance premiums. Insurance is a particularly important budget item.

Insurance is a necessity that constitutes a fixed charge on income. It is least expensive when acquired at a young age and is an important means of protecting and generating an "estate" if untimely death intercedes. It can cover the loss of a home, personal and property damage involving automobiles, unexpected disability, and accidents or injuries occurring at work, at home, or elsewhere. Comprehensive coverage should be planned for and acquired, and a reasonable budget should be maintained for insurance premium costs.

Although the statistics compiled by the AOA provide a composite representation of the mean income earned by optometrists, individual circumstances can vary. No matter what the actual income is, however, it should be adequate to satisfy three criteria:

- The income is adequate for the practitioner's budgetary needs, which are based on financial records maintained by the practitioner, and satisfies the practitioner's obligation for a home, cash reserve, and insurance protection.
- The income will grow above the eroding effects of inflation and taxation.

- The income will be sufficient to allow for investing or participation in a tax-deferred retirement plan.

Budgeting of income for the rental or purchase of a home is one of the first concerns of a young practitioner.

The Home

The choice of a home is usually based on considerations of personal taste. The selection of a home, because of its potential as an investment, only peripherally enters into the process despite the assurances of real estate agents that "buying is better than renting." For some individuals, buying is not better than renting, for purchasing a home incurs an obligation that extends beyond the cost of a mortgage to include the expenses of furniture, appliances, repairs, remodeling, insurance, taxes, and similar items. There is also the investment of capital in a home—capital that could be used for other purposes, such as the generation of income. Whether the purchase of a home is a good choice depends on the practitioner's circumstances and the economic burden that the payment of home-related expenses represents. If a practitioner makes the choice to purchase a home, however, the decision to do so will exert a significant effect on the practitioner's estate plan.

The purchase of a home provides some unique estate planning benefits:

- The home, if well chosen, can appreciate by as much as 8–12% annually. This return on capital is rather substantial, and, since a home increases in value with inflation, the eroding effects of inflation are neutralized.
- Interest on a home mortgage is deductible on the owner's personal income tax return.
- The payment of a home mortgage, because it is also a return of principal, actually increases the value of the home to the owner—for each payment made, the debt is reduced, thereby increasing the owner's equity or value in the home.
- Taxes on a home are also deductible.

Therefore, a home does provide what can be considered an investment return, thereby providing a benefit to the estate plan. There are also some disadvantages to home ownership that must be considered:

- A home is not a liquid asset and cannot be disposed of quickly; months are usually required before a sale can be transacted.
- The costs required to maintain a home can exceed budgetary expectations and capabilities.
- A home must be held for a number of years before a sizable financial return can be realized.
- If the selection of a home is not wisely made, it can actually decrease in value.

The cost of a home occupies a central position in the budget of a homeowner. The down payment required to secure a home mortgage is generally 5–10% of the home's cost. The size of monthly mortgage payments will be considered by the mortgage company and should be no more than 28% of the homeowner's net income. Payments might be the same from month to month, which is the traditional method of amortized mortgage payment, or they might vary in accordance with the lending rate offered by the mortgage company. Variable-rate mortgages have a ceiling beyond which they cannot increase, and they can require "balloon" payments after several years, which could have a large negative impact on budgetary planning.

One other aspect of home ownership that has significance for estate planning is the title. The title to real estate is of particular significance for married couples, because the title to real estate can be divided or undivided among the owners. An undivided interest has several advantages, because of the right of joint survivorship. A form of title known as "tenancy by the entirety" considers both spouses to be owners of the entire estate, with the right of joint survivorship. Upon the death of either spouse, the survivor is considered to be the owner of the home.

Another important consequence of an undivided title involves the rights of creditors. If the title is tenancy by the entirety, creditors cannot satisfy their claims out of the real estate, unless both owners have become debtors. Therefore, if an optometrist borrows from a bank to finance a practice and is not able to repay the debt, the creditor can proceed against any collateral that the optometrist has used to secure the loan; unless the optometrist's spouse has also signed the loan agreement, the bank may

not collect the amount due from the optometrist by selling the house. This is because the spouse has an undivided interest in the realty, and because this interest was not used as collateral for the loan, it cannot be used to collect the debt of the optometrist. For practitioners who are in community property states, there are special considerations that require consultation with a lawyer whenever property transactions are anticipated.

Besides the acquisition of a home, estate planning also requires the accumulation of a cash reserve for emergencies.

Cash Reserve

A cash reserve provides needed security for a practitioner, particularly in the event of emergencies or other situations that call for the immediate use of cash. The cash reserve can be likened to a piggy bank that is dutifully filled with an allowance, usually cited as 10% of net income, until 4–6 months' worth of gross income has been accumulated. After this goal has been attained and insurance needs have been fulfilled, income can be used for investment.

There are several means of accumulating liquid assets that can serve as a cash reserve: savings accounts, interest-bearing checking accounts, certificates of deposit, whole life insurance policies, and credit cards.

Savings Accounts

Savings accounts are a traditional method of accumulating a cash reserve that allows savings to grow, although at a rather modest rate that might not be able to keep up with inflation. Even so, the return of interest is guaranteed, and savings accounts have the advantage of liquidity, which means money can be withdrawn on demand. In addition, most savings accounts are insured up to a certain maximum, either by the Federal Deposit Insurance Corporation (FDIC) or the Federal Savings and Loan Insurance Corporation (FSLIC).

Interest-Bearing Checking Accounts

Beginning in the 1980s, interest-bearing checking accounts—known as negotiated order of withdrawal

(NOW) accounts—have offered an alternative means of accumulating income in an on-demand cash reserve. The interest paid on NOW accounts is offset by service charges that can be avoided only if a minimum balance is maintained in the account each month. As a result, larger sums have been deposited in checking accounts and smaller amounts into savings accounts.

Certificates of Deposit

Although not truly a cash reserve, certificates of deposit (CDs) are another means of setting aside cash in an interest-bearing account so that it is available in times of emergency. The interest paid on CDs is higher than that for savings accounts or interest-bearing checking accounts, but to receive the interest payment the CD must be held for a specified period of time, which might be as short as 6 months or as long as several years. The longer the period, the higher the interest paid. If the CD is cashed in before the period has run, a penalty must be paid, so CDs do not have the liquidity of savings accounts and NOW accounts.

Whole Life Insurance Policies

Whole life insurance policies acquire cash value in addition to providing insurance protection. Over a number of years, the cash value can accumulate to a nice sum. This money can be withdrawn or borrowed, with or without an interest charge, depending on the type of policy and its provisions. The capacity to withdraw or borrow the cash value of a policy should be considered when purchasing whole life insurance as part of an estate plan.

Credit Cards

Although credit cards cannot properly constitute part of a cash reserve, they can provide a source of income—borrowed money—in an emergency. A line of credit is established, based on the income of the cardholder, and the cardholder can draw cash up to the credit ceiling as long as periodic payments are made to reduce the balance. Interest rates, though high, have not been subject to the same fluctuations as the prime interest rate in re-

cent years, and they do not usually compare unfavorably with the interest rates charged by commercial banks. For a practitioner, credit cards are a necessity, providing identification, immediate credit, and a means of recording professional expenses for tax purposes. They can be abused, however, by individuals who do not have the discipline to restrict their use.

Insurance Coverage

If a practitioner can realize an adequate income, acquire a satisfactory home, and make systematic contributions to a cash reserve, there is still one prerequisite remaining—adequate insurance coverage. This last step is a sizable one, requiring an understanding of the basic types of insurance and their proper use in an estate plan.

Although the fundamental purpose of insurance is to provide financial protection against disaster, insurance can also be used as an estate planning device. Some typical uses of life insurance are:

- For payment of the costs of death, including estate taxes and the immediate expenses incurred by the estate
- To create a "nest egg" for the spouse or family of the deceased
- To provide cash to pay the mortgage balance on a home through the purchase of a mortgage rider
- To fund a cross-purchase agreement between partners or stockholders of a professional association or corporation
- To protect a practice against the death of a "key person"

The primary purpose of life insurance is to provide money in the event of death. In return for payment of premiums, the insurance company agrees to pay the face amount of the policy to the beneficiary on the insured's death. Although some types of life insurance, such as universal life policies, are often referred to as "investments," life insurance primarily provides protection, with some use for estate planning.

There are four types of insurance that should be acquired by a practitioner—life, disability, professional liability, and personal (health, automobile, home). Each type of insurance should be thoroughly understood before it is purchased.

Life Insurance

There are two basic types of life insurance—term and whole life. Term, as the word implies, provides only death benefit insurance coverage for a specific period, usually 1–5 years. The cost of term insurance is initially less expensive than whole life coverage, but the cost increases with age. Term policies generally are not available after age 65. Whole life policies provide both insurance and investment return, thereby acquiring a "cash value" that can be borrowed against. The premium is based on the age at which the policy is taken out and does not change. Ordinary life policies require payment for the insured's whole life; limited payment life policies limit premiums to a certain age, at which time the insurance coverage becomes permanent. Universal life is popular with professionals because it combines insurance with reasonable investment return and permits tax-free withdrawals (up to the amount contributed). A maintenance fee is charged by the insurer.

Because of its lower cost, term is often the first life insurance that is purchased. An alternative is whole life, with a mortgage payment rider if the insured is a homeowner. This rider is actually a decreasing term policy that pays to the beneficiary the amount owed on the home mortgage at the time of the insured's death. Later in life, term policy holders can convert to a whole life policy or purchase a whole life policy such as universal life.

Life insurance proceeds paid at the death of the insured are for the face value of the policy, plus any cash value if a whole life policy was purchased. Payment can be in a lump sum, over a fixed period of time, in fixed installments, or for the life of the beneficiary (as with an annuity).

When attempting to determine the amount of life insurance to purchase, there are several factors to be considered, including the earning power of the practitioner, the earning capacity of the spouse, educational obligations to the children or spouse, and the amount of debt that has been acquired. In general, these considerations tend to indicate that life insurance protection should equal 5–7 years' worth of gross income plus 5–7 years' worth of debt (such as loans and mortgages).

Disability Insurance

Serious disability is a much more likely possibility than premature death, yet disability insurance is far less likely to be planned for than life insurance. Policies are expensive, and the benefits vary considerably from policy to policy. There are five essential elements of a disability insurance plan:

- How long is the elimination period (the period of time before benefits are paid)?
- How long does coverage continue (does it extend to age 65)?
- What is the definition of disability? (Is the definition "inability to perform the duties of one's regular occupation"?)
- What is the cost? (Are the policy benefits worth the cost?)
- What is the provision for renewability? (Is the policy "guaranteed renewable and noncancellable"?)

Disability insurance pays the disabled policyholder a guaranteed monthly income, which is expressed as a percentage of earned income before disability. The percentage is usually limited to 60%, and proof of income will be needed.

Office overhead insurance is used to cover the expenses of running a practice when a practitioner is disabled. There are several important provisions:

- The practitioner must be disabled as defined in the policy.
- The benefits paid are limited to actual overhead expenses.
- The elimination period is brief (usually 2 weeks).
- The benefits are paid for a stated period of time (18–24 months).

The purpose of this insurance is to pay for the operating expenses of a practice, such as staff salaries, utilities, and office rent, during temporary disability. Office overhead insurance does not pay for non-overhead items like laboratory bills and the costs of a substitute practitioner.

Professional Liability Insurance

Professional liability insurance protects practitioners against the costs of defending liability claims. A typical insurance policy will cover claims arising out of negligence, defamation, product liability, premises liability, or vicarious (employee) liability. There are two basic types of policies:

- Occurrence policies cover liability claims that arose when premiums were paid—even if the claim was filed after payments for premiums ended.
- Claims-made policies cover only claims that are brought while premiums are being paid. A "reporting endorsement" must be purchased to provide coverage after premiums are no longer being paid.

Extra coverage is usually needed for professional employees (e.g., optometrists, opticians), to cover embezzlement, and for injuries to employees (if there is no worker's compensation).

Coverage under a professional liability insurance policy typically provides for the costs of defense, including attorney's fees and court costs, and for the cost of any judgments or settlements, up to the policy limit. The insurance company can reserve the right to settle the claim without the consent of the insured.

The amount of insurance coverage should be at least $1 million per claimant—the purchase of an extra $1 million is worth the usually modest cost.

Fire Insurance

Beginning practitioners, who usually lease office space in a building, should obtain fire insurance coverage of office contents. Insurance should be purchased for the replacement value (rather than fair market value) of contents. Receipts, photographs, and other documentation of insured items and their value should be retained. If a practitioner owns a building, adequate coverage is needed for partial and full loss. Because buildings appreciate in value, insurance coverage for 80% of the building's fair market value will provide coverage in the event of a 100% loss. Because of appreciation, it is also necessary to adjust insurance limits periodically.

Personal Insurance

Personal insurance should be purchased to protect health, home, and vehicles.

Health insurance will be needed until age 65, when Medicare eligibility is attained. Major medical coverage is often a beginning point for young self-employed practitioners, but employed optometrists might be able to secure health insurance as a benefit of employment.

Homeowner's insurance covers injuries occurring on the property; damage from fire, lightning, and other perils; and loss of personal property. In the event of total loss, the personal effects are valued as a percentage of the coverage on the home (usually 50–60%). There is a limit to the value of individual items unless they are "scheduled." Items of special value (such as jewelry, works of art, and antiques) should be appraised and listed on a schedule for their fair market value. Of course, an extra premium is paid for these items.

Vehicles should be adequately insured for the following types of coverage:

- Liability—this offers protection if the owner or other insureds cause an accident that results in personal injury to others, property damage, or both.
- Collision—the insurer pays for damage to the insured vehicle (less the deductible), even if the insured is at fault.
- Comprehensive—this provides coverage for events other than collision, such as fire, theft, and similar perils; deductible coverage is probably the best way to purchase this type of insurance.
- Medical payments—this insurance pays for the medical expenses incurred by the insured (and passengers) as the result of an accident, no matter who is at fault. Coverage is usually limited and restricted to the immediate expenses resulting from the accident.
- Uninsured motorist—this provides coverage for personal injuries caused by an uninsured motorist; property damage is not covered.

Policy limits for vehicles are typically listed as two figures, such as $250,000/$500,000, which means that coverage extends to a total of $250,000 per person injured and to a total of $500,000 for the event that resulted in injury. Coverage should be adequate to protect the policyholder (and family) in the event an accident occurs. Generally the policy limits are increased as the policyholder's economic status improves over the years.

Once the four basic requirements of estate planning have been satisfied, income can be used for investment.

INVESTMENT

Many variables must be considered when making investment decisions, which are educated projections of the potential economic performance of selected items. Inflation and interest rates must be considered, because they will affect how quickly investments will grow, how much buying power the earned income of a portfolio will achieve, and how much buying power the earned income of a portfolio will have at retirement. Safety and risk are also major factors that must be considered when choosing an investment. As a rule, the safer the investment, the lower the reward. Although with very risky investments it is possible that a large windfall profit could result, it is more likely that all or much of the investment will be lost. (Otherwise, those offering the investment opportunity would not be willing to reward the investor so greatly for assuming the high risk.) Another variable that must be weighed is liquidity—the ease with which the investment can be converted into cash. Liquidity affords an investor the opportunity to change investments, typically to better ones, without incurring a significant loss. Investments without liquidity can take months to convert to cash and can result in a loss, such as the sale of real estate in a down market.

There are three general characteristics of an investment, and each will affect the decision-making process:

• Will the investment produce income? Different investments will produce income in different ways—mutual funds, stocks, and bonds will offer dividends; rental property (e.g., an apartment building) will produce cash payments.

• Will the investment appreciate? Some investments might not produce an income while they are owned but will increase in value with profit being realized only when the investment is sold. This type of investment is usually considered speculative in nature and includes gold, gems, or collectible items, which might or might not increase in value as anticipated. Appreciation of these items is usually better during periods of inflation.

• Will the investment be convertible? How quickly can an investment be sold (turned into cash without a loss in value)? If convertibility is a major concern, investments of a more speculative nature, such as real estate and collectibles, are not a good choice since they will often take longer to liquidate.

There are three basic levels of investment: short term (< 2 years), intermediate term (2–5 years), and long term (> 5 years). These different levels of investment must be considered when designing an investment plan. In fact, an investment portfolio can be regarded in the same way as a house, with the foundation needing to be strong enough to protect the upper structures. The foundation should be built on the four fundamentals of estate planning, with appropriate protection afforded by basic insurance and ready cash reserves that can be drawn on as necessary. Funding for minor emergency situations should be afforded by CDs, savings accounts, and cash value in whole life insurance policies. These types of investments have very little risk and can be readily converted into cash if the need arises. Only after this protection is obtained should an investor go on to riskier investments that can yield higher returns. Stocks, bonds, and mutual funds are among the more popular types of investments. These three types of investment differ significantly, and their differences should be understood by the investor (Table 32.2).

Another type of low-risk investment that can be used is a tax-deferred retirement plan, such as an individual retirement account (IRA) or a pension plan. These investments grow in value over time and provide income at retirement. The riskiest type of investments (such as tax-sheltered limited partnerships in oil, dairy, or equipment leasing companies, or collectibles such as art, gold, coins, and

Table 32.2. Types of Investments

  I. **Stocks.**   Stocks are issued by corporations to obtain money to finance the start-up or operation of the corporation. The traditional method of earning money from the stock market is to "buy low and sell high." Of course, the successful investor must not only determine that a particular company is solvent and well structured but also that it faces favorable market conditions and industry prospects. There are two types of stock, common and preferred.

      A. **Common stock** holders are the owners of the corporation and are entitled to share in the profits, called dividends, of the company. When a corporation first sells its stock the price is set, but afterward the value of the stock is based on the prosperity of the company. If the company is well run and profitable, the value of the stock increases; if it is mismanaged and suffers a loss, the value decreases (and there is no dividend).

      B. **Preferred stock** is a more stable investment, because dividends are fixed in advance and thus, unlike common stock dividends, which depend on the generation of profits, fluctuations in dividends are minimal. A preferred stockholder is more of a financial backer than an owner, and the stockholder's investment is better protected than with common stock.

 II. **Bonds.**   Bonds are long-term obligations that pay back a stated amount, the principal, at the end of a term of years (usually 20 or 30 years) and another stated amount, the interest, each year. Bonds are issued to obtain financing for long-term capital investments. The usual sources of bonds are corporations, public utilities, and federal, state, and local governments. The interest paid on a bond is based on interest rates at the time of issue. If interest rates are high at the time of issuance, but they subsequently fall, the bond issuers will want to redeem the bonds because money can be borrowed at lower cost. For this reason, investors may demand "call protection" for high-interest bonds, which prevent the bonds from being redeemed for a period of years.

      The bond market constantly adjusts the value of outstanding bonds to compensate for changes in interest rates. If interest rates go up, the value of outstanding bonds goes down, and if interest rates go down, the value of outstanding bonds goes up. No matter how much of a "discount" is placed on the market value of a bond, however, it is redeemable at maturity for the full face value.

      Bonds may be held until maturity or they can be bought and sold like stocks, through brokers. Some bonds are tax exempt, such as bonds issued by municipalities; others, such as U.S. Treasury bonds, are exempt from state and local income taxation only.

      Whether taxable or tax exempt, the interest on a bond will automatically be paid if the bond is issued in registered form (i.e., the owner's name and address is on the bond), but if the bond is in bearer form (i.e., no name is on the bond) a coupon has to be clipped off and sent in to receive payment.

III. **Mutual funds.**   These large investment funds were created to allow small investors to enjoy the advantages of professional money management, risk reduction, and investment mobility. Mutual funds are large investment units, composed of the funds of thousands of individuals, which purchase a highly diversified portfolio containing a wide variety of investment vehicles. The size and diversity of these funds protect against large changes in value even when economic indicators shift suddenly. Mutual funds may be classified on the basis of their purpose. Growth funds are used for long-term investments that will appreciate over time; income funds are used to provide more immediate financial return. Funds can also be classified by type of investment, such as specialty funds (which concentrate on certain industries) and balanced funds (which invest in bonds as well as stocks). There are also load and no-load funds. In load funds, a sales charge must be paid at the time the investment is purchased, whereas for no-load funds there is no sales charge.

      Mutual funds are used for long-term investment, and the type of fund in which to purchase shares is dependent on the investor's goals.

---

antiques) should be considered only after a proper foundation has been achieved because they are speculative investments and might yield little return. An investment portfolio, based on the retirement plan of the investor, can be built to include all these items. It is the ability of these investments to provide for retirement that is the guiding force behind the strategy.

PLANNING FOR RETIREMENT

It is essential that retirement planning begin well ahead of retirement, preferably soon after graduation from optometry school. There is a sizable financial benefit to be derived from beginning retirement planning early in a career (Table 32.3). Retirement planning is an essential part of an estate

Table 32.3. Accumulating and Depleting a Retirement Fund

The annual investment needed to accumulate a $100,000 fund for retirement is determined by the amount contributed each year and the percentage return on the investment. The following table illustrates the amount of money, interest rate, and length of time the money would have to be invested to accumulate $100,000.

Interest Rate	5 yrs	10 yrs	15 yrs	20 yrs	25 yrs	30 yrs
5%	$17,236	$7,572	$4,414	$2,880	$1,966	$1,433
6%	$16,736	$7,157	$4,053	$2,565	$1,720	$1,193
7%	$16,254	$6,764	$3,719	$2,280	$1,478	$989
8%	$15,783	$6,392	$3,410	$2,024	$1,267	$817
9%	$15,332	$6,039	$3,125	$1,793	$1,083	$673
10%	$14,890	$5,704	$2,861	$1,587	$924	$553

The length of time required to deplete a retirement fund depends on the amount withdrawn each year and the investment return being earned. The following table illustrates the number of years needed to deplete a $100,000 retirement fund, based upon a regular monthly withdrawal.

Monthly Withdrawal	Interest Rate of Investment					
	5%	6%	7%	8%	9%	10%
$600	23	29	*	*	*	*
$700	18	20	25	*	*	*
$800	14	16	18	22	30	*
$900	12	13	14	16	19	26
$1,000	10	11	12	13	15	17
$1,200	8	9	9	10	10	11
$1,400	7	7	7	9	9	9
$1,600	6	6	6	7	7	7

*Withdrawals can be made indefinitely at this rate.

plan. It is almost certain that any Social Security benefits or employee pension plan payments will be inadequate to satisfy the retiree's needs, especially if the retiree is fortunate enough to be healthy and to live for many years.

There are three key elements involved in planning for retirement: forethought, patience, and specific goal setting. The investor must be able to project expenses and monetary needs 30–40 years into the future. Some expenses, such as housing, food, and taxes, will most likely decrease. A retiree might wish to spend more time traveling, however, and that would be an increased expense. Medical costs could also increase at retirement. In addition, retirement needs will have to take into account the effects of inflation, which will increase retirement costs and necessitate a higher retirement income.

The investor must estimate these specific retirement needs, set financial goals that will obtain the necessary financial resources, and have the patience to follow the plan over several decades. In constructing a retirement plan, an investor must consider the financial benefits to be derived from Social Security, work-related pension plans, insurance plans, and personal investments.

Social Security

At present, full eligibility for Social Security begins at age 65, and partial eligibility can be elected at age 62. A retiree receives monthly benefits, which are based on the years of contribution to Social Security by the retiree. An estimate of these benefits can be obtained at any time by directing an inquiry to the Social Security Administration. These payments are modest, however, and inadequate to fund a retirement plan. After retirement, a retiree might work part-time, but this earned income can be taxed if the retiree earns in excess of a certain amount (currently $25,000 for single retirees and $32,000 for married couples).

Work-Related Pension Plans

Pension plans are tax-deferred retirement plans in which a certain amount of an employee's income is deducted, placed in an investment account, and allowed to grow without taxation until withdrawal at retirement. These plans are usually available to the employees of corporations (including professional associations and professional corporations and S corporations) and of incorporated multidisciplinary practices (such as health maintenance organizations). There are two main types of plans: defined contribution and defined benefit.

Defined contribution plans permit a specified amount (20% of income, up to $30,000) to be placed in the pension plan each year. These plans can be funded with stock bonuses, profit sharing, and matching contributions from the employer. The most frequently used plan is a 401(K), which permits a limited amount (set by the employer) to be contributed annually (25% of income, up to $7,000) to the pension fund.

Defined benefit plans are based on actuarial projections and allow contributions (up to 100% of income or, as of 1995, a maximum of $120,000) to be placed in the pension plan each year for the purpose of paying a stated benefit during retirement. The amount of the benefit is set by the retiree, and the amount contributed each year is based on this benefit and the anticipated years of retirement that the retiree will have.

Personal Investments

There are several plans available to self-employed professionals, including IRAs, simplified employee pension individual retirement accounts (SEP-IRAs), and Keogh plans.

Individual retirement accounts allow up to $2,000 per year to be placed in a designated custody or trust account established for this purpose. The two big advantages of an IRA are that the yearly contribution can be deducted from income taxes and the contribution earns tax-free interest until it is withdrawn at retirement, disability, or death. Another advantage is that the contributor can choose the type of investment (within certain limits) for the IRA funds. The contributor is eligible to start withdrawing income from the IRA at age 59½ and must do so by age 70. If income is needed before eligibility is attained, other than for disability or death, income tax and a 10% penalty must be paid on the amount withdrawn. Anyone can set up an IRA—employers or employees—and IRAs can be established even if the contributor also participates in other types of retirement plans. Although the annual contribution to an IRA is limited to a maximum of $2,000, if such an account is begun early in a professional's career and is diligently contributed to, a sizable nest egg can be realized at retirement.

SEP-IRAs are like IRAs. A self-employed practitioner or the qualified employee of a professional association or professional corporation can contribute to a SEP-IRA (up to 15% of income to a maximum of $30,000), and the contributions will be tax deferred until withdrawn at retirement, disability, or death. Like an IRA, the contributions are invested and grow tax free until withdrawn between the ages of 59½ and 70.

Keogh plans are like pension plans and allow nonincorporated, self-employed individuals and their employees to participate in defined benefit and defined contribution retirement plans. Defined benefit plans permit 100% of income, up to $120,000, to be contributed annually to the Keogh account. Defined contribution plans allow 25% of income (up to $30,000) to be contributed annually to the account. There are a number of rules that must be followed to determine eligibility, vesting of benefits, and the size of annual contributions.

Insurance Plans

When whole life insurance policies are purchased, they provide not only death benefits but also cash value, which can be withdrawn and used as retirement income. The cash value of a policy depends on the investment of the premium payment by the insurer and the length of time premiums have been paid. If money is borrowed against the cash value of a policy, an interest charge might have to be paid. At death, the amount borrowed will be deducted from the death benefit paid to the policy beneficiary. The cost of whole life insurance is higher than term coverage because of the accumulation of cash value. Whole life policies constitute a type of forced savings plan, which might be preferable for individuals who cannot follow an established budget or investment plan. Whether whole life or term policies are preferable for a given individual depends on that individual's needs, abilities, and retirement plan.

A whole life insurance policy can also be converted into an annuity. Rather than pay the policy proceeds to the beneficiary at death, an annuity pays an income (usually monthly) to the policyholder for the remainder of the policyholder's life. Various types of annuities can be purchased. An annuity with an "installments certain" clause ensures that a certain number of payments will be made to the heirs if the beneficiary dies before receiving them. An annuity with a refund clause allows the heirs to receive income equal to the amount contributed by the policyholder to the annuity if the policyholder dies prematurely.

When considering these various means of funding a retirement plan, the investor should consider the following questions:

- Do I have clear goals in mind as to what I hope to achieve with my retirement fund?
- Will the income from the retirement fund be adequate for my needs?
- Is the retirement plan performing up to my expectations?
- Is the retirement plan set up for maximum tax benefits, both for myself and my heirs?
- Am I sufficiently familiar with the specifics of my plan?
- Have I discussed my retirement plan with my spouse?
- Am I reviewing and monitoring my retirement fund regularly?

Of course, planning is only half of the effort in building an estate; execution of the plan is also necessary. The actual execution of a plan usually requires the advice and assistance of a financial advisor. The wise investor will obtain a knowledgeable professional advisor to assist in the efforts to acquire an adequate retirement fund.

LAST WILL AND TESTAMENT

A good estate plan provides for the transfer, with minimum taxation, of an estate to the desired heirs. Federal law imposes a unified transfer tax on lifetime gifts and property that passes at death. A carefully drawn will is essential, not only to minimize taxes, but also to ensure that the decedent's estate passes to the appropriate individuals at death.

Wills

A person who leaves a will is said to die testate; if there is no will, the person is intestate. In such a case, state law (referred to as statutes of "descent and distribution") will determine the manner in which the property is to be divided. Relatives of the decedent are specified in these statutes, beginning with spouse and children and, if there are none, to parents and siblings and others of more remote blood relation. If there are no heirs that can be found, the property escheats (reverts) to the state.

The purpose of a will is to direct how the estate of the decedent is to be distributed. The person given the responsibility of seeing that the estate is properly divided is called the executor. The will should identify this person and describe the powers to be exercised by the executor in carrying out the will's provisions. The will must be submitted to probate court, where a judge will ensure that it is indeed the last testament of the deceased and oversee the executor's administration of the estate.

Wills should provide for the distribution of the estate if both spouses die in a common disaster. Some states have adopted the Uniform Simultaneous Death Act (all joint property is halved).

Wills also need to provide for minor children when both parents die at or about the same time. A trust is often used for this purpose. In this case, the executor transfers the estate proceeds into the trust, which is then administered by the trustee in accordance with the trust instrument's provisions (e.g., for the support and education of the children). A guardian can also be named in the will to serve as the "parent" for the children; however, the probate court is not bound by the will's choice and can select another individual if the judge is convinced it is in the child's best interests to do so.

Complex wills should be drafted by a competent attorney. Holographic (handwritten) wills are enforceable as long as they have been properly executed (signed). The signing of the will must be witnessed. The number of required witnesses varies from state to state but is usually two or three people. These individuals should be readily identifiable and relatively easy to contact for purposes of attesting to the will's authenticity.

The estate is subject to both federal and state taxes, which are determined and paid during the probate process. There are some important ways in which the estate can be reduced for purposes of determining the tax so that the heirs can inherit more of the estate and the state and federal government will receive less.

Estate and Gift Taxes

The federal estate tax is imposed on the gross estate of the decedent at death. This consists of:

- Property that the decedent owns at death
- Transfers of property that are effective at death (e.g., annuities)
- Transfers occurring within 3 years of death (except certain gifts)
- Life insurance proceeds paid because of death
- Property owned in joint tenancy (e.g., a house)
- Payments from qualified retirement plans (e.g., IRAs)

Generally, the estate's value is the fair market value of the property that composes the estate at the date of death. The taxable estate is the gross estate, less:

- Administration and funeral expenses
- Claims against the estate
- Casualty and theft losses (if any)
- Charitable deductions (if any)
- Marital deduction (if married)

Table 32.4. Use of the Unified Gift and Estate Tax Credit

Gifts made during year: $570,000
Less annual exclusion: $10,000
Total taxable gifts: $560,000
Gift tax owed: $178,000
Less unified credit: $178,000
Net gift tax: $0

The marital deduction is allowed for the value of property in the estate that is passed to a surviving spouse. Therefore, it is limited only to the gifts and bequests made to the spouse, with no monetary limit. The marital deduction is an important estate planning device since it allows the property transferred to the surviving spouse to be excluded from estate taxes.

Life insurance is subject to special provisions. If the policy was given to a surviving spouse, and the decedent retained no incidents of ownership after the gift, the life insurance proceeds will be excluded from the taxable estate. If the gift occurred within 3 years before death, however, it will be included in the taxable estate.

For a home owned as tenants by the entirety or as joint tenants with right of survivorship, one-half of the fair market value of the home will be included in the taxable estate.

The estate tax is also affected by gifts made by the deceased. A gift tax is imposed on gifts that exceed $10,000 per individual (the "annual exclusion"). A gift to a spouse that qualifies for the marital deduction is excluded from taxation. For gifts in excess of the annual exclusion a return must be filed, using Form 709, by April 15 of the year following the year the gifts were made. The gift tax is computed on the return. However, there is a unified credit that can be applied to the gift tax. This credit is $192,800, which provides a dollar for dollar reduction in the gift tax. An example of how this credit can be applied is provided in Table 32.4.

The unified credit is also applied to estate taxes. It can be used to provide a dollar for dollar reduction in the estate tax (Table 32.5). Because of this credit, federal estate tax is applied only to estates that have a net worth in excess of $600,000. However, if the unified credit has been

Table 32.5. Use of the Unified Credit
to Offset Estate Taxes

Taxable estate of: $1,000,000
   Federal estate tax: $345,800
   Less unified credit: $192,800
   Net estate tax: $153,000

Table 32.6. Deduction from Unified Credit
of Previous Credit Claimed for Gifts

Unified Credit: $192,800
   Less previous credit claimed: $92,800
   Unified credit for estate taxes: $100,000

used for gifts, the amount so used must be deducted and cannot be used for reduction of estate taxes (Table 32.6).

Other credits that can be applied to the federal estate tax include:

- Credit for state death taxes
- Credit for gift taxes (for gifts included in the taxable estate)
- Credit for foreign death taxes

Expert advice is needed to plan for estate transfers at death. A competent attorney or financial advisor should be consulted.

CONCLUSION

Estate planning is a complicated but important part of a practitioner's life. It is essential to begin planning early in a professional career, to secure competent technical advisors for guidance, and to develop the estate in a stepwise, orderly fashion. Consistent effort, applied over the course of a professional career, will result in the development of a sizable estate for retirement, protect against disability, and ensure that the estate is passed as desired to loved ones at death.

BIBLIOGRAPHY

Blackman IL. Transferring the Privately-Held Business. Chicago: Probus Publishing, 1993.

Brosterman R, Adams K. The Complete Guide to Estate Planning (rev ed). New York: Mentor, 1990.

Brown J. The basics of estate planning. Colorado Med 1984;12(6):24–8.

Commerce Clearing House. Federal Estate and Gift Taxes Explained. Chicago: Commerce Clearing House, 1995.

Commerce Clearing House. Social Security Benefits Including Medicare. Chicago: Commerce Clearing House, 1995.

Crumbley DL. Keys to Estate Planning and Trusts. New York: Barron's, 1993.

Esperti RA. The Handbook of Estate Planning. New York: McGraw-Hill, 1991.

Kapoor J, Dlabay L, Hughes R. Personal Finance. Homewood, IL: Irwin, 1993.

Leimberg S. The Tools and Techniques of Employee Benefit and Retirement Planning. Cincinnati: National Underwriter, 1990.

Lochray P. Financial Planner's Guide to Estate Planning (3rd ed). Englewood Cliffs, NJ: Prentice-Hall, 1991.

Index

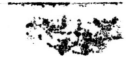